The Trials of Psychedelic Therapy

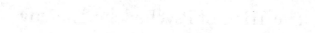

THE TRIALS *of* PSYCHEDELIC THERAPY

LSD Psychotherapy in America

MATTHEW ORAM

Johns Hopkins University Press
Baltimore

Johns Hopkins University Press
2715 North Charles Street
Baltimore, Maryland 21218-4363
www.press.jhu.edu

Library of Congress Cataloging-in-Publication Data

Names: Oram, Matthew, 1984– author.
Title: The trials of psychedelic therapy : LSD psychotherapy in America /
    Matthew Oram.
Description: Baltimore : Johns Hopkins University Press, 2018. | Includes
    bibliographical references and index.
Identifiers: LCCN 2017056668 | ISBN 9781421426204 (hardcover : alk. paper)
    | ISBN 9781421426211 (electronic) | ISBN 142142620X (hardcover : alk.
    paper) | ISBN 1421426218 (electronic)
Subjects: | MESH: United States. Food and Drug Administration. | Mental
    Disorders—drug therapy | Lysergic Acid Diethylamide—therapeutic use
    | Psychotherapy—methods | Hallucinogens—therapeutic use | Pharma-
    ceutical Research—history | Drug and Narcotic Control—legislation &
    jurisprudence | History, 20th Century | United States
Classification: LCC RC483.5.L9 | NLM WM 402 | DDC 616.89/18-dc23
    LC record available at https://lccn.loc.gov/2017056668

A catalog record for this book is available from the British Library.

CONTENTS

For almost ten years this project has evolved through different forms and traveled with me through four universities in three countries, and through many major milestones and upheavals in my life. I have been very fortunate to receive support and guidance from many talented and generous individuals—mentors, colleagues, friends, and family—without whom it would not have been possible.

The project began as my doctoral dissertation at the University of Sydney. Prior to this my growing interest in history cemented into grand ambitions thanks to the rigorous and stimulating supervision of my honors research by Günter Minnerup and the encouragement of Anne O'Brien, at the University of New South Wales. At the University of Sydney, Alison Bashford and Stephen Robertson expertly guided my inexperienced enthusiasm through every aspect of my academic development. Alison saw potential in my ideas, brought me in, and supported my work to its conclusion and beyond, always generously and responsively providing her time and advice, without ever alluding to the demands it placed on her busy schedule. She particularly helped me gain confidence in my work and to see above the minute detail and look at the big picture of my topic and candidature. Stephen's exceptionally close readings of my drafts shaped my development as a writer, and his comments and advice were crucial in honing my arguments and thinking. Also at Sydney I am indebted to the personal support and guidance of Judith Keene, as well as other faculty members of the Department of History who provided support and review of my work, including Warwick Anderson and Stephen Garton. The friendship and support of Micaela Pattison, Dave Earl, and others in the history postgrad community was crucial in these years and has meant a lot.

During my doctoral work I relocated from Sydney back home to Christchurch, New Zealand, and in February 2011 a major earthquake destroyed my office, along with much of my research material. My recovery from this event was significantly helped by the generosity of the University of Sydney's School of Philosophical and Historical Inquiry. Subsequently, I worked from space in the Department of History of the University of Canterbury. Special thanks go to Jane Buckingham for inviting me to engage with the department and offering me access to the workspace, as well for her continued support over the years. Thanks also to Peter Field, Judy Robertson, and the other staff and students of the department for making me feel welcome. The department, with which I held no formal ties, was in no way obliged to offer me a place to work. Its generosity saved my project at a difficult time, when I was close to abandoning it. Thanks to Jeremy Greene, Hans Pols, and Catharine Coleborne for their valuable feedback as the dissertation came to a conclusion, encouraging and advising me on developing the work into a book.

The revision of my dissertation into this book was made possible by a 2015 AMS History of Medicine and Healthcare Postdoctoral Fellowship from AMS (Associated Medical Services, Inc.), which I undertook at the University of Calgary. The content is solely my responsibility and does not necessarily represent the official views of AMS. Bringing me to Canada, the fellowship provided me with a plethora of opportunities to advance my work and academic experience in a new context. Thanks go to Frank W. Stahnisch for introducing me to the scheme and for hosting and supporting me at the university, as well as to Beth Cusitar, Donna Weich, and the Department of Community Health Sciences, Cumming School of Medicine. I was lucky to also be affiliated with the Calgary Institute for the Humanities. Thanks go to Jim Ellis, Sharla Mann, Caroline Loewen, and the other fellows for providing an ideal context for my writing. Thanks to Aleksandra Loewenau for her postdoc camaraderie, as well as to the graduate students of the history of medicine program. Final revisions were made at the University of Saskatchewan. Deep thanks go to Erika Dyck for providing me with this opportunity, for her advice and support during my time in Canada, and for the fun times together with our families.

Research for this project benefited greatly from the assistance of many archivists, librarians, and others throughout North America. Special thanks goes to Stephanie Schmitz, archivist for the Psychoactive Substances Collection at Purdue University Libraries, for her significant help as well as friendship over many years. At Purdue, thanks also to Lauren Haslem, Kristin Leaman, and Emma Meyer for their fast and diligent help preparing, copying, and checking material over the years. Though I never met them, thanks also to David Nichols, Betsy Gordon, and all of those who donated material for their foresight and work in developing this fantastic collection that has been so important to my work. I am extremely grateful to Richard Yensen and Donna Dryer for inviting me into their home and generously sharing their stories, materials, and hospitality with me, the fruits of which have added much to the book. Thanks also to William Richards for taking an interest in my work and sharing some enlightening memories with me. Thanks to Emmy Savage for kindly providing a photo of her father. Daniel Carpenter and John Swann took time to advise me on possible research collections to consult, and the anonymous reviewers for Johns Hopkins University Press and elsewhere have provided valuable feedback that has greatly improved my work. At the press, thanks to Matt McAdam for taking on my project, to Carrie Watterson for her careful copyediting, and to all the other staff who helped to bring the book to fruition. Thanks also to Jackie Wehmueller for a stimulating initial conversation that sparked things off.

An abridged version of chapter 2 was previously published as "Prohibited or Regulated? LSD Psychotherapy and the United States Food and Drug Administration," *History of Psychiatry* 27, no. 3 (2016), pp. 290–306. Copyright © 2016 Matthew Oram. Reused by permission of Sage Publications. Further material in the book appeared in "Efficacy and Enlightenment: LSD Psychotherapy and the Drug Amendments of 1962," *Journal of the History of Medicine and Allied Sciences* 69, no. 2 (2014), pp. 221–250. Reused by permission of Oxford University Press.

To those who appear in my narrative, I hope I have been fair and accurate in my assessments and portrayals of your work. I have certainly tried my very hardest. I hope that this book brings greater recognition to the important research and therapy to which many of you dedicated your careers.

Finally, the various stages of this work would certainly not have been possible without the generous and unfaltering support and encouragement of my family, particularly my parents Anne and Richard, as well as Theresa, James, Zina, Margaret, Rob, Bob, Trevor, Sandy, Bill, and Cher. I met my wife, Amy, partway into the project, and for seven years it has existed alongside our relationship. In addition to her endless patience and support, she agreed to take a foolhardy venture in moving to the other side of the world with an eight-month-old and an uncertain future so that I could work on the book. I am endlessly grateful for her hard work caring for Elias with no support in a foreign environment so that I could follow my dreams. I hope I can, in at least some small way, repay this sacrifice. And, to Elias, thank you for your tolerance of our many moves and for being such a charming companion on our adventures.

AA	Alcoholics Anonymous
CIA	Central Intelligence Agency
DEA	Drug Enforcement Administration
DMT	dimethyltryptamine
DPT	dipropyltryptamine
ECT	electroconvulsive therapy
FDA	Food and Drug Administration
IND	Notice of Claimed Investigational Exemption for a New Drug (Form FD 1571)
LSD	lysergic acid diethylamide
mcg	micrograms
mcg/kg	micrograms per kilogram of body weight
MDA	methylenedioxyamphetamine
MDMA	methylenedioxymethamphetamine
MMPI	Minnesota Multiphasic Personality Inventory
MPRC	Maryland Psychiatric Research Center
NDA	New Drug Application
NIDA	National Institute on Drug Abuse
NIMH	National Institute of Mental Health
PHS	Public Health Service

The Trials of Psychedelic Therapy

Introduction

Mysticism, Clinical Science, and the FDA

> The question may well be raised how it is that after a decade of research on the therapeutic value of LSD, the matter is still hotly debated, while only a few years of research . . . were required to establish the general effectiveness of tranquilizers and their acceptance.
>
> Charles Savage, c. 1960

On 4 August 1965, Sarah reported to cottage 13 of Spring Grove State Hospital, just outside of Baltimore, Maryland, to receive the psychedelic drug LSD, or lysergic acid diethylamide.[1] Sarah was suffering from terminal cancer and hoped LSD could help bring peace to her final days. As a member of the hospital's professional staff, Sarah was familiar with the institution's large research program investigating the therapeutic potential of LSD with alcoholic and neurotic patients. However, she had not been directly involved with it. In fact, she had been "violently opposed" to LSD, dismissing claims of its benefits to patients and ridiculing the mystically oriented treatment procedure. Nevertheless, she now believed LSD could help her to become more "acutely aware of the world" and make the most of her remaining days. Her friend, psychologist Sidney Wolf, a member of the psychedelic research team, had suggested the treatment. He believed that, behind her guarded facade, Sarah had led an unhappy life and was a "frightened, unstable individual." He concluded that LSD therapy could help her to attain insight into her life, resolve inner conflicts, and "gain the inner strength necessary to . . . die with dignity." Further, he hoped the psychedelic experience could help her to "understand the purpose of life, love and death."[2]

To prepare for her LSD session, Sarah underwent approximately thirty hours of intensive psychotherapy with Wolf. During this, the pair deeply explored Sarah's low self-esteem and poor relationships with her mother and husband, and together they "began to expose unresolved conflicts, unfulfilled needs, crippling fears, and a psychological foundation that was shaky, hollow and rotten." By the end of her preparation, Sarah had gained profound insight into herself and her past, and her relationships with her husband and children had greatly improved. She had also come to peace with her troubled relationship with her mother. Sarah's husband and children also met with Wolf, and, after discussing their anxieties regarding the procedure, gave their full support.[3]

Sarah arrived on treatment day feeling confident, eager, and at peace. As her car pulled up to the cottage, a group of colleagues associated with the research program—psychiatrists, psychologists, and secretaries—gathered on the front lawn to wish her well as she made her way to the specially furnished treatment room. As the drug began to take effect, she reclined on a sofa wearing eyeshades and headphones, which played a carefully curated selection of music. Soon she began to feel "fused to the music" and was transported into experiences where she reassessed her life, values, and concept of self and discovered new perspectives:

> Mainly I remember two experiences. I was alone in a timeless world with no boundaries. There was no atmosphere; there was no color, no imagery, but there may have been light. I was in a kind of maelstrom, bodiless, lofted and buffeted. Suddenly, I recognized that I was a moment in time, created by those before me and in turn the creator of others. This was my moment and my major function had been completed at and by my birth. By being born, I had given meaning to my parents' existence. Why then the rat race, the need to achieve, to attain the meaningless goals we spend our lives chasing?
>
> Again in the void, alone without the time-space boundaries. Life reduced itself over and over again to the least common denominator. I cannot remember the logic of the experience, but I became poignantly aware that the core of life is love. At this moment I felt that I was reaching out to the world—to all people—but especially to those closest to me. I wept long for the wasted years, the search for identity in false places, the neglected opportunities, the emotional energy lost in basically meaningless pursuits.[4]

In the late afternoon, as the drug effects began to diminish, Wolf took Sarah outside to walk among the trees on the hospital grounds. She communed with the natural setting, stretched, and "took a deep breath for the first time in months." Her colleagues again gathered around, and all were moved to tears by her transformation.[5]

Immediately after her treatment, Sarah took a two-week lakeside holiday with her family, where, as Wolf later recollected, she "experienced a joy, an intimacy of contact, a freedom of relationships and a freedom to live that [she] had never known before."[6] On her return, Sarah described her psychedelic experience as having had a profound positive effect on her mental state, her experience of her illness, and her relationships:

> What has changed for me? I live a different value system. I am no longer on the merry-go-round chasing a tarnished brass ring. I am living now, and being. I can take it as it comes. Some of my physical symptoms are gone. The excessive fatigue, some of the pains. I still get irritated occasionally and yell. I am still me, but more at peace. My family senses this and we are closer. We no longer talk about the issues that were opened, but should we want to, the avenues of communication are open. All who know me well say this has been a good experience.[7]

These positive results were supported by data from psychological tests, which were performed one week prior to her session and two weeks after. They showed a significant reduction in depression and a general lowering over several other ratings of psychiatric pathology. Five weeks after her treatment, Sarah died when her condition suddenly worsened.[8] Wolf described the scene at her deathbed as free of the desperation and denial that frequently accompanied terminal illness: "There was such peace and acceptance that no one suffered."[9]

Sarah's treatment was a particularly successful case of "psychedelic therapy," a form of psychiatric treatment originally developed in Canada in the 1950s. Most commonly used to treat alcoholism, psychedelic therapy used a high dose of LSD, within a framework of brief, intensive psychotherapy, to elicit a mystical "psychedelic" experience. This experience had the power to reorient patients' perceptions of themselves and their place in the world, in ways that could lead to lasting positive changes in their values, attitudes, and behavior. By 1965, a Canadian pioneer of the treatment, Abram Hoffer, reported data from eleven North American studies showing that, out of a total of 269 alcoholic patients, just over 50 percent were "much improved" and only 30 percent had not improved to some degree.[10] LSD had been used in widespread clinical research in the United States since 1949, in the context of the breakthrough era of psychopharmacology research, which saw the development of the first effective drugs to treat psychosis, severe depression, and anxiety.[11] Many psychiatrists believed LSD would join these drugs in revolutionizing the discipline. Researchers found success treating not only alcoholism and distress associated with terminal illness but also a variety of neurotic illnesses, and narcotic addiction.

Yet in 1965, despite more than fifteen years of clinical research in the United States, LSD remained officially an investigational new drug, not approved for sale or use beyond clinical research. Over the decade, LSD psychotherapy research declined, before coming to a close in the 1970s. This book explores why LSD failed to live up to its promise of at least entering, if not revolutionizing, mainstream psychiatry.

In the mid-1960s, LSD was of course not only a promising tool of psychiatry. Recreational use of the drug increased over the decade hand in hand with the rise of the politically and socially rebellious youth countercultural movement. Preaching a utopian vision of peace and love, members of the counterculture believed that the "consciousness-expanding" effects of LSD had the potential to liberate American society by facilitating a spiritual revolution.[12] To mainstream Americans, the drug represented escapist hedonism that could corrupt the minds of youths, threatening the nation's social fabric. Inflamed by sensationalist media reports, LSD use became a major public and political controversy, and the dominant perception of the drug shifted from an unconventional but promising tool of medicine to a dangerous drug of abuse. Less than one month before Sarah's treatment, Congress passed the Drug Abuse Control Amendments of 1965, beginning the drug's criminalization. By 1970, the Controlled Substances Act listed LSD in its most restrictive category of regulation—Schedule I—alongside heroin and marijuana. The established narrative of the history of LSD psychotherapy has followed the close correlation between the decline in research and the rise in controversy and prohibitive legislation surrounding LSD to conclude that, intentionally or unintentionally, the government backlash against nonmedical use of LSD killed medical research with the drug.[13]

This, however, was not the case. Through a close analysis of the provisions and enactment of the various regulations that impacted LSD over the 1960s and early 1970s, this book will reveal that the federal government never significantly restricted psychedelic research. In fact, it actively supported research for much longer than has been recognized. Further, where research has often been depicted as coming to a close in the mid- to late 1960s, limited research with LSD and other psychedelics continued until 1976, long after both the apex of the controversy over LSD's nonmedical use in the late 1960s and the drug's prohibition.[14] This later research was still focused on establishing treatment effectiveness, which remained a contentious issue. Considering this, perhaps the most significant question in the history of LSD psychotherapy research becomes not why did research end but why, despite more than twenty-five years of study, were researchers still trying to prove LSD's efficacy? Why, in 1976, was LSD still an "investigational new drug"? The answer to this question lies in a close examination of the later research with LSD.

LSD research beyond the early 1960s has been consistently overlooked largely because of the manner in which historians and other commentators have interwoven different elements of the drug's history in the postwar decades. There are three primary narratives in the history of LSD: medical research, public nonmedical use, and clandestine research by the US Central Intelligence Agency (CIA) and military. The first two of these narratives, and to a somewhat lesser extent the third, have been depicted as inseparably entwined. CIA and military research with LSD began alongside psychiatric research in the early 1950s, exploring the drug's potential as a mind-control device, truth serum, and chemical weapon. The CIA, in addition to conducting its own research, provided funding to many extramural psychiatric researchers, both with and without their knowledge. Authors such as Martin Lee and Bruce Shlain have therefore argued that CIA funding propelled the psychiatric LSD research of the 1950s.[15] The common narrative then connects this psychiatric research, as well as self-experimentation by distinguished intellectuals, through clear links to the development of the LSD counterculture from the early 1960s—medical use transforms into nonmedical use, leaving medical use behind.[16] The figures at the center of this story are psychiatrist Humphry Osmond, author and intellectual Aldous Huxley, psychologist Timothy Leary, and author Ken Kesey.

Osmond was a pioneer of LSD research in Canada in the 1950s. With his colleagues—particularly Abram Hoffer—he developed both a biochemical theory of the origins of psychosis influenced by his study of mescaline (a hallucinogen produced by certain cacti, most notably the peyote cactus) and psychedelic therapy for the treatment of alcoholism. He also famously coined the word "psychedelic"—meaning "mind-manifesting"—as a term to describe LSD and similar drugs in 1956, in a rhyming couplet sent to Huxley: "To fall in Hell or soar Angelic / You'll need a pinch of psychedelic."[17] As well as being one of the most significant early LSD researchers, Osmond influenced nonmedical interest in psychedelics by administering Huxley his first dose of mescaline in 1953. Based on this experience, the renowned English author of *Brave New World*, who was by now based in Los Angeles, wrote

The Doors of Perception (1954) and, after further experimentation with LSD, *Heaven and Hell* (1956). These essays recounted his experiences and discussed their implications for understandings of consciousness, visionary experience, and religion. Huxley's final novel, *Island* (1962), offered a vision of a utopian society where psychedelics were used for spiritual purposes in rite of passage rituals. Although he did not encourage widespread casual nonmedical use of LSD, and this did not occur until more than a decade after his first psychedelic writings, Huxley's works heavily influenced the intellectual direction and cultural vision of the 1960s counterculture movement.[18]

Leary, together with his colleague Richard Alpert (later known as Ram Dass), has most prominently played the pivotal role in the transformation of the drug's image from medical tool to social threat over the 1960s. Leary had arrived as a lecturer in psychology at Harvard University in 1959, on the back of significant work in the fields of personality assessment and behavioral change. The next year he sampled psilocybin mushrooms while vacationing in Mexico. The profound experience revealed "reality" to be merely a social fabrication and convinced him that the future of psychology lay with the drug. On his return, Leary quickly gathered a group of graduate students and junior faculty to explore the effects of psilocybin, and early research included treating prisoners with the drug to lower recidivism rates. Yet Leary's methods were always unorthodox—with researchers taking the drugs alongside their subjects—and their work devolved into heavy informal use of psilocybin and LSD, under only the loosest guise of research. The research loci also shifted from the university to Leary's large home-turned-commune, which became a drop-in center for those interested in psychedelics. Concern grew in the university administration and reached a head in May 1963 when the *Harvard Crimson* reported that faculty member Alpert—the cohead of the psilocybin project—had supplied the drug to an undergraduate student, going against a promise made to the university. Alpert was subsequently fired, as was Leary, although in his case the official reason was failing to fulfil teaching obligations. The controversy received coverage in several major national newspapers.

The dismissals were no setback for the pair, who saw the potential of psychedelics as much more significant than academic research. They, particularly Leary, began to publicly endorse widespread use of psychedelics and became figureheads of an emerging counterculture. They preached a psychedelic philosophy that borrowed heavily from Eastern religions, and in turn religious movements developed around them that promoted psychedelics as sacraments. Over the decade, Leary's attempts to lead the youth away from traditional American values and lifestyles—to "turn on, tune in, drop out"—garnered him increasing notoriety.[19] According to lore, President Richard Nixon declared him "the most dangerous man in America."[20]

In the case of Kesey it was the research subject, rather than the researcher, who broke LSD out of the confines of the scientific world. Kesey first tried LSD as a volunteer for a study on the effects of various hallucinogenic drugs at the Veterans Administration Hospital in Menlo Park, California, while he was a graduate student in creative writing at Stanford University. He took a strong liking to the drugs and self-experimented with them while working as an orderly at the hospital. These experiences influenced his writing of the critically acclaimed and highly successful novel *One Flew Over the Cuckoo's Nest* (1962).[21] As famously recounted in Tom Wolfe's *The Electric Kool-Aid Acid Test* (1968), Kesey used his royalties to fund a commune from which a distinct West Coast form of psychedelic culture emerged.[22] Compared to the psychological, philosophical, and spiritual focus of Leary's East Coast movement, Kesey's group—the Merry Pranksters—adopted a brash, chaotic style, characterized by bizarre costumes, swirling fluorescent colors, and experimental rock music. The Pranksters confronted mainstream America while traveling the country in an elaborately decorated bus and hosted large public parties—"Acid Tests"—in California, replete with free LSD, experimental light shows, and, often, house band the Grateful Dead.

These individuals were indeed the most influential figures in shaping public perceptions of LSD, and their narrative thread accurately portrays the evolving role that LSD played in American society. However, it does not tell the full story of LSD's medical use. The medical and nonmedical histories of LSD were certainly entwined, yet they are—to a significant extent—separable. This book does not deny that controversy tarnished the reputation of LSD and that some researchers were unable to continue or initiate LSD research under the new regulations of the 1960s. Instead, I argue that these developments did not end research and that the research that remained was the most significant yet conducted. While the controversy and regulation certainly impacted research, the demise of LSD psychotherapy can be understood as distinct from it. Following this narrative provides different—perhaps greater—implications for the history of clinical science, regulation, and therapeutics in American psychiatry.

This book explores how the rise, decline, and ultimate fall of LSD psychotherapy research was primarily shaped by the changing context of pharmaceutical research and development in the period. As well as an era of social and cultural upheaval, the 1950s and 1960s was a time of transformation for pharmaceutical research and development, from an age of empirical research and limited government oversight to one of sophisticated controlled clinical trials and complex federal regulations.[23] The initial successes of LSD psychotherapy in the 1950s reflected the loose regulation of pharmaceutical research and development in that decade, which allowed psychiatrists to freely explore methods of treatment that blended biological and psychological techniques. The passage of the Kefauver-Harris Drug Amendments of 1962 significantly changed this context.[24] Reflecting both advances in the science of clinical evaluation and rising concerns over the need to protect the public from unscrupulous research and development, the amendments introduced federal oversight of premarket clinical drug research by the Food and Drug Administration (FDA) and required proof of effectiveness for a drug to be approved for sale. Although not specifically targeting LSD, these provisions dramatically altered the landscape and prospects of LSD psychotherapy research in the United States.

First, they transformed a field that had progressed in a disorderly fashion with numerous small and varied studies into a smaller number of formal clinical trials. Second, the requirement that drug efficacy be demonstrated through controlled clinical trials made mandatory a method of drug evaluation ill-suited to accommodate LSD psychotherapy's complex method of using drug effects to catalyze a psychological treatment. The difficulties in balancing scientific standards with the clinical requirements of treatment left researchers unable to clearly demonstrate treatment efficacy. More than this, the studies conducted after 1962 in fact did establish a consensus in the eyes of many in the medical mainstream: that LSD psychotherapy was ineffective. However, the negative results from many of the controlled studies were based on problematic research. These studies were conducted by several of the most experienced and prominent psychopharmacology researchers of the era, who designed trials with high standards of scientific rigor. Yet, in doing so, they subverted the established treatment methods, ultimately testing techniques that the pioneers of LSD psychotherapy would never have expected to be therapeutic. This critique was lost in a medical context increasingly focused on accumulating data, rather than honing technique and studying patient responses. Funding and support for research subsequently dried up, and research dwindled and died.

Several other authors have noted the difficulty of evaluating LSD psychotherapy through controlled clinical trials. Most significantly, in *Psychedelic Psychiatry* historian Erika Dyck has explored how the work of Canadian psychedelic therapy pioneers Osmond, Hoffer, and their colleagues was undermined by debates over the need for controlled studies of their treatments, as well as the negative results of a further Canadian study that was controlled but evaluated a treatment method that was almost guaranteed to fail. In this and other works, such scientific debates have been presented as hurdles that frustrated researchers before moral panic and criminalization made any scientific arguments—for or against LSD's therapeutic use—irrelevant.[25] However, by revealing that criminalization did not end LSD research—at least in the United States—and by exploring the later clinical research in depth, this book shows that debates over efficacy and research methodology were not just contributing factors in LSD psychotherapy's demise but the terminal factors.

From this perspective, the story of LSD psychotherapy becomes less about the stifling of science by reactive politics and more about the complex ways in which clinical science and regulation have shaped modern medicine. It is a story of the evolving standards of scientific evidence, a unique treatment that casts light on the limitations that strict research standards can impose and the hidden biases in dominant research methodologies. In unforeseen ways, the Drug Amendments of 1962 would not simply ensure accurate evaluation of new drug therapies but effectively require that they conform to specific concepts of treatment efficacy, with significant implications for psychiatry. Through this lens, LSD psychotherapy is therefore a story of a promising treatment for devastating illnesses lost in debates over how to understand and evaluate treatment effectiveness. While patients and therapists were overwhelmingly convinced of the value of LSD therapy—in terms of personal growth and meaningful experience, as well as the reduction of symptoms of pathology—growing mistrust in the validity of subjective experience and evaluation left such convictions invalid in the absence of specific forms of data.

The intent of the Drug Amendments of 1962 was both simple and unquestionably desirable: to ensure that clinical research was conducted in a safe and scientifically sound manner and that drugs that came to market were effective. The amendments famously passed on the back of the thalidomide tragedy. Although FDA medical officer Frances O. Kelsey had refused to approve the sedative's New Drug Application (NDA) due to her skepticism of its safety data, widespread distribution of the drug under the guise of research had resulted in thousands of pregnant women receiving it as a treatment for morning sickness. When the dramatic birth defects thalidomide caused were discovered in 1962, the danger of leaving the conduct of premarket drug research largely up to the discretion of researchers and pharmaceutical companies became starkly apparent. Senator Estes Kefauver had been investigating numerous aspects of the pharmaceutical industry since 1959, and in 1961 had introduced a bill to amend the 1938 Federal Food, Drug, and Cosmetic Act to require—among numerous other provisions—proof that new drugs were effective as well as safe. The bill had languished because of strong opposition; however, in 1962 the renewed public and political concern over drug safety allowed a new version of the bill to pass.[26]

The amendments required that drug effectiveness be demonstrated through "adequate and well-controlled investigations."[27] In practice, the randomized double-blind placebo-controlled trial (usually referred to as simply the randomized controlled trial) became the model against which the FDA judged the adequacy of a clinical trial's design.[28] This was simply the state-of-the-art methodology for clinical research, which had gained favor among medical elites over the 1950s as a way of minimizing bias in research. In its purest form, the method involved randomly assigning patients to receive either the experimental treatment or a placebo, with both researchers and patients "blind" to the assignment until after the conclusion of the trial. Researchers also placed emphasis on the need for large patient populations and sophisticated statistical analysis to determine the validity of results. This technique theoretically allowed the objective assessment of drugs, as all nondrug factors that could influence the outcome of a treatment—by producing a placebo effect—were equally present in the experimental and control groups. This ensured that any statistically significant difference in the results between the groups could only be due to the drug.

While this methodology was aimed at ensuring objectivity in research, the unique case of LSD will show how problematic this notion was. The design of the randomized controlled trial was based on the assumption that a drug's therapeutic effectiveness resulted from a direct biological action, which operated independently of nondrug influences, including the patient's knowledge of its ingestion. However, LSD psychotherapists considered LSD to have no inherent beneficial effects. Instead, with the active cooperation of the patient, they used the drug to craft a subjective state of consciousness that could be beneficial as part of a psychotherapeutic process. This made establishing a double-blind with an inert placebo impossible and complicated the notion of distinguishing between "specific" pharmacological treatment effects and "nonspecific" extrapharmacological placebo effects.

LSD psychotherapy was ultimately a form of psychotherapy, rather than a drug treatment in any conventional sense. Historians have long been interested in the relationship between psychodynamic and biological forms of psychiatry in the mid-twentieth century. These have often been represented as distinct and competing paradigms: psychodynamic psychiatrists saw mental illness as a product of psychological stresses, often originating in childhood, which could be resolved only through psychotherapy, particularly psychoanalysis. Biological psychiatrists treated mental illness with drugs and somatic therapies, as they believed it to have origins in the brain, as opposed to the mind. Psychodynamic psychiatry was in ascendency in the years following the Second World War, but biological psychiatry grew to dominate after the breakthroughs in psychopharmacology of the mid-1950s.[29] While accurate in a broad sense, other scholars have drawn attention to how the practice of midcentury psychiatry could be highly eclectic, with psychiatrists often embracing treatments that were seemingly incompatible with their theoretical orientations: barbiturates and amphetamines were also used to facilitate psychotherapy, and some psychoanalysts even provided psychodynamic explanations for the effectiveness of electroconvulsive therapy (ECT) and lobotomy.[30]

LSD psychotherapy clearly demonstrates this lack of a clear division between biological and psychodynamic forms of psychiatry in the 1950s. But more importantly, the trajectory of psychedelic therapy research after the Drug Amendments of 1962 shows how regulation later influenced these two forms of psychiatry to split. The amendments required evidence of the efficacy of psychiatry's drug treatments, while leaving psychotherapies unregulated. By effectively requiring the randomized controlled trial as the method of efficacy evaluation, the regulation cast drug efficacy as an objective biological phenomenon. Subsequently, drug-assisted psychotherapy disappeared from psychiatry's treatment landscape as psychopharmacology became synonymous with biological psychiatry. Where the division between biological and psychodynamic psychiatry had previously existed mainly among theorists, the amendments now required treatments to either be purely biological or psychological. The initial rise and subsequent demise of LSD psychotherapy not only reflects broad trends in the evolving relationship between psychology and biology in twentieth-century psychiatry but also reveals the role of regulation in inadvertently influencing this.

This argument is explored through closely following LSD psychotherapy research as it evolved from the start of the 1950s through 1976 and how it was impacted by federal regulations enacted in those years. Published research reports, conference proceedings, and researchers' personal papers chart the development of treatment methods; the evolution of research methods; and the successes, frustrations, and debates that resulted. FDA files and congressional hearings reveal the complex regulatory processes that impacted the scale and nature of LSD research, as well as the skeptical yet supportive approach of the FDA and National Institute of Mental Health (NIMH) toward the research. Further, the book explores the work and careers of many researchers who profoundly shaped the history of LSD psychotherapy in the United States but whose roles have so far gone unacknowledged. Of chief importance among these are psychiatrists Charles Savage, Albert Kurland, and Jerome Levine.

Savage had the longest and most successful LSD research career of anyone in the United States. Among the first in the country to explore the therapeutic potential of the drug, Savage began his psychedelic career studying the effects of mescaline in 1949 and published his initial report on LSD 1952. His work with the drug continued with little interruption until 1973. His early research was eclectic, exploring LSD's potential as both a stand-alone drug treatment and a facilitating agent in psychoanalysis. From the late 1950s he began exploring psychedelic therapy and was a central figure in the establishment and refinement of that method in the United States. In 1965 he joined the then-small team at Spring Grove and helped to expand its studies into the country's most significant LSD program. Research methodology was a particular focus of Savage's, and he was a prominent figure in the research community, well respected by members of the FDA and NIMH, as well as other scientists. He was not, however, a public figure, and his publications and presentations appear to have been confined to the scientific community. His career trajectory mirrors the focus of this book, as it charts the development of the various forms of LSD psychotherapy, the evolving standards of research, and the frustrations they led to, while engaging little with the public controversy that raged over its nonmedical use.

Kurland, with psychologist Sanford Unger, founded the Spring Grove psychedelic research program in 1963 and continued to lead it until its eventual demise in 1976. Despite launching in the same year that the FDA first gained oversight of premarket clinical drug research and that LSD first became the subject of a major national scandal—as Leary and Alpert were fired from Harvard—over the decade the Spring Grove program would continuously expand. Beginning as a controlled study of the effectiveness of psychedelic therapy in the treatment of chronic alcoholism, the program grew to encompass four major clinical research areas—psychedelic therapy for alcoholism, neuroses, anxiety and depression associated with terminal cancer, and narcotic addiction—conducted by a large team that included many of the most experienced and innovative national and international psychedelic researchers. It was the largest and longest LSD research program in the United States, outlasting all others. Kurland held many powerful positions in the bureaucracy of psychiatric research in Maryland, and his strong leadership underlay the successes of the research program. Yet despite the researchers' attempts to balance the clinical needs of treatment with scientific rigor in their clinical trials, research difficulties undermined their work, and they disappeared into almost complete obscurity.

Levine appears more briefly, and near the end of the narrative, yet plays a crucial role. After conducting a small study of LSD in the treatment of narcotic addiction, Levine was hired by the NIMH in 1964 to oversee national efforts to evaluate the effectiveness of the drug. As part of this role, he conducted his own major clinical trial of LSD in the treatment of alcoholism. The study found negative results, which Levine and his colleagues claimed could be considered definitive, given the sophisticated design of the trial. Despite significant flaws in the treatment method the researchers employed, the study was lauded and won a major award. By the time these results were published in 1970, Levine had risen to the rank of chief of the NIMH Psychopharmacology Research Branch, which administered federal funding for drug research in psychiatry. Given his experience and position on the drug, under Levine there was little likelihood of continued federal support for LSD psychotherapy.

By exploring the fascinating and significant work of these and other researchers, this book disentangles LSD's medical from its nonmedical history. While the narrative that emerges may seem somewhat divorced of the cultural context of its age—particularly the significant baggage attached to the drug—it highlights the complexity of drug regulation and its relationship to medicine. Drugs are seldom simply legal or illegal—medicines or narcotics— but rather are regulated in different ways depending on the context of their use. Many other drugs, including opiates, amphetamines, and barbiturates, have maintained dual lives as illegal street drugs and valuable and legitimate tools of medicine. That recreational use of LSD was the subject of controversy and federal prohibition does not automatically explain the drug's fall from medicine. Instead, following LSD research in the insular world of pharmaceutical research and development reveals the struggle for psychology to retain its legitimacy in an increasingly biological field of psychiatry and the significant and complex public policy challenges for regulating treatment effectiveness in the best interests of public health.

CHAPTER ONE

Free Experiment

Explorations in LSD Psychotherapy

I remember very well earlier meetings of the American Psychiatric Association, and the American Psychoanalytic Association, when we got the first reports of some of the individuals who had had personal analysis. I can still remember one of the first Americans who went over to see Professor Freud, and came back and reported in some detail the various steps in the treatment. I can remember the half a dozen or maybe a dozen of us who clustered around and listened to these amazing experiences, little realizing that 25 or 30 or 35 years later they would seem so unnecessary to talk about in a public meeting.

Perhaps some of you will remember this meeting in a similar way 30 years from tonight.

Karl Menninger, 1955

Karl Menninger, one of the most prominent figures in American psychiatry and psychoanalysis in the mid-twentieth century, captured something of the excitement and promise of LSD research in the 1950s when he spoke at the first US conference on the drug, a 1955 round table entitled "Lysergic Acid Diethylamide and Mescaline in Experimental Psychiatry," held at the annual meeting of the American Psychiatric Association. LSD had arrived in the United States in 1949 at a particularly opportune time. Half a decade before the psychopharmacology revolution began with the discovery of chlorpromazine's antipsychotic effects, treatment options in psychiatry were limited. The discipline was characterized by eclectic and divergent biological and psychological approaches, and it was open to unconventional experimentation that could shed new light on the causes of mental illness or offer relief to its sufferers. To many researchers from varying backgrounds, LSD, a powerful and mysterious tool, presented such an opportunity.

Over the 1950s little stood in the way of researchers' investigations with LSD, and three broad frameworks for understanding its effects and use emerged. First, many viewed LSD as a "psychotomimetic": a "madness mimicking" drug that produced an artificial psychosis that could reveal the biological origins, or psychological dynamics, of psychotic illnesses such as schizophrenia. Second, psychoanalytically oriented researchers found that LSD unlocked the unconscious mind, allowing deeper penetration into the psychological roots of their patients' psychopathologies. They began employing LSD in what came to be called "psycholytic" (mind loosening) therapy. Finally, other researchers began exploring the transcendental, even mystical, experiences that some subjects were having under the drug. They developed "psychedelic" (mind manifesting) therapy as a unique form of psychotherapy focused on a single transformative, subjective experience with the drug. This therapy in particular, which seemed to have unprecedented effectiveness in the treatment of chronic alcoholism, seemed poised to be a true breakthrough for psychiatry.

The psychiatric and regulatory context of the 1950s encouraged free and innovative experimentation. This period would come to a sudden close, as the Drug Amendments of 1962 ushered in new era of highly regimented and regulated pharmaceutical research and development. Nevertheless, it was perfecting and evaluating the treatment methods and results of this early time that would occupy researchers' efforts over the 1960s and into the 1970s.

An Ideal Context

The story of LSD's discovery has been frequently told, to the point that it has reached an almost mythic status.[1] Its intrigue is to some extent due to the fortuitous nature of the discovery. Partly it is simply the story of a momentous event: the creation of a drug that would fascinate chemists, psychiatrists, intelligence and military agencies, and individuals all over the world. By the end of the 1960s, LSD was simultaneously considered a powerful therapeutic device, the most dangerous drug known to man, and a key symbol of liberation for a mass social movement. The story also appeals because of the personality and achievements of the inventor, Swiss chemist Albert Hofmann. Hofmann not only synthesized the drug and discovered its dramatic effects but also immediately recognized the wide range of implications it could have, rather than dismissing it as a toxic substance. He remained a proponent of the potential benefits of psychedelics to individuals and society until his death at the age of 102 in 2008, despite his condemnation of their widespread recreational use.

Hofmann was a chemist in the pharmaceutical department of Sandoz Ltd. in Basel, Switzerland, where he had been experimenting with alkaloids of

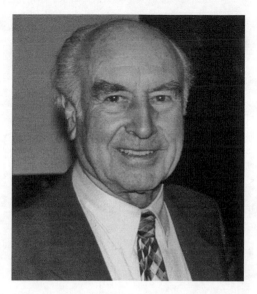

Albert Hoffman in 1993. Photograph by Philip H. Bailey, CC-BY-SA-2.5 (http://crea tivecommons.org/licenses/by-sa/2.5), via Wikimedia Commons.

ergot, a fungus that grows on rye. Famous for producing mass poisonings throughout European history when baked into bread, ergot had also been used for hundreds of years in obstetrics, to induce contractions and control bleeding after birth. In 1938 Hofmann synthesized d-lysergic acid diethylam- ide (or LSD-25, so called as it was the twenty-fifth in a series of substances produced) in search of a circulatory and respiratory stimulant. On animal testing, the substance proved of little interest and was abandoned. But, in 1943, for reasons he could never explain, Hofmann's interest returned to LSD. After synthesizing a new batch on 16 April, he began to feel odd and returned home, where he "sank into a not unpleasant intoxicated-like condition" and with eyes closed "perceived an uninterrupted stream of fantastic pictures, extraordinary shapes with an intense, kaleidoscopic play of colors."[2] He rea- soned that the only explanation for this condition could be the LSD, which he must have somehow accidentally ingested. Hofmann decided to experi- ment further, and three days later he ingested 250 micrograms (mcg) of LSD, believing this to be the smallest amount that could possibly have an effect. The dose turned out to be in fact very strong, overwhelming him with fear as his surroundings distorted into sinister forms and he lost all control over his mind. However, as the effects diminished, they became pleasant, as they had been the first time. Despite the largely terrifying experience, Hofmann con-

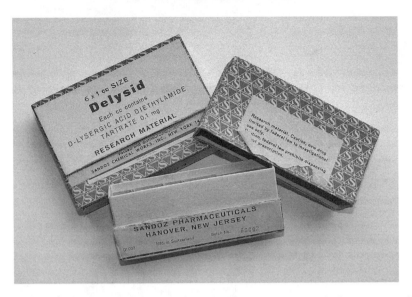

Empty boxes of Sandoz Delysid branded LSD, from circa 1960. The boxes originally held six ampoules, each containing 100 micrograms of LSD. Photo by Jon Hanna & Erowid (2009). Courtesy of Erowid Center's Myron Stolaroff Collection (sci6000).

cluded that the potency and dramatic effects of the drug would be of interest to pharmacologists, psychiatrists, and neurologists.[3]

Psychiatrist Werner Stoll, the son of Hofmann's superior, Arthur Stoll, performed the first clinical tests with LSD at the University of Zurich. Stoll's report, published in 1947, outlined the profound mental effects of the drug, as observed in volunteers, patients, and self-experiments. He noted that, in addition to visual, mood, and cognitive changes, many subjects experienced an upsurge of repressed memories.[4] Sandoz soon began distributing the drug free of charge to international researchers under the trade name Delysid, indicated for "analytical psychotherapy," "to elicit release of repressed material and provide mental relaxation, particularly in anxiety and obsessional neuroses," and for "experimental studies on the nature of psychoses."[5]

When the drug reached the United States in 1949, two factors influenced its quick uptake in psychiatry: the loose regulation of pharmaceutical research and development, and the eclectic nature of postwar psychiatry. Under the Federal Food, Drug, and Cosmetic Act of 1938, for a drug to be marketed in interstate commerce, a sponsor (usually the manufacturer) was required to submit a New Drug Application to the Food and Drug Administration to provide proof that the drug was safe when used as directed. The nature and extent of premarket clinical research was, however, largely at the discretion of the manufacturer. The manufacturer was free to distribute new drugs to qualified researchers so long as they were labeled for investigational use. The manufacturer simply had to obtain a written statement from researchers that they had adequate facilities to perform research with the drug and that all research would be under their direction.[6]

Sandoz, other than providing the broad indications for use, appears to have done little to direct or control research with LSD in the years prior to 1962. Such relationships where pharmaceutical companies supplied drugs to researchers with no funding or oversight were common in the mid-twentieth century. Researchers benefited from the freedom to pursue their own interests and publish any findings without censorship. Pharmaceutical firms benefited as a wide variety of research was undertaken at minimal cost to the company. Such research could potentially find new uses for a drug, help establish its efficacy and safety, or be used as advertising.[7]

LSD researchers, therefore, had great autonomy over their work, which could be conducted almost casually, with little planning or funding required to conduct studies with small numbers of patients. This meant that researchers could easily explore hunches, suggestions, and unconventional uses for drugs, and follow leads when they got unexpected results. With no required methodologies for research, psychiatrists could evaluate their treatments as they considered appropriate and leave others to decide for themselves ultimately how useful they were. This form of research would have its downsides, as it would lead to debates over efficacy and encourage researchers to work independently rather than build on each other's work. Further, with little oversight, the safety of patients depended largely on the experience, skill, judgment, and personal ethics of the individual treating psychiatrist.[8] Despite these drawbacks, the format was incredibly productive, encouraging great exploration and innovation.

Yet this freedom of research was not enough in itself to ensure significant interest in LSD. Indeed, despite its similar effects, peyote, and its active component mescaline (first synthesized in 1919), had attracted only limited and sporadic interest in the United States since it first came to the attention of Western scientists near the end of the nineteenth century. In 1896, prominent Philadelphia physician Silas Weir Mitchell had first published an account of self-experimentation with peyote, describing colorful visions but also physical discomfort. He had noted its potential value for psychological research, though he failed to see a therapeutic application. Further studies in the first half of the twentieth century continued to focus primarily on exploring and describing the drug's effects.[9] In a 1934 study, researchers had administered mescaline to psychiatric patients, exploring its influence on their emotional state and rapport. The schizophrenic and neurotic patients mostly became more withdrawn and anxious, and the authors did not suggest a therapeutic use for the drug.[10]

However, in the 1950s, freedom of research met with a psychiatric field eager to explore new treatment methods that blended psychological and biological elements. LSD arrived in the United States to a psychiatric landscape dominated by inpatient treatment in large state hospitals, which by 1940 held a total population of 480,000. These hospitals were plagued by underfunding, overcrowding, and insufficient staffing, and they housed a core population of severely chronically ill patients.[11] From the mid-1950s, treatment in these institutions would be revolutionized by the discovery of a range of new drugs that appeared to alleviate the specific symptoms of major mental illness: tranquilizers chlorpromazine and reserpine for psychoses, antidepressants imipramine and iproniazid, and the minor tranquilizer meprobamate for anxiety. Prior to this, biological treatment options were limited and could be dangerous.

Drug therapy was primarily limited to powerful sedatives, most significantly barbiturates in the mid-twentieth century, as well as stalwarts including paraldehyde and chloral hydrate. Rather than specific treatments for mental illnesses, these drugs were simply tools to increase the comfort and manageability of patients, by calming agitation and inducing sleep. The stimulant amphetamine became popular as a specific treatment for depression from the late 1930s. Its major market was in the treatment of depression's milder forms in outpatient rather than hospital settings, and it was most commonly prescribed by general practitioners.[12] For more severely ill hospital patients, the more dramatic somatic treatments—including insulin coma therapy, electroconvulsive therapy, and psychosurgery—held out the only hope of cure. Inducing hypoglycemic comas, inducing physical convulsions, and performing brain surgery each presented significant risks to patients, and in the case of psychosurgery caused permanent changes that could fundamentally alter personality and impair mental functioning. These treatments have often been represented as brutal, overused, and unscientific tools of punishment and control. However, while such problematic use occurred, these were at the same time mainstream treatments supported by the science of the day that offered hope for patients who were otherwise unreachable. That many psychiatrists deemed such dramatic and hazardous treatments justified simply reflects the severity of the problem of chronic mental illness before the advent of modern medications: faced with significant patient distress and a hopeless outlook, any chance of benefit was worth significant risk.[13]

While sedation, somatic therapies, and the hope of spontaneous recovery were the mainstays of hospital treatment, in the years after the Second World War psychoanalysis and other psychodynamic approaches came to dominate psychiatric theory. Two factors are commonly cited for this. First, an influx of European analysts fleeing Germany and Austria following the rise of the Nazi Party helped to raise the popularity and status of these treatments in the United States.[14] Second, the high rate of psychiatric casualties among military personal during the war, despite an extensive program of screening recruits for predisposition for mental illness, suggested that environmental stress had a greater impact on mental health than presumed factors such as personality or even history of illness.[15] In addition, military psychiatrists successfully treated soldiers suffering from neurotic conditions through early intervention and noninstitutional treatment: instead of being sent to far-away hospitals and separated from peers, patients progressed through a series of more local treatment stations until they improved, with a focus on rest, psychotherapy, diet, and a chance to normalize. Finally, the war created a greater population of psychiatrists, as demand grew and treatment proved successful. Army medical personnel assigned to psychiatry grew from 35 at the time of America's entry into the war to 2,400 at its conclusion, a number greater than the 2,295 total members of the American Psychiatric Association in 1940.[16]

After the war, psychodynamic psychiatry made its greatest impact on psychiatry's professional organizations and educational institutions. By 1955, nearly all psychiatric residents were being instructed in psychodynamic principles, and analysts held the top positions in the American Psychiatric Association.[17] The first edition of the association's nosological text, *Diagnostic and Statistical Manual: Mental Disorders* (*DSM-I*), published in 1952, while not explicitly stating a particular theoretical framework, was couched in dynamic terms, describing mental illness as resulting from difficulties of adaption. The large section on "psychoneurotic disorders" defined the illnesses as arising from individuals' attempts to handle anxiety that was frequently held in the unconscious by "psychological defense mechanisms" and that arose from "threats within the personality" such as "supercharged repressed emotions."[18]

Shifting away from psychiatry's traditional focus on severely ill, usually psychotic, patients, psychodynamic psychiatrists concentrated their attention on those with neuroses. War experience influenced this development not only by providing positive treatment experiences but also by expanding the potential patient population and suggesting a change in the locale of treatment. With the unexpected rate of cases of psychiatric disorders among prescreened military personnel, psychiatrists realized that mental illness affected, at least potentially, a far greater population than had previously been thought. These casualties seemingly showed that mental illnesses were not discrete diseases caused by genetic or biological factors but existed on a spectrum from health to severe illness, that environmental influences could precipitate a shift on this spectrum, and that early intervention could prevent the slide into severe illness, which was much more difficult to treat. This theory led to a push for psychiatrists to identify and treat patients in the community, to prevent them from reaching the point where they needed traditional hospital treatment.[19]

Despite the dominance of psychodynamic theory in postwar American psychiatry, psychotherapy was impractical as a primary treatment in hospital settings. The classical psychoanalytic method was a grueling process, with patients ordinarily seeing their analyst five times per week, often for years, and it required from the patient high motivation and—aside from their specific neuroses—relatively high mental functionality: as dean of the Los Angeles Institute of Psychoanalysis Ralph R. Greenson commented in 1959, "Actually, one has to be a relatively healthy neurotic in order to be psychoanalysed without modifications and deviations."[20] Hospital patients were mostly too mentally withdrawn or disorganized to engage in psychotherapy, and regardless hospitals simply could not accommodate the amount of individual time between psychiatrists and patients that psychotherapy required. Therefore, while somatic and psychodynamic treatments can seem at odds on a theoretical level, for pragmatic reasons psychiatrists often used them alongside each other. Indeed, historian Mical Raz has found that not only was opposition to psychosurgery among psychodynamic psychiatrists less common than is often portrayed, but many saw the treatments as complementary, and patients often received psychotherapy after lobotomy. Furthermore, psychosurgeons and analysts alike frequently explained the efficacy of lobotomy through psychodynamic theory.[21]

Increasingly, psychiatrists also looked to drugs as tools to enhance psychotherapy, rendering it more widely applicable and effective. The first to be widely used were the barbiturates. Their use would provide a direct precedent and blueprint for early explorations of LSD's therapeutic potential. William Bleckwenn, of the Wisconsin Psychiatric Institute, published the first indications that barbiturates had therapeutic potential greater than simple sedation in 1930. Bleckwenn had been exploring using the barbiturate sodium amytal to induce sleep in psychotic patients. He observed that in the hours after waking, even patients who were normally so catatonic as to require tube feeding could display "striking periods of normal existence," where they were able to calmly answer questions about their illness and families. He tried conducting psychotherapy in this period and reported excellent results. Erich Lindemann, of the Psychopathic Hospital of the State University of Iowa, then tested whether the effects of sleep or the action of the drug caused this lucid period in patients by administering smaller doses that would not induce sleep. He similarly found that severely disturbed and often mute psychotic patients would temporarily become "friendly and emotionally warm" and could articulate their fears and delusions. Lindemann suggested that this otherwise unattainable information could be used to break down patients' defenses and facilitate psychotherapeutic progress.[22]

During the Second World War, American military psychiatrists Roy Grinker and John Spiegel then developed a systematic psychotherapeutic treatment called "narcosynthesis" that utilized the barbiturate sodium pentothal to treat the frequent and debilitating cases of "war neuroses." Caused by the stresses of war, this condition was marked by severe anxiety, as well as extreme agitation, amnesia, muteness, hysteria, somatic ailments, and even near paralysis.[23] The first part of the therapy involved using the barbiturate to produce a powerful abreaction in the patient—an emotional reliving of past traumatic events. In a private, semidarkened room, the therapist administered the drug until the patient reached the desired semiconscious, dreamlike state of "narcosis." The therapist then encouraged the patient to talk about the traumatic wartime experiences. To facilitate the emotional reliving of these events, the therapist evoked battles in which the patient had been involved. As Grinker and Spiegel described in 1944, if resistance was high, or recall difficult, the therapist would dramatically play "the role of the fellow soldier, calling out to the patient, in an alarmed voice, to duck as the shells come over, or asking him to help with a wounded comrade."[24] With persistent use of this technique, even complete amnesias surrounding a traumatic experience could be reversed. Patients often responded by not merely describing a traumatic scene but by acting it out, moving around the room responding to events and communicating with absent friends. During this behavior the therapist continued applying encouragement and stimulus to help patients fully relive their experiences and provided support and comfort as traumatic scenes unfolded.

After the abreactive experience had concluded, the second part of the treatment commenced. During the abreaction, the traumatic emotions attached to the patient's wartime experiences were detached of their excess anxiety by the sedative qualities of the drug. As a result, after the drug had worn off the memories and emotions released could be more easily worked through with the aid of brief psychodynamic therapy sessions. The goal of this therapy was "to release unconscious psychological tensions, to strengthen the ego forces and decrease the severity of the superego's pressure."[25] Grinker and Spiegel noted that in severe cases it was unlikely that the treatment would allow patients to return to combat, and reclassification for limited duty was often the goal. Nevertheless, they showed great optimism about the efficacy of the treatment, arguing that results could be improved with better resources, and they provided case descriptions of many successful treatments.[26]

After the conclusion of the war, American psychiatrists in hospital and private practice began widely experimenting with narcosynthesis. Many found it to be an aid in establishing dialogue with patients, deepening insight, and speeding the process of psychotherapy. In 1948 narcosynthesis was even featured in the prominent and influential film *The Snake Pit*. During her hospitalization for mental illness, the main character, Virginia Cunningham (played by Olivia de Havilland), undergoes the treatment, emotionally recounting events in her past, and she appears to be reliving them at times. Previously repressed material comes to light, which her psychiatrist sees as significant to the cause of her illness. It is one of a variety of treatments that together eventually lead to her successful recovery.[27] Summarizing the field for prominent journal *Diseases of the Nervous System* in 1949, psychiatrist Leonard Tilkin found that narcosynthesis was "rapidly gaining support as a respected and valuable psychiatric treatment." Researchers reported greatest success in treating severe anxiety states and hysterical reactions, as well as promising results in the treatment of alcoholism. Perhaps somewhat naïvely, Tilkin went so far as to state, "The future of narcosynthesis is infinite, and the possibilities endless."[28]

Over the 1950s, other drugs would also become frequently used as facilitators in psychotherapy. Indeed, historian Nicolas Rasmussen has found that, in the early 1950s, pharmaceutical firm Burroughs Wellcome even advertised its stimulant Methedrine (methamphetamine) for such a use, under the heading "Release the Story for Analysis." According to the advertisement, intravenous administration of the drug produced in patients a "spontaneous, free flow of speech," featuring "previously withheld information," and also facilitated abreaction.[29] Similarly, historian Andrea Tone has found that researchers and manufacturers claimed that the early minor tranquilizers mephenesin and meprobamate (Miltown) were useful adjuncts to psychotherapy, but because of their relaxing rather than stimulating properties.[30] LSD would begin its medical life as just one of many tools explored to render psychotherapy more efficient and effective.

Early Research

Initial research with LSD followed Sandoz's recommendations and reflected the eclectic context of US psychiatry, as researchers explored the drug's implications for their biological or psychodynamic theories and treatments. Max Rinkel, at Boston Psychopathic Hospital, first brought LSD to the United States in 1949 in the hopes of creating an experimental "model" psychosis to advance research into the nature, biological basis, and treatment of schizophrenia. Administering the drug to healthy volunteers, including staff and students of the hospital, Rinkel found LSD produced a variety of symptoms that confirmed he had found his psychotomimetic: paranoia, hostility, hallucinations, inappropriate laughing, and strange physical sensations. These symptoms lasted several hours before disappearing. By the next day, all subjects were able to return to work, although one who had had a particularly harrowing experience did remain "somewhat depressed" for the day.[31]

Such psychotomimetic research would continue over the decade; meanwhile, psychiatrists also quickly began exploring the drug's therapeutic potential. Following the model of narcosynthesis, psychodynamic psychiatrists in the 1950s explored the power of the drug to deepen and quicken psychotherapy, through its power to break down patients' defenses, release repressed memories, and deepen psychological insight. Despite the dramatic effects of LSD, what came to be known as "psycholytic therapy" was not a radical form of treatment. Incorporating LSD into treatment did not present any challenges to the theoretical basis of psychoanalysis or require any fundamental changes to the therapeutic procedure. It merely provided a tool to aid the process. During the 1950s, psychodynamic therapists in the United States and Europe reported great success using LSD with their patients. However, as psycholytic therapy was simply conventional forms of psychotherapy facilitated through LSD, it never developed into a truly distinct, standardized

treatment: particular theories and methods varied according to the psychotherapeutic schools to which the researchers ascribed. This would ultimately
influence its demise in the 1960s.

Psychiatrists Anthony Busch and Warren Johnson published the first US
report describing the use of LSD in a psychotherapeutic context in 1950. At
the St. Louis State Hospital in Missouri, the researchers had been experimenting with ways to open up their chronically psychotic patients to psychotherapy. They had tried forms of narcosynthesis, as well as interviewing patients
during insulin coma therapy or after electroconvulsive therapy. Although
helpful, they found these methods had drawbacks: "speech difficulties" under
sodium amytal and mental confusion surrounding the somatic treatments.
Having noted cases of patients uncovering their internal conflicts while in
a state of "toxic delirium," the researchers took up Sandoz's suggestion to
use LSD to produce this state. For a first trial they chose twenty-one female
inpatients, eighteen of whom were diagnosed as schizophrenic and three as
manic. The patients had been hospitalized for between one and thirty-one
years. They were given small doses of between 30 and 40 mcg of LSD, the
effects of which were found to last up to eight hours. Busch and Johnson
described the mental effects of the drug as "those of excitation," with patients
becoming more active, engaged, and emotional, and displaying "greater
verbal expression of psychopathology." Although patients would occasionally become confused or disoriented and experience visual hallucinations,
euphoria was also common.[32]

The usefulness of the drug reaction varied widely between patients. Some
(including all of the manic patients) became disturbed and needed hydro-
therapy to calm their excessive excitation. Others became coherent, expres-
sive, and more focused on their problems. Encouraged by the latter reaction, the researchers decided to try using LSD with eight patients who were
already receiving psychotherapy. Four were outpatients, and the group included patients diagnosed with schizophrenia and psychoneurosis. Results
for this group were more uniform, and the researchers found the treatment
"profoundly influenced the course of their progress." Two patients improved
to the point where treatment was discontinued. Approaching treatment from
a psychodynamic perspective, Busch and Johnson indicated that LSD "disturbed the barrier of repression and permitted a re-examination of significant experiences of the past, which sometimes were relived with frightening
realism." Several of the patients had been unable to reach such abreactive
experiences under sodium amytal. Subsequently, the patients were often able

to reevaluate the emotional meaning of their symptoms, more realistically orient their thoughts "in relation to real rather than fancied problems," and display emotions more appropriately.[33]

This therapeutic process was therefore essentially identical to Grinker and Spiegel's narcosynthesis. The researchers simply saw LSD as an improvement on barbiturates, as it offered more clarity and depth in the emotional recall of past experiences. Busch and Johnson concluded that LSD could be useful in shortening the duration of psychotherapy and "for more readily gaining access to the chronically withdrawn patients."[34] While technique and theory developed over the next decade, this basic aim and theory of efficacy remained the defining feature of psycholytic therapy.

Charles Savage, who would become a leading figure in LSD research, published the second report of LSD's therapeutic use in 1952. He had begun working with mescaline in 1949 at the Naval Medical Research Institute in Bethesda, Maryland, in search of a facilitating agent for psychotherapy. However, his interest in psychedelics and the implications of hallucinations for psychiatry had begun even earlier, during his postgraduate studies. Born in Berlin, Connecticut, in 1918, Savage completed a bachelor's degree in psychology at Yale University in 1939, before undertaking a master's degree in psychology, alongside his medical degree, at the University of Chicago.[35] There, Savage studied under the German-born psychologist Heinrich Klüver, a pioneer in mescaline research.[36] In 1928, Klüver had published *Mescal: The "Divine" Plant and Its Psychological Effects*, in which he attempted to clearly delineate and categorize the drug's effects. He identified common elements in visions, such as specific geometric patterns, as well as changes in visual sensation and perception, and explored the nature of the "mescal psychosis." Klüver concluded that mescaline had wide implications for the study of psychology, including studying visual perception, dreams, hallucinations, synesthesia, and the "role of visual elements in thinking and the psychogenesis of 'meaning.'" Although he was skeptical of French researcher Alexandre Rouhier's suggestion that the drug may aid psychoanalysis—as he believed mescaline visions were not closely related to personality—Klüver did consider it "possible that some day the study of mescal effects will give us information about . . . 'the hinterland of character.'"[37]

Savage's 1943 master's thesis explored the phenomenon of "hypnagogic hallucinations"—visual hallucinations and other sensory illusions experienced while semiconscious, transitioning into or out of sleep. Savage personally experienced this phenomenon most nights and was curious as to

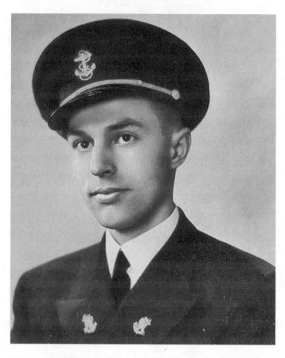

Charles Savage in naval uniform while a student at the University of Chicago in the 1940s. The navy funded Savage's medical education, and he subsequently served with the navy—first as a psychiatric resident and later as a research psychiatrist—from 1947 until 1952. Photograph courtesy of Emmy Savage.

the meaning behind the visions. Through a review of literature on the topic, he considered that the visions could relate to unconscious wishes as well as misinterpretation of sensory stimuli. He argued that analysis of the visions could aid psychotherapy—as in the manner of dream analysis—and that the visions were related to other forms of hallucination, including psychoses, and therefore could aid in the study of the origins of schizophrenia.[38] Influenced by Klüver's work, Savage moved on from this research convinced that mescaline held even greater potential in these areas, and he left the university determined to find opportunities to study the drug.[39] After graduating with his medical degree in 1945, Savage interned at the University of Chicago Clinics before commencing psychiatric residency, first at Yale and then in the navy. He also began his training in psychoanalysis through both the Washington-Baltimore Psychoanalytic Institute and the Washington School of Psychiatry, from which he would graduate in 1954 and 1957, respectively. During this time he trained under prominent Washington analysts, including

German émigrés Edith Weigert and Frieda Fromm-Reichmann, as well as Ernest Hadley and Merton Gill.[40]

In 1949, now certified and in the role of research psychiatrist at the Naval Medical Research Institute, Savage found his first opportunity to study mescaline. There he began exploring numerous drugs to aid psychotherapy, including barbiturates, harmaline, scopolamine, cannabis, and cocaine. Mescaline indeed showed the greatest promise, but treatment was complicated by patients' frequent experience of intense nausea. He therefore soon switched to LSD after hearing about the drug.[41] His 1952 report explored the effects of LSD in healthy individuals and its usefulness in treating depression. Despite administering only a very low 20 mcg dose to the healthy study participants, Savage observed a wide variety of effects. Subjects often experienced euphoria and feelings of omnipotence but also anxiety and tension, particularly when trying to resist the effects of the drug. Their minds became consumed in a "flight of ideas," and all sensory perceptions were distorted, as they saw the "walls seem to pulsate and melt and . . . apparently teem with insects" or heard the sound of a motor running as a symphony. One subject became convinced that under LSD's effects he could send out "impulses" that could control the mind of anyone else who had taken the drug. Savage noted that the subject was "unaware of the bizarre nature of this idea."[42]

Savage's use of LSD with depressed patients veered from the narcosynthesis model, where the drug was used purely as a facilitating agent for psychotherapy. Instead, Savage assessed whether LSD-induced euphoria could be therapeutic in itself, as well as whether the drug could facilitate psychotherapy, by administering low doses of between 20 and 100 mcg to patients daily for one month. The study included fifteen inpatients diagnosed with "depressive reactions," but most were also diagnosed with schizophrenia, involutional psychoses, or schizoid personalities. The study was loosely controlled, with the progress of each patient compared to that of an untreated patient who had a similar diagnosis, over the six months after treatment. This was not only the first use of a control group in LSD research but was also a very early example of controlled research in psychiatry. The results were disappointing. Half of the LSD patients improved to the point of recovery from their depressive symptoms; however, this rate of improvement was not superior to that of the control group. Further, LSD could increase symptoms of anxiety, weight loss, and insomnia, and psychotherapy was needed to maintain patients' improvements. The effects of LSD were also frequently too "disorganizing" to improve communication during psychotherapy sessions. Nevertheless, Savage found that analyzing patients' hallucinations provided "therapeutically valuable insights into unconscious processes."[43]

This last observation sustained Savage's interest in the drug. In 1953, having left the navy, Savage joined the National Institute of Mental Health, where he began investigating the implications of LSD for schizophrenia. As part of this he explored the LSD induced "psychosis" through the lens of psychoanalytic theory, particularly the ego psychology of Paul Federn. He observed that LSD produced profound disturbances in subjects' "ego feeling"—their conscious experience of their own mind, as well as their body in its association with the outside world—and "ego boundaries"—the boundaries between conscious and unconscious parts of the mind, and the self and the external world. He argued that accurate sensory perception was needed to maintain ego feeling and ego boundaries; therefore, the alterations of perception produced by LSD led to depersonalization, loss of touch with reality, hallucination, and delusion. Savage concluded that the LSD model psychosis closely related to endogenous psychoses and allowed easier study of psychotic processes, as well as the experimental study of psychiatric theory, with his observations seeming to support current theories in ego psychology.[44]

Savage also collaborated with NIMH colleague Louis Cholden and Albert Kurland, director of research at Spring Grove State Hospital in Maryland, to study the effects of LSD in patients with chronic schizophrenia. Their research, published in 1955, resulted in several significant findings. First, they discovered that the double-blind placebo-controlled experimental design was not useful with LSD: with an initial four patients who had been administered LSD or placebo in such a fashion, it was obvious who had received LSD. Second, patients developed a rapid tolerance to the drug. On the second consecutive day of LSD administration, the effects of the drug were diminished, and on the third day the drug appeared to produce no effect. It then took four to six days for this tolerance to completely disappear. Last, they found that the clinical effects of LSD in patients with chronic schizophrenia varied widely: some patients showed only minimal behavioral changes, others had their normal symptoms intensify, and some significantly improved.[45]

One particularly dramatic case of improvement occurred with a woman who had been hospitalized for more than fifteen years and had been mute and catatonic for "some" years. Shortly after LSD administration she began alternately crying and laughing. When asked why she was crying, she cryptically replied, "You should never leave the farm." After calming down she "began to walk about the ward studying the walls and the windows as though she were seeing them for the first time" and talked, although she was often incoherent and seemed to be responding to hallucinations. Later in the day she played basketball for the first time, continued to laugh, smile, and talk, and even took part in a hospital dance. However, the next morning she awoke "her old catatonic self, unable to speak, unable to show interest in anything about her, and quite withdrawn."[46] Because of the rapid onset of tolerance, any positive reactions such as this could not be maintained. Thus, LSD was of little use as a chemotherapeutic treatment for schizophrenia.

While Savage's research was still hovering between psycholytic and psychotomimetic understandings of LSD, New York psychiatrist Harold Abramson developed psycholytic therapy into its mature format. Born in 1899, Abramson received his medical degree from Columbia University in 1923. Initially his interests focused on immunology and physical chemistry, and in the late 1920s and 1930s he taught and worked in these fields at Johns Hopkins, Harvard, and Cornell Universities. In the 1940s, he became a leading allergy researcher at Mount Sinai Hospital, New York, where he was a pioneer of aerosolized medications, and was the first person to administer penicillin this way.[47] Through his private medical practice Abramson also developed an interest in psychiatry and psychotherapy, and pursued training in the disciplines. Despite his enthusiasm, he found his new field lacking in the laboratory research he was used to. Accordingly, on reading about LSD he became interested in its potential for bringing the laboratory to psychiatry.[48]

Starting in 1951, Abramson and his colleagues conducted a wide variety of research with LSD at Mount Sinai Hospital and at the Biological Laboratory in Cold Spring Harbor, New York. Their work investigated not only LSD's therapeutic potential but also a range of its physiological and psychological effects, such as its effects on perception, spatial relations, motor performance, and mathematical ability.[49] Much of this research was funded by the CIA, as part of its secret MK-ULTRA program of research into mind control. According to author John Marks—who played a major role in publicly exposing the program in the 1970s—Abramson was one of a number of researchers who performed LSD research for the CIA, as well as reported to the agency the results of their own work and other developments within the field. The CIA funded this research to glean information on how the drug could be used for purposes such as disturbing memory, eliciting information, increasing suggestibility, altering sex patterns, discrediting individuals by producing unusual behavior, and creating dependence.[50]

It is unclear precisely what role the CIA played in shaping Abramson's research and the extent to which it veered into unethical and sinister territories. Although the CIA clearly had sinister intentions in supporting Abramson's and his colleagues' research, their published studies simply systematically explored the effects of the drug, providing information relevant to a wide variety of research interests. Although the researchers obviously would not have published any overtly unethical research they conducted, many of their reports do furnish information relevant to CIA interests seemingly without treating the participants unethically: published studies on the effects of LSD on recall, personality, and concentration all reported employing paid, adult volunteers and simply compared standard psychological tests performed prior to and after LSD administration. The volunteers were screened for psychotic illness; had a high average level of education; and included graduate students, scientists, engineers, nurses, hairdressers, and housewives.[51]

In fact, as Abramson later described at a conference, the experiments took place at his home on Long Island following a communal dinner, a setting he considered ideal for a favorable reaction. Indeed, he had found out the hard way that disruptions in the setting could cause negative reactions: unannounced visits from medical colleagues had led to severe anxiety reactions that required psychotherapy to resolve, such as when one visiting psychiatrist pondered out loud, "Do you think these ergot drugs produce chronic brain damage?" By carefully crafting the setting to produce beneficial drug responses, Abramson's Friday night experiments gained an exciting reputation in his neighborhood, with locals eager to participate and those who did often repeating the experience: one subject participated eighty times.[52]

Regardless of the dubious ethical nature of some of Abramson's research, CIA interests likely lay in the psychological rather than psychotherapeutic aspects of his work. For therapeutic purposes, Abramson used low doses of LSD (20–50 mcg) in the context of ongoing "quasi-Freudian" psychoanalysis, to open patients up, move past psychological blocks, and aid in the recall of repressed memories. To avoid anxiety reactions, he recommended a two-week preparation period, during which the therapist discussed with the patient the variety of effects the drug could produce and emphasized its therapeutic benefits. The LSD interview then generally lasted for four hours, during which the therapist would meet any anxiety in the patient with confident reassurance that any unusual phenomena experienced were part of the therapeutic process. Abramson found that LSD enhanced, or reinforced, patients' egos, allowing them to better face and integrate unconscious material. It helped them to identify conflict situations in their lives and adapt their responses to these situations in more suitable ways. He called this process "hebesynthesis," and the benefits often lingered in subsequent therapy sessions. Further, he found that LSD improved on narcosynthesis, that patients remained conscious and cooperative and could recall the content of their sessions afterward, that the drug could be repeatedly administered without addiction, and that patients usually enjoyed the experience.[53]

To demonstrate the effectiveness of his LSD treatment, Abramson included in his reports lengthy transcripts from LSD sessions, rather than quantitative data on the number of patients treated, their diagnoses, number of sessions given, or results. These patients were generally neurotic outpatients already undergoing psychoanalysis (often for several hundred hours), who had reached a block or were unable to confront and resolve an important psychological conflict. Abramson discussed the results of the LSD sessions in terms of progress in therapy, such as insights gained and conflicts resolved, rather than in terms of more general measures such as "recovered" or "improved." This format mirrored the focus on case studies in psychoanalytic texts, including the works of Freud.

Abramson's most detailed report included the transcript of a four-hour LSD session, which, in typical Freudian fashion, focused on sex, childhood, and the patient's relationship with her mother.[54] The forty-year-old female patient had been in therapy with Abramson for the past four years, with more than three hundred regular sessions. Although her analysis had made great strides in improving many areas of her life, she had great difficulty opening up and talking about sexual anxieties that troubled her. In the interview she admitted that it was these problems that had prompted her to seek analysis, yet she had avoided the topic so far out of fear. A recent dream involving two dogs engaged in a sexual act brought the issues to the fore, but she anxiously refused to delve into the dream's meaning. Abramson had conducted previous successful LSD sessions with her, and he thought the drug could help her to discuss and resolve her sexual anxieties. Soon after ingesting 40 mcg of LSD, the patient revealed that she was primarily disturbed by her frequent desire to masturbate and her belief that this could indicate that she was a lesbian. This interpretation was based on her feeling that she should be fully satisfied by her sex life with her husband—and therefore not desire to masturbate—and on her frequent difficulty at achieving orgasm through intercourse alone, as she considered clitoral stimulation to be a lesbian and childish method of gratification. She acknowledged that her idea of what it meant to be a lesbian was likely wrong and that she had never felt attracted to women. Nevertheless, her anxiety over her sexuality remained.

Over the session, Abramson and the patient uncovered the apparent root of her mental correlation between masturbation and female homosexuality. She recalled that as a child she had first experienced sexual pleasure in the bathtub, and that after seeing her domineering and sexually repressed mother self-administering a douche—which she initially mistook as an enema—she frequently masturbated while fantasizing about receiving an enema from her mother and strongly feared that she would be punished if her mother caught her in the act. As an adult, she still masturbated with water; therefore, although she no longer thought of her mother, masturbation remained associated with feelings of guilt and retained unconscious ties with female attraction and childhood. This was an Oedipal analysis, as her "masculine" mother substituted for her emasculated father as the object of her sexual desire as she entered the genital phase of development, and she was left without a feminine woman to identify with.

The effects of LSD were not obvious in the transcript, except where Abramson specifically asks the patient how she is feeling. At one point she describes that she feels drunk but that she can also think clearly, is aware of everything she is saying, and believes that she will remember it all. Despite the apparently mild effects, Abramson frequently inserted notes into the transcript testifying as to how the patient's easy discussion of sexual topics, recall of past events, and integration of new insights is strikingly different from her past three hundred therapy sessions without LSD, which acted as a "control" for the effects of the drug. He considered the session a great success, with the patient overcoming her fear of homosexuality.

By 1955 LSD research had become significant enough to warrant a separate round table discussion at the prominent annual meeting of the American Psychiatric Association, as mentioned at the beginning of this chapter. The session featured papers by eleven LSD and mescaline researchers, which, although often very short, give a good indication of the state of research at that time. While researchers such as Abramson had been exploring LSD's therapeutic potential, the predominant interpretation of the drugs' effects was still as psychotomimetic: conference chair Louis Cholden stated that the purpose of the symposium was "to utilize the tools of lysergic acid diethylamide and mescaline in a multi-faceted assault on the problem of the psychoses . . . [based on] the conceptual construct that these drugs have a meaningful relationship to the naturally occurring psychotic states."[55] Much of the meeting was therefore concerned with the method of action of the drugs, their relation to endogenous psychoses, and other drugs used to treat these illnesses, rather than their therapeutic potential. Nevertheless, several researchers—including Abramson and Savage—moved away from a narrow understanding of LSD and mescaline as psychotomimetics and discussed their therapeutic potential, as well as aspects of their effects that would become an increasing focus of research over the later 1950s and 1960s.

In addition to Abramson, who summarized his work, Ronald Sandison, from Powick Mental Hospital in Worcestershire, England, also stressed the psychotherapeutic value of LSD. Throughout the 1950s and early 1960s, Sandison was a pioneer and leading figure in psycholytic therapy, a term he would coin in 1960.[56] Sandison had established a specialist unit for treating psychoneurotic patients at the hospital, with a highly structured LSD psychotherapy treatment procedure based on Jungian analytical psychology. He administered weekly doses to patients—varying from 25 to 400 mcg, depending on their reaction and the desired effect—to produce abreaction and manifestations of the "psychic unconscious" that could be analyzed in the same way as dreams, fantasies, and paintings. Sandison encouraged patients to reach "primal or regressive" experiences through the drug, and experiences such as being born could seem so real as to tempt "one to think that the patient has vividly stored memories of his own birth." Such dramatic occurrences led Sandison to assert that "if anyone wants confirmation of the great analytical principals laid down by Freud and Jung, let him study patients having LSD. The classical complexes and archetypes show in their abundance."[57] Sandison had so far treated approximately ninety patients with LSD, and found 55 percent had recovered from their neuroses, and only 12 percent had failed to show any improvement.[58]

Savage presented a paper exploring how extrapharmacological factors could influence the effects of LSD, an understanding critical to the progress of LSD psychotherapy research. While throughout he still referred to LSD as producing a psychosis, he described successfully using the drug to unblock a patient undergoing psychoanalysis, which helped advance her treatment. He also recognized that the drug did not always produce a psychosis, and, in investigating what determined the patient's reaction in a given LSD session, he highlighted the importance of many variables, which he grouped under the umbrellas of the "mental set of the individual" and the "experimental setting." The "mental set" included factors such as the patient's personality structure and motivation for taking the drug, while the "experimental setting" included environmental stresses, the presence or absence of other persons, and the nature of interpersonal interactions.[59] The manipulation of these factors would come to be recognized by LSD psychotherapists as the key for producing a therapeutic drug response—particularly in psychedelic therapy—and the term "set and setting" would be popularized in the 1960s by Timothy Leary and his cohort.[60]

Lastly, novelist and intellectual Aldous Huxley presented his interpretation mescaline's effects to the psychiatric community, based in part on his own experiences with the drug. The visionary experiences he described, while not immediately concerning psychiatric research and treatment, would become a major component of psychedelic therapy as it developed over the second half of the 1950s. Huxley explored the similarities between the "classic mescaline experience"—as he experienced it and as described by notable nineteenth-century researchers Silas Weir Mitchell and Havelock Ellis—and the spontaneous experiences of history's visionaries, such as William Blake. To Huxley, mescaline seemed to open usually inaccessible parts of the mind:

> Let us use a geographical metaphor and liken the personal life of the ego to the Old World. We leave the Old World, cross a dividing ocean, and find ourselves in the world of the personal subconscious, with its flora and fauna of repressions, conflicts, traumatic memories and the like. Travelling further, we reach a kind of Far West, inhabited by Jungian archetypes and the raw materials of human mythology. Beyond this region lies a broad Pacific. Wafted across it on the wings of mescaline or lysergic acid diethylamide, we reach what might be called the Antipodes of the mind. In this psychological equivalent of Australia we discover the equivalents of kangaroos, wallabies, and duck-billed platypuses —a whole host of extremely improbable animals, which nevertheless exist and can be observed.[61]

From these kind of visionary experiences, Huxley suggested, came the descriptions of the "Other World" found in religion and folklore—the worlds of gods, often described as "of surpassing beauty, glowing with color, bathed in intense light," featuring "buildings of indescribable magnificence" and "fabulous creatures . . . superhuman angels and spirits, who never do anything, but merely enjoy the beatific vision."[62] Audience member Roland Fisher dismissed Huxley's experience as "99 per cent Aldous Huxley and only one half gram mescaline. . . . [S]ome of us are visionaries and others just dry scientists." In an indirect response, Huxley criticized the use of the term "hallucinogen" to describe LSD and mescaline, because of its "pejorative overtone": "To call an experience a hallucination is, implicitly, to condemn it as unreal and in some way discreditable." Instead, he argued, the notion of what was "real" needed to be more critically examined: rather than impose visual distortions, the drugs could unleash latent potential in the mind, allowing the user to see the world as it was, "fresh, living, blazing with color and charged with infinite significance."[63] It was in this transformative power that psychedelic therapists would find LSD's greatest therapeutic potential.

Psychedelic Therapy

Huxley's experience and the mystical turn in LSD and mescaline research came by way of Canada. Beginning in 1953, a team of Saskatchewan-based psychiatric researchers led by Humphry Osmond and Abram Hoffer developed a unique method of using LSD-induced mystical experiences to treat chronic alcoholism, in what they called psychedelic therapy.[64] The therapy involved the deliberate manipulation of set and setting to produce the so-called psychedelic experience, and its theoretical basis combined ideas ranging from the study of mysticism and traditional Native American use of peyote to observations of the circumstances under which chronic alcoholics spontaneously quit drinking. Psychedelic therapy was a psychological treatment, but, unlike psycholytic therapy, it did not emerge from other psychotherapeutic forms but morphed out of psychotomimetic research. Rather than psychoanalysts, both Osmond and Hoffer were biologically oriented psychiatrists. However, when it became apparent that the drug effects they were observing could have therapeutic potential, they did not turn down the opportunity to explore this. While much of the early research was performed in Canada, the theories and methods of psychedelic therapy quickly crossed the border to the United States, and the treatment was well established there by the start of the 1960s.

Born in England, Osmond began his research career in the years after the Second World War at St. George's Hospital in London. There, with colleague John Smythies, Osmond began investigating chemically induced hallucinations and noted the similarities between the effects of mescaline and the symptoms of schizophrenia. After discovering that mescaline was chemically similar to adrenaline, they put forward an argument that schizophrenia was a biochemically induced illness, the result of a fault in the metabolism of adrenalin, which produced a psychoactive chemical.[65] In 1951 Osmond moved to Saskatchewan to take up the role of clinical director of the Saskatchewan Mental Hospital in Weyburn, where he used LSD to continue this line of research with his new colleague, Abram Hoffer, who was director of psychiatric research for the province's Department of Public Health. Before studying medicine, Hoffer had earned a PhD in agriculture, and his interest in biochemistry remained when he later specialized in psychiatry. Together they utilized the psychotomimetic effects of LSD not only to study potential biochemical processes involved in the cause of schizophrenia but also to further their understanding of the nature of the illness by taking the drug themselves. They believed that experiencing the LSD model psychosis had clinical applications, as it improved their understanding of patients' inner lives, thereby increasing their empathy with patients and improving their therapeutic relationship.[66]

The idea of using LSD to treat alcoholics came to Hoffer and Osmond in the early hours of one morning in 1953, after the two had had been unable to sleep while traveling on business. Discussing problems facing psychiatry, their minds turned from schizophrenia to the large population of alcoholics in their hospital, for whom there was no effective treatment. They considered that in Alcoholics Anonymous (AA), "hitting bottom" was often regarded as a crucial prerequisite for recovery. Although what constituted "bottom" was subjective to the individual, it was commonly experiencing delirium tremens. Caused by withdrawal from alcohol after long bouts of heavy drinking, the condition was characterized by tremors, hallucinations, and agitation and was fatal in approximately 10 percent of sufferers.[67] While it may have been an effective turning point for many chronic alcoholics, it was a dangerous and unpredictable event to wait for. Hoffer and Osmond postulated that LSD's psychotomimetic effects could be used to mimic delirium tremens, causing patients to artificially hit bottom. Not only would this be safer, but it could also be performed earlier, and in a controlled supportive environment where the experience's potential for positive impact could be enhanced.[68]

On their return, Hoffer and Osmond immediately tested the hypothesis, treating two alcoholic patients with LSD at the Saskatchewan Mental Hospital, with success for one.[69] On the basis of this, their colleague Colin Smith undertook a larger study with twenty-four alcoholics at the University Hospital in Saskatoon and published results in 1958. To establish efficacy, Smith included in the study only patients with the most severe problems and poor prognoses: most had failed AA and had further psychiatric complications. This helped to accurately determine efficacy, as these patients were less likely to spontaneously improve or manifest a placebo response. The study was uncontrolled, and patients were given a strong dose of LSD (200–400 mcg) or mescaline after two to four weeks of psychotherapy. The patients were accompanied throughout the session, which included a long interview focusing on their problems and strong suggestions from the therapist to stop drinking. Over the subsequent days the patient and therapist further discussed the LSD experience, before the patient was discharged and encouraged to join AA. Follow-up, through AA, ranged from two months to three years and found half of the patients either improved or much improved.[70]

Smith considered as critical to the success of the treatment both an intense drug reaction and the psychotherapeutic regimen it was enmeshed in. While the theory was to help patients hit bottom, he made no effort to scare the patient into the psychotomimetic reaction. Instead, he used a "technique of exhortation, persuasion and suggestion" to help patients increase their self-understanding, gain a new perspective on their drinking habits, and develop the motivation to quit.[71] This effect was displayed in one patient, who after 300 mcg of LSD commented, "This treatment has brought back many thoughts. When I think of it, what a fool I made of myself these last 22 to 23 years. . . . I wanted to stop drinking for a long time, but it's lack of willpower. I started drinking at 18. My stepfather was a heavy drinker. I drank to get even for I felt the more we had the less he had. . . . This is an experience worth going through. I feel I can stay away from alcohol now."[72] Early on, the Saskatchewan researchers began realizing that although the treatment was working, great numbers of the patients were not experiencing the model delirium tremens they set out to create. Instead, patients were having experiences that were "exciting and pleasant, and yielded insight into their drinking problems," with some even "escaping into a spiritual or religious type of experience."[73] They soon learned that this kind of treatment had a precedent, as members of the Native American Church of North America used peyote to commune with God and combat drinking.[74] The researchers would also point to renowned psychologist William James's observation that powerful religious conversion experiences could cure alcoholics, as discussed in his 1902 work *The Varieties of Religious Experience*. Such an experience had also famously led Bill W. to quit drinking and develop AA in the 1930s.[75]

Osmond took a particular interest in the transcendental effects that LSD and mescaline could produce. In addition to harnessing them clinically, he began exploring their nonmedical significance with Huxley. Huxley had long had a keen interest in mysticism, and he contacted Osmond in 1953 after reading reports of his early research. Osmond subsequently visited Huxley and administered him mescaline. The next year Huxley published *The Doors of Perception*, an account of this experience that would influence not only LSD researchers but also the psychedelic counterculture of the 1960s.[76] Osmond presented his new multifaceted understanding of the effects of LSD and mescaline to the scientific community in 1957, at a meeting of the New York Academy of Sciences. He connected the Saskatchewan research to cultural and intellectual traditions varying from the relatively recent work of figures such as William James and Carl Jung to the ritualistic and religious use of drugs by cultures throughout time, commenting that "we are the latest of generations of experimenters who, from before the dawn of history, in every part of the world, have sought for means by which man could alter, explore, and control the workings of his own mind, thus enlarging his experience of the universe."[77] Osmond believed the drugs had uses in studying psychotic illnesses, performing psychotherapy, training mental health workers, and "exploring the normal mind under unusual circumstances." Their mystical effects also had social, philosophical, and religious implications, as they could "help us to explore and fathom our own nature," through their ability to strip users of their acquired beliefs and "see the universe again with an innocent eye."[78] In light of their variety of effects and uses, Osmond considered "psychotomimetic" too narrow a term for LSD and similar drugs, and instead proposed the term "psychedelic." Meaning "mind-manifesting," the name was designed to "include the concepts of enriching the mind and enlarging the vision" and to escape the negative connotations of terms such as "psychotomimetic" and "hallucinogen."[79] While Osmond intended the term to encompass all the possible effects of the drugs, it soon came to represent their transcendental or mystical qualities.

In the mid-1950s, the Saskatchewan researchers were not the only researchers exploring the psychedelic effects of LSD and their therapeutic applications. In British Columbia, American Alfred (Al) M. Hubbard had been simultaneously developing a treatment for alcoholism that similarly focused on the patient attaining a psychedelic reaction, but with more advanced techniques for ensuring that this happened. Contact between Hubbard and the Saskatchewan researchers led to a refining of their therapeutic method. Hubbard, a lay therapist working under the medical guidance of psychiatrist J. Ross MacLean at Hollywood Hospital in Vancouver, was a mysterious character who had been a US Office of Strategic Services operative during the Second World War before becoming one of LSD's greatest advocates during the 1950s.[80] He made up for his lack of background in medicine or psychology by obtaining a PhD in Bio-Psycho-Dynamic Sciences in the mid-1950s, although it was most likely purchased from a diploma mill.[81] Despite his suspect credentials, Hubbard was skilled in the use and manipulation of LSD's effects. In 1957 he visited the Saskatchewan researchers to demonstrate his therapeutic method. His innovation was to manipulate the set and setting of the patient, through the use of a specially designed treatment room and visual and auditory stimuli, to help the patient relax and to foster the psychedelic experience. The room was not a clinical environment but instead used furnishings such as drapes, sofas, and rugs to create a comfortable, tranquil atmosphere. Music, photographs, artworks, flowers, and other items were used during the sessions to help patients relax, direct their emotions, explore their enhanced perception, and focus toward a spiritual experience.[82]

Adopting these changes, Nick Chwelos led a new study at the Saskatchewan Hospital with sixteen alcoholics. Results, published in 1959, found that, after an average follow-up period of six months, all but one patient was improved and ten were much improved. In addition to incorporating visual and auditory stimuli, the new method involved a greater emphasis on the nature of the therapist's attitude toward and interaction with the patient: the therapist should present an accepting attitude, encouraging patients toward self-acceptance while stressing that they had the power and responsibility to change the pathological attitudes that became apparent. The researchers also emphasized the need for the therapist to have had personal experience with LSD to understand patients' drug experiences and effectively direct them toward a therapeutic response.[83] The exact nature of the psychedelic experience, because of its individual, subjective, and otherworldly nature, was difficult for patients or researchers to easily describe. Similarly, the mechanism by which the experience could help alcoholics was highly complex but could be seen as involving a change in their perception of themselves, their drinking, and their relationship to others. The researchers explored how some of the common experiences, such as "being able to see oneself objectively," a "feeling of being at one with the universe," and a "change in the usual concept of self," had a therapeutic effect:

> Because the drug makes him feel he is infinite in essence it is much easier for him to accept himself completely and it readily becomes evident that he can only accept the outside world to the exact degree that he accepts himself. The patient feels, at the same time, that this is not only true in the LSD experience but also outside it; that this process is only telescoped under LSD. He then sees that lack of faith or acceptance that he is essentially infinite is the exact coun-

terpart of anxiety and that faith and anxiety cannot be experienced at the same time. He also sees that guilt is disrupting in that it is a denial of this infinite self which is the same for everyone. This equalizing effect tends to remove any form of pride, prejudice, guilt or anxiety. The person then sees that faith which is the acceptance of himself as infinite and love which is the acceptance that everything around him is equal to him in substance is the clue to a smooth, pleasant, useful LSD experience, and he generalizes this to everyday experience. The patient then ceases the tragedy of desiring to be other than he is in essence and realizes that he can only be other than he is in terms of his acts. The energy diverted from attempts to alter his basic nature can now be used to alter his feelings and acts in a way which makes his life more peaceful and satisfying and his outlook more compassionate.[84]

With Chwelos's study, the psychedelic therapy paradigm had fully developed: a single, high-dose LSD treatment, embedded in a framework of psychotherapy, utilizing visual and auditory stimuli, with a therapist acting as supportive and encouraging guide rather than analytic interviewer, to produce a psychedelic experience that could fundamentally change an alcoholic's attitudes, perspective, and behavior, leading to sobriety.

In the United States, interest in the psychedelic effects of LSD began to grow near the end of the 1950s in California. Rather than simply replicating the Canadian psychedelic therapy method, much of this psychedelic research was exploratory in nature, approaching the effects of LSD from philosophical and religious, as well as psychiatric, perspectives. Philosophical and religious perspectives were most notably explored by Aldous Huxley and philosophers Gerald Heard and Alan Watts, who shared Huxley's interest in the relationship between psychedelic and religious experiences, across cultures and throughout history.[85] This intellectual interest was not divorced from clinical research, as Huxley and Heard, as well as Los Angeles psychiatric researcher Sidney Cohen, were members of the Commission for the Study of Creative Imagination, a collective formed to share and support psychedelic research, which also included Hubbard, Hoffer, Osmond, and other researchers from Canada, the United States, England, and Mexico.[86] Through the collaboration of intellectuals and clinical researchers, the psychedelic theory and method soon migrated out of Canada.

Cohen and his research partner, psychologist Betty Eisner, were early adopters of some of the Canadian researchers' techniques, at the Los Angeles Veterans Administration Neuropsychiatric Hospital. Their use of LSD sat somewhere between psycholytic and psychedelic therapy. Patients with a wide variety of diagnoses were treated, in multiple sessions, with doses building up to 125 mcg, and the goal was more effective psychotherapy through conventional channels such as abreaction and enhanced insight and recall. However, elements of psychedelic therapy were also present—music, mirrors, and photographs were used to aid relaxation, direct emotions, and promote insight, and a therapist who was personally experienced with the drug was present for the length of the drug reaction. The researchers further noted that the drug could produce an integrative experience where the patient was "able to see himself in proper perspective and in relation to his environment," a key factor in the therapeutic potential of the psychedelic experience.[87] Eisner and Cohen's own personal experiences with the drug had also been in the psychedelic realm: both first tried it in 1955, with Eisner reporting "being drawn into a mystical experience—the sense of unity with all things in the universe," and Cohen, who expected to be catatonic, writing, "I seemed to have finally arrived at the contemplation of the eternal truth. . . . At one moment I was a timeless spirit."[88] The pair was also notable for administering LSD to AA founder Bill W., who likened his experience to the religious revelation that had led to his sobriety.[89]

Psychedelic therapy reached its mature form in the United States through the research of Savage, James Terrill, and Donald Jackson at the Mental Research Institute of the Palo Alto Medical Research Foundation. The trio first presented its work in 1960 to a daylong symposium on LSD held at Napa State Hospital, which received considerable local attention and was broadcast on the radio. Terrill had administered LSD to both volunteers and psychiatric patients in an atmosphere and physical environment similar to that of the Canadian researchers. He found that patients had a wide variety of reactions (including transcendental), which were heavily influenced by set and setting. In therapeutic sessions, beneficial results came from changes to patients' value systems, rather than through the traditional channels of psychotherapy, and were "in the direction of a higher valuation of esthetic, creative, philosophic and perhaps even religious interests."[90] Jackson echoed this and discussed how the transcendental reaction could "lead to a lessening of alienation, to a rediscovery of the self, to a new set of values, to the finding of new potential for growth and development and to a new beginning. This may be followed by a change in behavioural patterns, as in the cessation of drinking."[91]

Savage drew on his experience with twenty alcoholic patients to explore how LSD could promote sobriety. The patients had been treated with 150–500 mcg of LSD in a psychedelic therapy setting, and 50 percent had stopped drinking.[92] Like Hoffer and Osmond, Savage discussed psychedelic therapy's precedent in the Native American use of peyote to cure or prevent alcoholism, which, he argued, worked by giving not only a renewed connection with religion but an increased faith in and identification with their culture in the face of European domination. He also similarly explored the theories of William James as an explanation for both the causes of alcoholism and LSD's use in treating it, quoting his remark, "The cure for dipsomania is religiomania."[93] The LSD-induced religious experience seemed to Savage to produce a powerful feeling of forgiveness that could break the cycle of "drink to still guilt, and drink giving rise to guilt."[94]

Expanding this discussion, Savage went on to explore the manner in which LSD-induced mystical experiences could address the conflicts at the heart of alcoholism. James had postulated that alcohol's allure came from its "power to stimulate the mystical faculties of human nature."[95] It did this, however, only in a fleeting manner, leading the seeker of these experiences to destructive overindulgence. Drawing on the theories of psychoanalyst Erich Fromm, Savage argued that the need for mystical experience was based in feelings of alienation. LSD's more powerful mystical effects could more fully resolve these feelings, relieving the patient's desire to drink:

> Many drinkers drink because their lives have lost purpose and meaning. The old drunk might drown his sorrows; the modern drunk fills the emptiness of his existence.
>
> The alcoholic attempts to find himself, to fulfil himself with drink; but the attempt fails and now the guilt over drink and the wasted opportunity has him trapped. How then may LSD help with this situation? It may provide a genuine transcendental or mystic experience instead of the spurious one "bit of mystic consciousness" which the alcoholic has been seeking. The artificial distinction between subject and object, self and world, conscious and unconscious, ego, id and superego are all abolished. The person is at one with the universe. In his mystic selflessness he awakens with a feeling of rebirth, often physically felt, and he is provided with a new beginning, a new sense of values. He becomes aware of the richness of the unconscious at his disposal; the energies bound up in and by repression become available to him.[96]

In addition to confirming the therapeutic potential of psychedelic therapy, through their research, Savage, Terrill, and Jackson also discovered the dangers LSD could present when used in an uncontrolled setting. In 1958, the researchers had arranged for Hubbard to visit and give a demonstration session of his psychedelic therapy technique with one of their patients. When Hubbard failed to show up, two researchers attached to the project decided to experiment with the 200 mcg dose themselves. The researcher acting as "guide" was not well trained in this task, and the clandestine nature of the session—conducted without the knowledge or permission of the senior researchers—created a stressful setting that likely influenced the outcome. This outcome was, according to Savage, a "classic 'bad trip.'" The subject "was immediately plunged into hellfire, where he found himself roasting his father over a slow fire, basting and turning him with great glee. He found he was the infant Jesus, about to be sacrificed. He suffered from the eruption of abhorrent cravings, which he was unable to identify. He emerged from the session with the conviction, the 'insight' that he was no damned good." Despite the best efforts of Savage and his colleagues to treat the lasting negative impact of the session, the subject developed a hypomanic reaction, destroyed the project's records, and wrote to the US president describing his plan to enact "world peace through the 'Wedding of Heaven and Hell.'" The subject was removed from the project and assigned an independent psychiatrist, but the psychiatrist and patient developed an unhealthy relationship: they moved into a house in the country together—along with the patient's wife—and according to Savage both became "acutely psychotic." It took two years for the subject to completely recover. Besides the personal cost to the subject, the incident destroyed Savage and Jackson's relationship and the entire research program.[97] It would not, however, end Savage's psychedelic research career.

Conclusion

As the 1950s came to a close, the promise for LSD in psychiatry appeared to be only increasing. Through careful experimentation, North American and European researchers had observed the wide variety of effects the drug could produce; learned how to alter its effects by manipulating dose, set, and setting; and explored how the effects could be harnessed to better understand and treat mental illness. Over the decade, LSD research had thrived in an eclectic and innovative context of psychiatry in the United States and had been facilitated by the loose regulation of pharmaceutical research. While psycholytic and psychedelic therapy were distinctly different treatment forms, both involved using a drug to facilitate a psychotherapeutic process. They both, therefore, bridged any theoretical divide between biological and psychodynamic psychiatry. While the treatments were unconventional, their effectiveness seemed obvious to those who had explored them, and their success with chronic and otherwise refractory patients seemed to provide convincing evidence that the effects were genuine. The dramatic successes reported for treating alcoholic patients particularly suggested that the drug had significant public health implications. LSD seemed destined to join the ranks of other new drugs revolutionizing psychiatry.

CHAPTER TWO

Regulating Research

LSD and the FDA

As LSD has become a problem, the possibility has arisen that public reaction will discourage and dry up legitimate research into and therapeutic use of LSD. . . . If we in the Federal Government allow these legitimate uses to be interfered with, the loss to the Nation in hopes of potential aid for the handicapped would be serious indeed.

Senator Robert F. Kennedy, 1966

At a May 1966 congressional hearing, Senator Robert F. Kennedy questioned FDA commissioner James L. Goddard on the recent decline in the number of approved clinical LSD research programs. In April Sandoz Pharmaceuticals had voluntarily withdrawn its sponsorship of LSD research, and subsequently the number of programs had dropped from seventy to nine. After ascertaining from Goddard that the FDA had considered all of these programs worthwhile, Kennedy criticized the administration for doing too little to ensure their continuation: "If they were worth while I would think you would let them continue. . . . If it was helpful [research] 6 months ago, why is it not helpful now?"[1]

With the passage of the Drug Amendments of 1962, the era of unimpeded psychedelic research had come to a close. Where previously researchers could freely and easily source LSD and use it as they saw fit, research now required FDA approval. The amendments did not specifically control LSD; the FDA gained oversight of all premarket clinical drug research. However, the amendments' impact on the scale of LSD research was direct and immediate: in 1963 the previously widespread research had dwindled to just seventeen approved programs, recovering somewhat to seventy by 1966, before dropping again to nine. Those researchers who could not continue using LSD put the blame squarely at the feet of the federal government: Myron Stolaroff recollected that in 1965 Commissioner Goddard "brought a halt to all LSD research in the nation," and Harold Abramson described in 1967 how

LSD research was being "seriously hampered in the U.S. by the curtailment of Government approval," due to the government's inability to "distinguish between the medical use of LSD and the sociological problems engendered by *all* drugs that influence the mind."[2]

This decline in the scale of LSD research coincided with LSD's rising popularity as a recreational drug and ensuing controversy. It can therefore appear almost self-evident that the government deliberately restricted LSD research. The initial 1963 reduction came in the same year as the first significant scandal over LSD erupted, when Harvard psychologists Timothy Leary and Richard Alpert were dismissed from the university following concerns that their psychedelic research was little more than widespread use of the drugs. The second drop corresponded closely with the passage of the Drug Abuse Control Amendments of 1965, which began LSD's prohibition as a drug of abuse, as well as Sandoz's withdrawal of its research sponsorship, which the company blamed on the drug's increasing misuse and notoriety. Indeed, 1966 was a flashpoint for the LSD controversy, as nonmedical use of the drug broke out of niche circles to become increasingly widespread among the nation's youth, attracting growing concern from medical and law enforcement authorities. Reflecting this, Kennedy's hearings were one of three sets that year to focus significant attention on the drug.

FDA files documenting the regulation of LSD research in the 1960s reveal a different story. Rather than opposition to LSD psychotherapy research, the reduction in research in the 1960s simply reflected the formalization of pharmaceutical research and development in the United States that the Drug Amendments of 1962 ushered in, as well as actions of Sandoz. The FDA's evaluation of applications to conduct LSD research made by Sandoz, Abramson, and Stolaroff's research foundation, the International Foundation for Advanced Study, shows that when researchers were denied access to the drug—as was the case with Abramson and the foundation—it was done for clear reasons. Rather than intentionally thwarting research, the FDA evaluated applications to conduct research according to new, rigid criteria. Where the LSD controversy had its major impact was in influencing Sandoz to withdraw its sponsorship of LSD research in 1966. This made LSD's development into a marketable pharmaceutical much less likely, as researchers were not normally responsible for pushing drugs through the NDA process without the support of a pharmaceutical company. However, that research survived at all was thanks to the federal government: with Sandoz's withdrawal, the FDA teamed up with the National Institute of Mental Health and Veterans Administration

(VA) to voluntarily save research from complete extinction—even Kennedy's criticism of the FDA was misplaced.

Introducing Oversight

The research oversight provisions of the Drug Amendments of 1962 emerged as a result of FDA concerns that drug manufacturers were using the premarket phase of a drug's development for more than just research. From the mid-1950s, FDA officers had been aware of their inability to prevent widespread distribution of investigational drugs to physicians for the ulterior purpose of establishing their place in the market prior to official release.[3] The danger of this practice became evident in the case of thalidomide, the sedative found to cause severe birth defects when ingested during pregnancy. FDA medical officer Frances O. Kelsey had withheld approval of William S. Merrell Company's NDA for thalidomide in 1960, because of concerns over the safety data supplied. Nevertheless, the firm had distributed the drug widely to physicians recommending its routine usage. As a result, an estimated sixteen thousand patients received thalidomide. It was mostly luck that only seventeen confirmed cases of phocomelia were found in the United States: most of the patients who were pregnant did not receive the drug during the first trimester, when damage to the fetus occurs.[4] The thalidomide tragedy pushed through investigational drug reforms that the FDA had long promoted but that had previously languished because of public disinterest and political and industry opposition.[5]

To safeguard against dangerous and nonresearch investigational drug use, the Drug Amendments of 1962 provided that a drug manufacturer, or other investigative sponsor, would be permitted to use a drug without an accepted NDA in human research only after providing the FDA with details of preclinical research that justified such use. Assurance also needed to be given that patients would be under the personal supervision of the investigators, that the experimental drug would not be supplied to anyone outside of the investigation, and that data resulting from research would be recorded so that it could be reported to the FDA to determine the safety and effectiveness of the drug.[6] To enact these provisions, the FDA drew up new investigational drug regulations, which became effective on 7 February 1963. Earl Meyers, chief of the controls evaluation branch of the FDA's Division of New Drugs, described the intent of the regulations as ensuring that adequate preclinical research had been performed to justify clinical testing, that investigators were qualified to perform clinical research with the drug, and that a scientifically sound

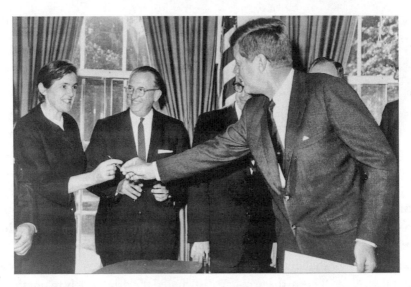

President John F. Kennedy handing FDA medical officer Frances O. Kelsey a pen he has just used to sign the Kefauver-Harris Drug Amendments of 1962 into law on 10 October 1962. Photograph courtesy of the US Food and Drug Administration.

program of research would be followed.[7] The regulations centered on the creation of the IND form, officially entitled Form FD 1571, or Notice of Claimed Investigational Exemption for a New Drug. Before commencing clinical research with an investigational drug, the potential sponsor needed to submit this form to the FDA. Approval of the IND was not required; research could start immediately on submission. However, if the FDA was not satisfied with the contents of an IND, the sponsor's exemption could be terminated.[8]

Following the intentions of the regulations, the information required on the IND form focused on drug data, the investigators, and the plan of research. Required data included the drug's chemical structure, the composition of the preparation, manufacturing and quality control standards, and details on preclinical investigations—including animal studies—that suggested reasonable safety for use in clinical studies. Details regarding the investigators included their names, qualifications, and experience, as well as a statement of the qualifications and experience that the sponsor considered necessary for investigators to evaluate the drug's safety. Investigators were also required to submit a separate individual statement with further details on their qualifications, facilities, plans, and responsibilities. The plan of investigation required designating the "phase" of the research: Phase 1 consisted of basic clinical pharmacology, testing issues such as toxicity, metabolism, absorption, and elimination. Phase 2 tested the drug in an initial small series of patients, while Phase 3 established the drug's safety and effectiveness in a large number of patients with a reasonably standardized treatment protocol. Further required details included the number of subjects involved, their selection criteria, the clinical trial design, testing methods, and the duration of treatment.[9]

For drugs that were already being used in human research, the FDA set a deadline for the submission of IND forms of 7 June 1963.[10] Shortly before the deadline, Sandoz Pharmaceuticals submitted INDs for the clinical investigation of LSD and psilocybin. Sandoz had isolated the psychedelic alkaloid psilocybin from a Mexican variety of mushroom (*Psilocybe mexicana*) in the late 1950s and had subsequently synthesized it and distributed it in a manner similar to its distribution of LSD.[11] FDA notes on the INDs suggest that they were very broad in their scope and light on details. Sandoz proposed Phase 3 clinical trials, which were already underway, as Phase 1 and 2 studies had been completed. The drugs were being investigated in the "treatment of varied psychotic and psychoneurotic disorders"—including chronic alcoholism and autism in children—as a facilitator of, and adjunct to, psychotherapy and as an analgesic for intractable pain. A proposed adult dose range for LSD was given, ranging from 1 microgram per kilogram of body weight (mcg/kg) once to twice a week to the unprecedentedly massive 200–300 mcg/kg in two doses over five weeks. A minute dose of 1–5 mcg per day, over an indefinite period, was indicated for children. The application emphasized that the determination of dosage and the duration of treatment would ultimately lie with the individual investigator.[12]

The INDs were more specific on who would be able to research the drugs under Sandoz's sponsorship: access was restricted to those working under grants from, or the authority of, the NIMH, state agencies, or the VA, with all research to be conducted in a hospital setting. According to the FDA, Sandoz made this decision to ensure that investigators were specially qualified and had adequate facilities for patient care.[13] It was also likely influenced by growing concern that the use of psychedelics was in some places veering from traditional medical research—introducing the possibilities of abuse and controversy, as most notably seen in the recent case of Leary and Alpert. Sandoz likely considered that having each research program specifically sponsored by a government agency would guard against this and reduce any possible liability or tarnish to the company's reputation if medical research with LSD became scandalized.

The FDA's pharmacology division made its initial review of the Sandoz

LSD and psilocybin INDs in August and September 1963. It found the INDs lacked the required level of toxicity data and recommended that "consideration be given to the termination of the clinical investigations."[14] However, the FDA's Bureau of Medicine considered the fact that the LSD IND was supported by a bibliography of more than one thousand scientific papers that detailed a wide variety of research, conducted over more than twenty years, that had resulted in no deaths or serious side effects. As there was in practice no serious concern over toxicity and the literature attested to promising effectiveness, the Bureau of Medicine decided that clinical investigation could continue, with a request for further data. Subsequent review of the research confirmed that there existed sufficient data to allow research under the Sandoz IND.[15]

Initially Sandoz sponsored seventeen LSD investigators. These researchers, some of whom had been working with LSD prior to 1962, investigated the drug's effects and applications in a wide variety of ways. Keith Ditman at the University of California, Los Angeles, had compared the effects of LSD to delirium tremens and reported on the positive benefits experienced by subjects given LSD in an experimental, rather than therapeutic, setting. Dietrich Heyder, of the Norfolk Mental Health Center in Virginia had found success using LSD with an otherwise treatment-resistant psychotherapy patient. Eric Kast, of Chicago Medical School, studied LSD's analgesic effects, and Lauretta Bender of Creedmoor State Hospital in California treated autistic schizophrenic children with the drug. Albert Kurland, of Spring Grove State Hospital in Maryland, and Harry Hook of Mendocino State Hospital in California, would go on to publish studies of psychedelic therapy in the treatment of alcoholism.[16] Sandoz added investigators to the IND over the next three years, reaching approximately seventy by 1966. The company also expanded the criteria for eligibility to include grantees of "approved national agencies" such as the National Science Foundation.[17]

With Sandoz's decision to restrict its sponsorship of research to hospital-based, government-endorsed studies, privately funded and private-practice researchers who had been using LSD found themselves cut off. However, nowhere in the new regulations did it say that only a drug's manufacturer could act as a sponsor, so independent researchers were free to submit their own IND forms for clinical research with LSD. Examining the independent INDs that were submitted by Harold Abramson and the International Foundation for Advanced Study reveals that the struggle to gain access to LSD in the years immediately following the Drug Amendments of 1962 was not due to any specific restrictions from the government but instead the result of Sandoz's own efforts to maintain control over all research, as well as the general difficulty in meeting the IND requirements as an independent researcher.

Harold Abramson

By 1963, Abramson was the director of research at the South Oaks Research Foundation, a division of the South Oaks Psychiatric Hospital in Amityville, New York. Founded in 1882, the private hospital averaged a population of two hundred patients and treated all psychiatric disorders.[18] Sandoz had initially listed Abramson as an LSD investigator in its IND, but he was quickly removed once the company decided to restrict its sponsorship to those working under the NIMH, state agencies, and the VA.[19] Abramson first contacted the FDA in May 1963, after finding that he could no longer source the drug from Sandoz. He believed that he had been deemed unqualified to perform research under the new drug rules. Having used LSD for more than ten years, Abramson wished to clarify his qualifications "in order to eliminate what at present is damaging to my position professionally."[20] The FDA's Bureau of Enforcement advised him to take up the issue with Sandoz, as it was a drug's sponsor, not the FDA, who initially determined the adequacy of researchers' qualifications. Subsequently, Abramson decided to become a sponsor for LSD research himself, and the FDA instructed him to submit an IND form.[21]

In November 1963, Abramson met with Frances Kelsey and Merle Gibson of the FDA's Investigational Drug Branch to discuss submitting an IND for LSD research. The FDA officers again emphasized that Sandoz's criteria for researching LSD under its IND had nothing to do with the new drug regulations. The decision was voluntary and had come out of discussion between Sandoz and the NIMH. Clearly taking Sandoz's criteria personally, Abramson suggested that the company might have denied him access to LSD because of his criticism of Sansert—another Sandoz drug he had experimented with. He had argued that Sansert could produce effects similar to those of LSD but with greater potential danger. Abramson also stated the he had been turned down for an NIMH grant because of the agency's skepticism of his animal research on fighting Siamese swordtails.[22] In 1954, Abramson had published research reporting that the fish uncharacteristically swam nose up, tail down, when exposed to LSD. This behavior increased with the concentration of LSD in their water. He had therefore suggested that by exposing the fish to human urine, this phenomenon could be observed as a bioassay for the presence of LSD. Considering LSD to produce a model psychosis, he had also suggested that exposing the fish to the urine of patients with schizophrenia might help uncover a naturally occurring substance causing the illness.[23]

Further defending his position to the FDA officials, Abramson attested to his extensive experience with LSD, through the military's Chemical Warfare Division, which had included self-experimentation and administering the drug to subjects for long periods. He had found that LSD was a very safe drug that was not addictive. He still had stock of LSD that had previously been supplied by Sandoz. He wished to use this in research treating mental illness, particularly schizophrenia. He also believed that LSD psychotherapy was valuable in the treatment of alcoholism. Abramson presented a drafted IND form to Kelsey and Gibson, but they told him that it was lacking in chemical control data, which he should request from Sandoz.[24]

Three days after the meeting, Abramson wrote to the US headquarters of Sandoz in New Jersey. He stated that he wished to become his own sponsor for LSD research. To do so, he requested that Sandoz provide him with the drug data required to complete sections 1–6 on the IND form. These sections covered preclinical data such as the drug's chemical structure, composition, and manufacturing controls, as well as details of animal and other research that indicated that it was reasonably safe to conduct human research. Only a drug's manufacturer could produce much of the chemical and manufacturing data, while the rest could theoretically be produced by any experienced scientist with supplies of the drug, but only at great expense and difficulty. Abramson appealed to Sandoz to "be kind enough" to supply the data, as it "can be obtained from no other source."[25] Sandoz's Leonard Achor replied coolly, repeating the company's criteria for LSD investigators and stating, "For the record, it is necessary to advise that Sandoz Pharmaceuticals will remain the sole sponsor of *LSD-25* in the United States as per Company policy. Accordingly, it will not be possible to supply you with the information contained in items one through six in the form #1571."[26]

Frustrated by this response, Abramson replied that Achor's statement directly contradicted advice he had received from the FDA's Bureau of Enforcement, that "anyone may become a sponsor for an investigational drug." If "for reasons which are obscure to me" Sandoz was unwilling to supply the data he requested, Abramson inquired whether the information was already filed with the FDA and whether it was in the public domain. If this was the case he could use it to become his own sponsor, thus "relieving Sandoz of any responsibility." He also drew attention to the implications of his situation for drug research more generally: "in this period of transformation" brought about by

the new regulations, it was important to make sure that "unnecessary obstacles" did not hamper "freedom of medical investigation."[27] In response, Achor
again emphasized that Sandoz would remain the sole sponsor for LSD. He
stated that the necessary data had been supplied to the FDA; however, it was
given in confidence and was "not, I repeat not, in the public domain."[28]

Reaching a dead end with Sandoz, Abramson forwarded his correspondence with the company to Kelsey at the FDA. He complained that "Sandoz
refused to acknowledge the right to self-sponsorship," which the FDA had
made clear to him. Unable to complete an IND, he asked how he could proceed. He pointed out that, as he already had stocks of LSD, he did not need
the company's cooperation to perform his proposed research.[29]

However, instead of the sympathetic support that Abramson was hoping
to receive, the FDA began to view him with suspicion. Kelsey had heard that
Abramson was "rather an LSD enthusiast," and Sandoz had confirmed that he
was no longer listed as one of their investigators. She therefore became concerned that Abramson was using the drug in human research without filing
an IND and decided to investigate. Sandoz had also informed Kelsey that it
had supplied LSD to Abramson prior to 1963 for animal use only.[30] This was
significant. If Abramson had obtained LSD for human use prior to the Drug
Amendments of 1962, Kelsey believed that the new regulations would likely
not apply to that stock and he would be free to continue human research with
it. However, as the LSD was for animal use only, human research with that
stock had not been covered under the previous regulatory scheme. Therefore,
he needed to submit an IND for the new use.[31] Kelsey decided to send an FDA
inspector to visit Abramson. The inspector was to examine his stock of LSD
to ascertain its quantity, manufacturer, and labeling, as well as to investigate
whether he was currently using the drug in human research. If there was any
evidence of this, a sample of the drug was to be taken, on which seizure could
be based.[32]

On 22 May 1964, New York FDA inspector Irwin Schorr telephoned
Abramson to arrange an inspection of his LSD stocks. Obviously taken by
surprise, Abramson took great offence and refused to comply without an official written request—that would be assessed by his lawyer—or a court order.
Abramson questioned Schorr's qualifications and jurisdiction, referencing
higher FDA officials he had consulted with, such as Kelsey. He objected to
being treated like a "criminal" and raved about his work for the Department
of Defense and his publications. He argued that he was "not just an 'ordinary
practicing doctor' but an expert on LSD" and that Schorr should have looked

him up in a "Who's Who." Schorr tried to emphasize that he did not wish to interrogate Abramson but simply inspect his stock of LSD. But this did not calm him. Instead, Abramson threatened to take the matter to his senator and told Schorr that if his IND was not approved, he would "take the matter to court."[33]

Three weeks later, Schorr and a partner visited Abramson at the South Oaks Research Foundation and issued him with a Notice of Inspection. Having been advised to cooperate by a senior FDA official, Abramson was now "extremely cordial." He described having received a "huge quantity" of LSD from Sandoz over the past thirteen years, though exactly how much he did not know. When his current stock was gathered together for inspection a week later, he was found to have 604.1 milligrams of LSD, which Schorr described as enough for more than twenty thousand doses. Abramson stated that he had not used the drug on humans since the new drug regulations. This was not because the FDA prohibited it but out of fear of malpractice suits, as his LSD was labeled for investigational use only. In fact, he believed that the government had no jurisdiction over his right, as a doctor, to "administer any drug to his patients in the course of treatment." If Abramson genuinely believed this, it is not clear why he had been fighting so hard to complete an IND. He may have believed that FDA approval would protect him from malpractice suits when using an investigational drug. Instead of human research, Abramson was presently using LSD with fish. Particularly, he described how his observation of the effects of LSD on fish had led New York State to experiment with using the drug to rid its streams of the "trash fish" carp. This use was not widely practiced, as apparently there was "much public objection to putting LSD into streams which run into the reservoirs of New York City."[34]

Regarding his IND application, Abramson complained about the need to supply preclinical data that Sandoz had already filed with the FDA. Since he was using Sandoz LSD, he logically argued that requiring him to provide the data himself was unnecessary. Nevertheless, Schorr told him that he needed Sandoz's written consent to refer to its data. Abramson again claimed that Sandoz's refusal to permit him to use its data was due to his falling out with the company over Sansert. He also reemphasized his qualifications and experience in the use of LSD and similar drugs, even offering to act as a consultant to the FDA on them. Schorr was sympathetic, stressing to Abramson that there were no doubts as to his qualifications and nothing personal in the delayed decision over his IND—"it was just a matter of law."[35]

Following the visit, Schorr reported to his superiors that he was satisfied that Abramson was not using his supplies of LSD on humans while his IND was under review. No sample for seizure was taken. He wrote that Abramson was "extremely anxious" to have his IND approved and resume clinical research with the drug and that he might test the law in court if the IND was terminated. However, in the interim, he considered it "doubtful that he would do anything to jeopardize his position as a prospective investigator/sponsor or doctor."[36]

On 11 May 1965 FDA commissioner George Larrick sent Abramson the results of his IND review. The review concluded that Abramson's IND "fails to contain sufficient data to support a conclusion that it is reasonably safe to initiate the intended clinical investigations with the drug." This determination was based on the application's lack of information on both preclinical investigations and the "methods, facilities, and controls used for manufacturing, processing and packing the investigational drug." The letter acknowledged that Abramson had referenced Sandoz's data in regard to these sections of the IND, but it stated that the FDA could not refer to data already on file "without written authorization" from the original submitter. Abramson was given ten days to remedy the situation; otherwise, his IND would be terminated.[37] No additional data was submitted. On 23 July Larrick sent notice to Abramson that his IND for LSD was terminated.[38]

In August 1965, FDA inspector Robert Dee visited Abramson to confirm that he was complying with his IND termination and to again inspect his supplies of LSD. With his lawyer present, Abramson expressed the great offence and humiliation he had experienced as a result of the FDA denying him approval to conduct clinical LSD research. He had found the process a "personal affront to his professional integrity." Abramson and his lawyer argued that the FDA had overstepped its jurisdiction by interfering with a physician's right to administer a drug that had been safely used for many years, and that it was unreasonable to require him to provide manufacturing data that the FDA already had on file. They again threatened to take the issue to court and to register a complaint with their local member of Congress. Abramson emphasized his embarrassment at meeting younger and less experienced physicians and psychologists who could use LSD simply because they worked in a state institution. He had also encountered embarrassing situations where patients had offered him black market supplies of the drug after he had been forced to deny their requests for LSD therapy.[39]

Dee found that Abramson was complying with the law by only using his

LSD in animal research. He had been investigating whether LSD could be used to rid swimming beaches of sharks. He had hypothesized that if sharks were fed carp laced with LSD, like other fish they would float vertically near the surface of the water and could then easily be captured or killed. However, tests had subsequently found that sharks did not react to LSD. Dee also found that Abramson's stock of LSD was largely unchanged since the previous inspection. As it had been obtained prior to the Drug Amendments of 1962 and was not being used in human research, it could not be seized. The matter was laid to rest.[40] Abramson continued his animal research with LSD, but he never resumed clinical research with the drug.[41]

The correspondence among Abramson, Sandoz, and the FDA reveals three distinct attitudes regarding who was entitled to perform research with investigational new drugs. Sandoz believed that it had the right, as the drug's manufacturer, to control access to the drug. Abramson, by contrast, thought that his rights as a physician came first: as a qualified and experienced physician, he was entitled to use drugs in treatment and research as he saw fit. The FDA's position was on the surface neutral—anybody could sponsor clinical research with a drug as long as they could complete the necessary paperwork showing that it was reasonably safe to do so. However, as a drug's manufacturer was the only party practically able to produce much of the necessary data and as the FDA held IND data in confidence—reading any subsequent applications with an artificial ignorance regarding the safety of the drug—in practice the manufacturer had great control over what research could be conducted with a drug. A manufacturer could not itself sponsor research without the FDA's approval, but it could prevent others from using its drugs in research that the FDA would otherwise approve. Sandoz used this power to maintain a monopoly over LSD sponsorship and limit research to government-sponsored, hospital-based projects. Despite Abramson's claim that Sandoz's rejection of his requests was personal, there is little evidence to support this—Sandoz set up clear company policy for how it wished LSD research to proceed, and Abramson did not meet the criteria. The FDA's policy protected the intellectual property rights and commercial interests of the manufacturer yet undermined the lofty ideals to which Abramson subscribed—freedom of research and the primacy of medical interests over commercial.

Ultimately, Abramson's inability to gain approval to conduct clinical LSD research under the Drug Amendments of 1962 was not due to any effort by the FDA to restrict such research. The FDA made no negative judgments on the validity of Abramson's qualifications, experience, plan of research, or facilities; it simply could not accept his application without the required pre-clinical data, regardless of the fact that this data was already on file.

The International Foundation for Advanced Study

The International Foundation for Advanced Study of Menlo Park, California, also submitted an independent IND to the FDA for clinical research with LSD (as well as psilocybin) in 1963. The FDA eventually terminated the IND in February 1965.[42] Like Abramson, the researchers struggled to provide the preclinical data required on the IND form without the cooperation of Sandoz. Although this problem alone would have resulted in the IND's termination, the FDA review also cited another issue—the qualifications of the investigators. A nonprofit organization founded to explore the potential of LSD, the foundation was at the forefront of establishing the Canadian "psychedelic therapy" method of LSD administration in the United States. Reflecting the unconventional nature of this form of drug research, the members of the foundation came from a variety of backgrounds: experience was a more relevant qualification than medical credentials. Prior to 1962, this situation had not proved problematic. However, after the IND rules of the Drug Amendments of 1962 formalized access to investigational drugs, the foundation's position became untenable.

The International Foundation for Advanced Study was founded by Myron J. Stolaroff in 1961. Stolaroff had achieved success as an engineer in the 1950s at the Ampex Corporation—a pioneering firm for magnetic recording—where he had risen to the position of assistant to the president for long-range planning. Outside of work, he was involved with the Sequoia Seminar, a spiritual group led by Stanford professor of business law Harry Rathbun. Through the group, Stolaroff came to know Gerald Heard, the Los Angeles–based British intellectual and author. An expert on mysticism and Eastern religions, Heard introduced him to the idea that LSD could be a profound spiritual tool and encouraged him to contact Al Hubbard in Canada, one of the pioneers of psychedelic therapy. Hubbard and Stolaroff first met in February 1956 and connected immediately. In April that year, Stolaroff traveled to Hubbard's home in Vancouver, where Hubbard administered him LSD for the first time. The 66 mcg dose, while relatively low, produced a profound experience and convinced Stolaroff that LSD was "the most important discovery man has ever made" and that he should devote himself to studying the drug.[43]

Stolaroff took LSD back to the Sequoia Seminar, out of which he formed a research group. Members took turns taking the drug, with the others present for support, and experiences were discussed at later meetings. However, some of the members found Hubbard's larger than life personality disagreeable and subsequently moved away from his guidance, much to Stolaroff's disapproval. Stolaroff also took LSD to Ampex, where he suggested that the drug's effects could be used to enhance problem solving, by creating a state of mind where "fresh ideas and perspectives flow unhindered."[44] His idea met with strong resistance.

In 1959, Stolaroff took a stronger than usual 150 mcg dose of LSD, which resulted in a powerful mystical experience. This convinced him to dedicate himself full time to the study of LSD. Subsequently, Stolaroff left his job at Ampex and his disappointing research group, and he self-funded the nonprofit International Foundation for Advanced Study, which he established with Hubbard. Together they collected a number of researchers, who came from a variety of backgrounds but had a common interest in psychedelic drugs, and set up specially furnished offices above a beauty parlor in downtown Menlo Park.[45] The researchers included Charles Savage, Stanford University professor of engineering Willis Harman, Stanford graduate student in psychology James Fadiman, and San Francisco State College associate professor of psychology Robert Mogar.

Savage, who joined the foundation as medical director in November 1961, was the most qualified, experienced, and esteemed member of the foundation. In addition to his previously discussed LSD research at the Naval Medical Research Institute, the NIMH, and the Mental Research Institute, Savage had also conducted research in California at the Center for Advanced Studies in the Behavioral Sciences, the Napa State Hospital, and the Palo Alto Veterans Administration Hospital.[46] As psychologists, Mogar and Fadiman were also qualified to perform LSD psychotherapy research, at least under medical supervision. Mogar brought to the group significant experience in evaluating therapeutic outcomes with objective rating instruments.[47] He was therefore useful in raising the scientific standards of the foundation's research. Nevertheless, Hubbard, Stolaroff, and Harman were objectively laypeople.[48]

The foundation justified the use of lay researchers on the grounds that there were simply not enough therapists who had both training in psychiatry or clinical psychology and experience with psychedelics. They considered psychedelic therapy to be an art that could be learned only through personal experience with the therapeutic process and believed orthodox training could in fact act as a hindrance. Savage indeed found value in Harman's background, even though it was not in psychiatry: he brought "to the

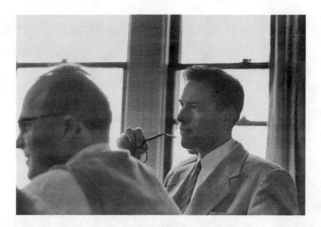

Charles Savage (*right*) circa 1958. This photograph was likely taken while Savage was a fellow at the Center for Advanced Study in the Behavioral Sciences, Stanford, California (1957–1958). Charles Savage Papers, courtesy of Purdue University Libraries, Karnes Archives & Special Collections.

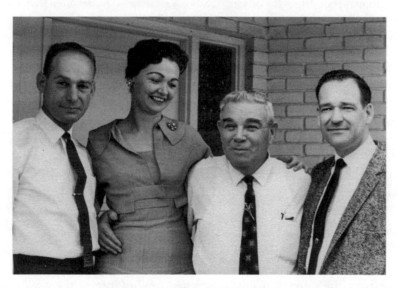

Left to right: Myron Stolaroff, Rita Hubbard, Al Hubbard, and Willis Harman. Undated, photographer unknown. Courtesy of Erowid Center's Myron Stolaroff Collection (sc5046).

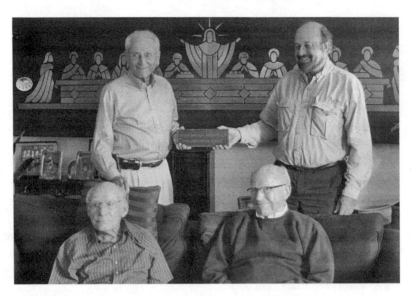

International Foundation for Advanced Study researchers at a 2010 reunion. *Clockwise from bottom left*: Myron Stolaroff, Don Allen, James Fadiman, and Robert McKim. Allen and McKim, like Stolaroff, Hubbard, and Harman, came from backgrounds in engineering. Allen and Fadiman hold the foundation's building plaque and stand in front of a Last Supper artwork that adorned the office. Photo by Jon Hanna & Erowid (2010). Courtesy of Erowid Center's Myron Stolaroff Collection (sci6001).

project a background in scientific method, research design, communication and statistical theory, as well as an interest in the scientific basis of values and beliefs." The researchers suggested that the situation was characteristic of revolutionary new treatments, comparing it to the early days of psychoanalysis, and that in the future those trained in psychedelic therapy would come from formal mental health backgrounds.[49]

By the time of the enactment of the Drug Amendments of 1962, research at the foundation was well established. The research program was broad, encompassing the study of many aspects and implications of the psychedelic experience in a variety of populations. The program was conceived as a direct continuation of the work of Hubbard, Humphry Osmond, and Abram Hoffer, the Canadian developers of psychedelic therapy, and in fact Hoffer and Osmond were on the foundations' advisory board. The foundation researchers' basic concept of the value of the psychedelic experience was that, "just as a single traumatic incident can have lasting untoward effects, so can a single propitious experience, if sufficiently profound, have lasting beneficial effects."[50] The transcendental psychedelic experience could allow patients to see themselves, and the world around them, from an entirely new perspective, resulting in lasting changes in their values and beliefs. These changes were usually "in the direction of aesthetic, creative, philosophic and religious interests; deeper realization of the vastness of the self; and increased feeling of oneness with other persons and with the universe in general."[51] These changes in the patient's "value-belief system" could in turn influence their behavior and personality. Changes in behavior and personality were typically "in the direction of increased self acceptance, reduced anxiety and guilt, reduction in feelings of inadequacy accompanying the increased self esteem, greater freedom to develop and use potential abilities, and increased ability to form satisfying relationships with and communicate with others."[52] Having observed this process, the foundation's research was directed at furthering the understanding of how positive changes in values, beliefs, personality, and behavior came about and interplayed, and how to maximize the likelihood of a given patient experiencing such changes.

The first publication to emerge from the foundation's work appeared in the *Journal of Neuropsychiatry* in 1962. Entitled "The Psychedelic Experience—a New Concept in Psychotherapy," the paper outlined the theory, method of treatment, and results attained with twenty-five outpatients. The male and female patients had come to the foundation's clinic requesting treatment for a variety of problems, categorized as marital problems, alcoholism, ineffectual personality, and neurosis, as well as one patient categorized as "near homicidal."[53] Preparation for the drug session lasted a minimum of two to three weeks, although sometimes months. During this time, patients explored their personal problems and goals for the psychedelic session with their therapist, who also instructed them to surrender totally to the experience, be receptive to insights that challenged their normal beliefs, and trust their unconscious and those around them. To aid in developing these states of "willingness and trust," the patient was administered inhalations of 30 percent carbon dioxide, 70 percent oxygen, which produced brief alterations in consciousness.[54] These experiences helped patients practice letting go and helped the therapist determine whether they were ready for their psychedelic session. The treatment session then lasted eight and a half hours and took place in a room that was comfortably furnished and featured a record player and art. The patient was administered 100–200 mcg of LSD, as well as 200–400 mg of mescaline. Ten milligrams of methamphetamine was given later in the day to intensify the session and improve the patients' ability to integrate their experiences. Of the twenty-five patients treated, the researchers classed twelve (48 percent) as "much improved," nine (36 percent) as "improved," and four (16 percent) as "no improvement."[55]

Following this experience, the foundation drew up proposals to expand its psychedelic research. The intended studies were significantly more advanced than any that had previously been conducted. The researchers proposed to study both the process and outcome of psychedelic therapy in a diverse population and to more specifically test its efficacy in treating alcoholism. Importantly, the studies were to be at least partially controlled, with significant numbers of subjects, objective and extensive outcome assessment procedures, and substantial follow-up periods. The complexity of psychedelic therapy's procedure and the dramatic effects of LSD had resulted in few prior researchers attempting controlled studies, but the foundation researchers devised creative ways to provide reasonable control without undermining the therapeutic method. The studies, therefore, would carry a scientific weight that could potentially convince skeptics of the validity of results.

In July 1962, the foundation submitted a research grant application to the Department of Health, Education, and Welfare (the parent department for the NIMH, through which its funding was accessed), for a study entitled "LSD-25: Value Changes in the Psychedelic Experience." Savage was listed as principal investigator, with Harman as co–principal investigator. The study aimed to demonstrate two hypotheses: first, that the psychedelic experience resulted in changes to subjects' value-belief systems, which in turn led to changes in behavior. Second, that these behavioral changes were toward Abraham Maslow's concept of the self-actualizing person, whereby "the person is in the process of developing to the full stature of which he is capable, with full use of talents, capacities, and potentialities, motivated not to satisfy some need, real or imagined, but activated by the sheer joy of growing and becoming."[56]

The study was to be partially controlled, with 120 subjects studied, only half of whom would receive LSD. These two groups were to be further divided: thirty of the LSD subjects would be psychiatric patients, with only "pre-psychotics" excluded, and thirty would be "normal" volunteers. These volunteers would be professionals interested in the potential of the experience to enhance self-understanding, awareness, and creativity. Thirty of the non-LSD control subjects would be undergraduate psychology students, expected to change little over the time. The other thirty would be graduate students taking a Stanford seminar entitled "The Human Potentiality." These students would control for the influence of exposure to new concepts for self-under-standing and new values, without the psychedelic experience. Results would be determined through administering a battery of psychometric tests—both purpose-made questionnaires and rating scales and conventional instruments such as the Minnesota Multiphasic Personality Inventory (MMPI)—before treatment and at various stages the over six months afterward.[57]

Savage recognized that this design did not control for whether the subjects' value changes arose from their drug experience or were impressed on them by the enthusiastic therapist while they were under a state of increased suggestibility. However, he argued that experience had shown that value changes were often not in the direction of the therapist's own values—indicating that it was not simply suggestion—and that it was hard to control this aspect "since a cold impersonal scientific attitude inhibits the psychedelic experience."[58] The design also did not control for the possibility that subjects who volunteered for LSD therapy were already disposed to value changes in the direction hypothesized. If the tested hypotheses were proven correct in this study, Savage suggested that these two issues could be satisfied with a further study that used an active placebo, such as scopolamine, in a double-blind design, and that randomly assigned patients between the treatment and control groups.[59]

In the same year, Savage drafted another application for a research grant to the Department of Health, Education, and Welfare on behalf of the foundation. The study proposed to test the efficacy of the foundation's psychedelic therapy procedure in alcoholic patients. The ambitious proposal was controlled, with two hundred patients divided into four groups: no treatment; treatment with only 30 percent carbon dioxide, 70 percent oxygen inhalations; psychedelic therapy with a low dose of psilocybin; and psychedelic therapy with a high dose of LSD. The low dose of psilocybin was intended to work as an active placebo, as it would produce a "pleasant aesthetic experience" but not a psychedelic reaction. Assignment to each of the four groups would be random and, in the case of the two psychedelic therapy groups, double-blind.[60] Another proposal expanded this design into a multihospital study, by having each of an undetermined number of hospitals replicate the trial. The researchers anticipated that the hospital staff would be junior and inexperienced with LSD, and they planned to train them simply by providing basic instructions and having them undergo a psychedelic experience at the foundation. To control for therapist skill, a further control group was added—fifty patients who would undergo the high-dose LSD treatment at the foundation with highly experienced therapists.[61]

Exactly what came of these applications is unclear. In 1966, the foundation researchers published a study that closely resembled the first proposed study of value-belief system and behavioral changes following psychedelic therapy, but with a more limited protocol: seventy-seven persons (one-third patients, two-thirds "normals" dissatisfied with life) received LSD therapy between July 1962 and April 1963 and were evaluated over six months. The researchers reported that most patients significantly benefited from the treatment. The report lists partial funding from both the private Ittleson Family Foundation and a Public Health Service fellowship, so the application may have been at least partially successful.[62] The proposed alcoholism studies appear not to have come to fruition.

The reason that the foundation was denied any further federal funding appears not to have been due to any objection to funding LSD research in general, or to the foundation's specific form of research. At June 1966 congressional hearings entitled *Drug Safety*, Representative Lawrence Fountain's Intergovernmental Relations Subcommittee questioned the FDA extensively regarding its regulation of LSD research. Subcommittee senior investigator W. Donald Gray inquired as to why the foundation was turned down for a grant and whether it was because the research was not "bona fide" or because some of the investigators were unqualified. Kelsey replied that the National Institutes of Health "think very highly and thought very highly of Dr. Savage." She could not remember whether she had been told a specific reason why the grant had been turned down but opined that "there are usually a great deal more applications than there are funds for." Gray added that the National Institutes of Health had informed him that the rejection "wasn't necessarily on the basis of the proposed research, but largely the fact that there was some question about the reliability of some of the people there."[63] The grant proposals listed Harman as co–principal investigator, and knowledge that fellow lay researchers Stolaroff and Hubbard directed the foundation could have influenced suspicion of the personnel other than Savage.

Despite receiving some funds from the Public Health Service, Sandoz excluded the foundation from its IND, likely because its research took place in an outpatient clinic rather than a hospital. Subsequently, the foundation submitted its own IND for LSD and psilocybin on 5 June 1963. On 7 October, FDA Division of Pharmacology reviewer William D'Aguanno wrote to Kelsey recommending termination of the IND, as "the animal data [supplied] are insufficient to support clinical studies." The IND had referred to Sandoz's IND for animal data, but, like Abramson, the researchers had not provided authorization from Sandoz to use this confidentially filed data.[64]

Despite this immediate recommendation, the FDA did not terminate the foundation's IND until February 1965. At the *Drug Safety* congressional hearings, Fountain questioned the FDA as to the reasons for this delay. He drew attention to numerous recommendations for termination from several different FDA officers, due primarily to the lack of preclinical and manufacturing control data, which had been given between the initial October 1963 review and final termination. Kelsey explained that they respected Savage as a "distinguished scientist" with great experience with LSD and had wished to avoid unnecessarily terminating potentially useful research. They therefore gave the foundation a chance to provide the necessary data, particularly on the nature of its stocks of LSD. The foundation claimed to have received its LSD from Sandoz, but the labels were missing, so the FDA was concerned as to its exact composition and condition. The researchers promised to collect all the necessary data and offered to suspend their clinical work while their IND was under review. However, they were unable to obtain the data.[65]

Ultimately, the final nail in the IND's coffin came with Savage's departure from the foundation: he left in September 1964, to take up a new role at Spring Grove State Hospital in Maryland, where he would continue his psychedelic research.[66] In addition to the foundation's difficulties in obtaining FDA approval for its research, Savage's departure was influenced by conflict with his old LSD research colleague from the Mental Research Institute, Donald Jackson. Savage and Jackson's relationship had soured since their research program came to an end after a member of the team underwent an unauthorized LSD session, resulting in an extended psychotic break. Jackson—who went on to pioneer family therapy and become a significant figure in American psychiatry before his death in 1968—was by now chief of the psychiatry division of the Palo Alto–Stanford Hospital Center, where Savage was also on staff. In mid-1964, Jackson had led departmental action against Savage, reporting concern over his activities to the executive committee of the hospital. Jackson was concerned about Savage's failure to properly attain membership with the San Mateo County Medical Society, the foundation's source of LSD—as he believed Sandoz LSD would no longer be available—whether members of the foundation were conducting medicine without a license, what promises they made to patients, and the size of fees charged.[67]

For Kelsey, with the requested data not supplied, Savage's departure was the deciding factor in termination.[68] Additionally, by 1964 the FDA was growing suspicious that the foundation was using LSD outside of legitimate research. In November an undercover agent was sent to the foundation to try to obtain

LSD treatment. He was unable to even attain a promise of treatment, but "the inference seemed to be that possibly it could be arranged." Like Jackson, the FDA was also increasingly suspicious of the foundation's stocks of LSD, with Commissioner Goddard suggesting that it had LSD "in a fruit jar buried in the ground."[69] At the December meeting of the FDA's Advisory Committee on Investigational Drugs, Kelsey reported that Hubbard's qualifications were "totally inadequate" and that—strangely, considering the sophisticated clinical trials proposed in its funding applications—the foundation's IND was "devoid of any reasonable investigation plan." Particularly, it lacked control groups. In response, committee member Sidney Merlis stated, "The sponsor should not be dignified by a site visit—it should be terminated."[70] The foundation researchers had attempted to bring credibility back to its organization by appointing Osmond as medical director. However, his location—by now at the New Jersey Neuropsychiatric Institute—suggested that this was a token position.[71]

Finally, on 6 January 1965 the FDA sent the foundation a notice of the deficiencies in its IND application. If corrections were not provided within ten days, the IND would be terminated. Besides listing deficiencies in the preclinical and manufacturing data provided, the FDA also judged the investigators and their plans to be inadequate: "In our opinion, the proposed co-investigators, Willis W. Harman, Alfred M. Hubbard and Myron J. Stolaroff, do not possess the necessary qualifications for undertaking the proposed clinical investigations; in addition, the data submitted do not support the use of psychotomimetic compounds in such syndromes or diseases such as asthma, colitis, psoriasis, etc. Furthermore, the supervision of the project in California by the principal investigator in New Jersey, is unsatisfactory."[72] The inclusion of asthma and other physical ailments in the foundation's investigative plans suggests that the researchers had proposed branching into psycholytic therapy: while not a common indication of psychedelic therapy, many psychoanalysts researched and treated asthma, believing it to be psychosomatic. On 2 February the IND was terminated.[73]

From its inception in 1961, the International Foundation for Advanced Study had led the field of psychedelic therapy research in the United States. Not only had the researchers been among the first to adopt the Canadian method, but they had attempted to advance the field by designing controlled clinical trials. While some of their plans were not realized, they accrued great experience with psychedelics, administering them to approximately 350 subjects, and published their findings in mainstream journals such as the *Inter-*

national Journal of Neuropsychiatry.[74] While several of the core researchers of the foundation had no formal training in medicine or psychology, they were not merely making excuses when emphasizing the importance of experience over medical credentials. LSD administration was known to cause few medical complications; its effects, contraindications, and dangers were all related to psychological factors. Additionally, medical training did not prepare a therapist for handling the powerful and variable effects of the drug, as carefully manipulating set and setting were not normal aspects of medical drug administration. Indeed, the experience and innovation of Hubbard was highly regarded by many psychiatrists researching LSD with whom he had collaborated, such as Ross MacLean, Osmond, and Hoffer in Canada.[75] However, with the formalization of drug research through the Drug Amendments of 1962, this was not a perspective that the FDA could support. Ultimately, without a medically qualified lead investigator such as Savage, the foundation would have been denied an IND for clinical research with any drug, let alone LSD.

Further Control

The first legislation to introduce specific control over psychedelics was signed into law in July 1965. The Drug Abuse Control Amendments of 1965 amended the Federal Food, Drug, and Cosmetic Act to prohibit the manufacture, sale, distribution, and possession (except for personal use) of depressant, stimulant, and hallucinogenic drugs outside of legitimate channels of commerce and research. Increased registration and record-keeping requirements were placed on those involved in the legitimate manufacture and distribution of these drugs.[76] For enforcement, the Bureau of Drug Abuse Control was established within the FDA. The bureau staffed offices nationwide with agents authorized to make arrests, carry firearms, serve warrants, and conduct seizures.[77]

This increased control over psychedelics reflected growing public and political concern over their nonmedical use. However, the legislation was primarily intended to target the abuse of amphetamines and barbiturates. In his hearings over the bill, Representative Oren Harris estimated that more than nine billion amphetamine and barbiturate tablets were produced annually in the United States, and that half found their way onto the black market.[78] The hearings, as well as the House and Senate reports on the bill, were almost exclusively concerned with the dangers of depressant and stimulant drug abuse, how these drugs entered the black market, and how best to prevent it.[79] Justification for including hallucinogenic drugs was given only in passing. FDA commissioner George Larrick referred to the abuse of hallucinogens around college campuses that had resulted in "rather extensive publicity a few years ago," most likely alluding to the Harvard scandal. Larrick described LSD as "capable of inducing lasting changes in the mental and emotional stability of some users." This had led some college students to become "disturbed to the point that they had to leave college or even enter mental institutions." He also stated that the drug could produce "strong suicidal tendencies." The FDA had successfully prosecuted two men under the existing provisions of the Food, Drug, and Cosmetic Act, for attempting to sell a large quantity of LSD to an undercover FDA agent in April 1963. The judge in the case had recommended legislation to specifically control drugs such as LSD.[80]

As passed, the amendments did not name any specific psychedelic drugs for control under its provisions but instead authorized the secretary of health, education, and welfare to add new drugs to the list of those controlled (initially only amphetamines and the chemical derivatives of barbituric acid) based on their "potential for abuse" due to their "depressant or stimulant effect" or their "hallucinogenic effect."[81] The addition of LSD to this list was delayed as the FDA commissioned an external committee to advise on the inclusion of further specific drugs under the amendments and built the capacity to enforce the law. In January 1966 the FDA published notice in the *Federal Register* proposing that LSD—as well as a number of other drugs—be controlled under the provisions of the amendments. After a further delay to allow public comment, the FDA published a final notice in March, bringing LSD under control as of 15 July that year.[82]

Although the 1965 amendments contained no provisions that directly affected LSD researchers working under an IND, the FDA's new responsibility to curb the nonmedical use of LSD through police action did have the potential to impact legitimate research, by influencing the FDA to more strictly control access to the drug. While LSD had not been the major focus of the 1965 amendments, by the next year controversy surrounding the drug was significantly increasing, and pressure was on the FDA halt the drug's spread. In May 1966 a special subcommittee of the Senate Committee on the Judiciary, chaired by Senator Thomas J. Dodd, diverted its hearings on a bill to liberalize penalties for narcotic addicts—favoring treatment over punishment—to consider whether further control of LSD was needed, including adding personal possession to the list of crimes under the Drug Abuse Control Amendments. Despite the subcommittee's strong preference, further criminalization did not immediately result from the hearings but instead would be enacted in 1968.[83] Nevertheless, testimony from the hearings provides a useful window into the increasing controversy surrounding LSD, changing medical perspectives on the drug, and the tensions that the FDA faced in regulating it.

Testimony from expert medical witnesses focused on the dangers of LSD's nonmedical use and the increasing frequency with which they were seeing LSD-related psychiatric admissions. Psychiatrist William Frosch from Bellevue Hospital in New York City reported that the hospital had recently seen admissions related to LSD double, to approximately four per week. These patients were primarily in their late teens or early twenties, came from middle-class backgrounds, had dropped out of school or college, and had some prior personality difficulties, as well as experience with other drugs. Reasons for admission were split roughly between acute panic reactions, reappearance of LSD-like symptoms long after taking the drug, and prolonged psychosis. Frosch described that patients in this last category had mostly been psychotic prior to ingesting LSD or otherwise had "severe personality disturbances." While attesting to the drug's danger, he was hesitant to state that LSD produced permanent damage and questioned whether the prohibition of personal possession would be an effective strategy for addressing the problem. Donald Louria, chair of the New York Council of Drug Addiction, who testified representing Governor Nelson A. Rockefeller, spoke more alarmingly of LSD's dangers. He asserted that the increasing use of LSD by young people represented a "crisis situation," that "people are violent under LSD," and that the state had seen cases of attempted homicide and suicide. He supported increasing federal penalties for LSD offenses but also testified that the drug had many potential legitimate uses, although "conclusive evidence" was lacking.[84]

The situation was similar in California, where psychiatrists Duke Fisher and J. Thomas Ungerleider from the UCLA Neuropsychiatric Institute testified to having seen seventy patients with LSD-associated psychiatric problems over the past seven months, representing 12 percent of patients seen in that period. Prior to September 1965, the clinic had only seen approximately one case every two months. In addition to the panic and psychotic symptoms that Frosch had witnessed, Ungerleider also reported that patients frequently displayed a "diminished interest in working and in living a productive life" and an increasing obsession with the philosophical significance of their LSD experiences.[85] Fisher was particularly concerned by the "missionary quality" of LSD users, who became insistent that everyone else should try the drug and share in their enlightened awareness. This had reached the extreme example of one mother who had given LSD to her twenty-three-month-old daughter, thinking that it would help her develop into a better adult. Fisher guessed that there might be one hundred thousand LSD users in Los Angeles and supported making personal possession a crime.[86]

Criminalization of LSD possession was further supported Captain Alfred W. Trembly, commander of the Narcotics Division of the Los Angeles Police Department. California had recently passed such legislation, and Trembly described some of the bizarre—although not necessarily dangerous—behavior from LSD-addled "teenagers, students, nonconformists, radicals, and beatniks" that police had encountered: two men found on the front lawn of a property eating grass and bark off the trees; a couple lying naked in an apartment building hallway, yelling for help while also shouting "GOD" and "LIFE," and spelling the words out; a young man whom officers had to retrieve from the ocean—praying on his knees while shouting "I love you, I love you"—after being reported for making obscene gestures; and a teenager who could not remove a rubber band from his arm, which he believed was tightening and would cut off his arm.[87] Trembly testified that the majority of individuals who came to police attention already had criminal records, as well as experience with other drugs. This suggested that the drug was already associated with criminality and should not be regulated differently than other narcotics. He also stressed the apparent ease with which "bathtub chemists" could manufacture LSD, with one recently investigated chemist allegedly having the capacity to produce between two hundred thousand and one million doses in a three-month period.

The subcommittee attempted to provide some balance to the negative depictions of LSD by also inviting the testimony of some of the drug's most outspoken advocates, including Leary, poet Allen Ginsberg, and Arthur Kleps, leader of the Neo-American Church, a new religious group that used LSD as a sacrament. These individuals challenged the prevailing depictions of LSD's dangers and testified to its remarkable potential for benefit, in terms of consciousness expansion and religious experience. Yet the subcommittee remained unmoved. Leary, who claimed to have personally taken psychedelic drugs 311 times over the prior six years and to have overseen more than three thousand administrations, argued that the drug was nonaddictive and had no known lethal dose, that there was no evidence it caused physiological or lasting psychological harm, and that cases of panic reactions and bizarre behavior were statistically rare and reflected poor training in the use of the drug. While occasionally using language that alienated and confused the subcommittee—such as testifying that the "so-called peril of LSD resides precisely in its eerie power to release ancient, wise, and I would even say at times holy sources of energy"—he also attempted to build bridges by arguing that he had never supported indiscriminate use and by agreeing that LSD needed to be regulated.[88] In fact, he praised the current legislation whereby manufacture and sale, but not possession, were regulated. He recommended that colleges offer training in the use of psychedelics and that, after physical and psychological evaluation, responsible adults should be licensed to use psychedelics for purposes including personal growth and spiritual development. Stronger psychedelics—such as LSD as compared to marijuana—would require more intensive in licensing, in the same manner as different licenses were required to operate a car versus an airplane. However, the subcommittee members did not seriously engage with these suggestions—whether or not they were realistic—but rather relentlessly pushed Leary to admit that the drug was dangerous. This he ultimately did, although he stressed that it was dangerous only when used improperly and qualified that it was less dangerous than "other forms of energy" such as alcohol or cars.[89] Ultimately, Leary made no headway in altering the subcommittee's perception of the drug as inherently dangerous and in need of prohibitive regulation.

When FDA commissioner Goddard testified before the subcommittee, he largely confirmed the negative perspective of medical and law enforcement witnesses. He submitted to the record a report of thirty-five "bizarre and often pathetic cases" involving psychedelics and young people that the FDA had investigated or was aware of, which included children who had eaten LSD-infused sugar cubes that they had found in their homes, adverse psychiatric reactions, and arrests where psychedelics were found alongside other illicit drugs.[90] Goddard had sent a letter warning two thousand college and university administrators of the "gravity" of the situation and urging them to report any illicit activities involving psychedelics to the FDA. The FDA currently had 49 cases involving LSD under investigation, had investigated approximately 360 cases since 1961—the first year that nonmedical use of the drug came to FDA attention—and knew of six clandestine manufacturers of the drug.[91] However, despite significant pressure from Dodd, Goddard argued against criminalizing personal possession—a move he feared would turn 10 percent of college students into criminals—and disputed the notion that LSD was more dangerous than heroin. Nevertheless, he described claims of LSD's "mind-expanding properties" as "pure bunk"—much to Dodd's de-

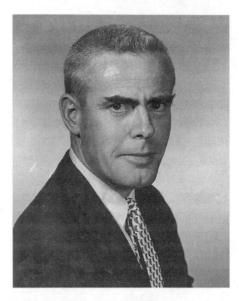

FDA commissioner James L. Goddard. As commissioner from January 1966 until July 1968, Goddard was responsible for the regulation of LSD during a period of increasing controversy and control over the drug, which saw Sandoz withdraw its sponsorship of research. Courtesy of the US Food and Drug Administration.

light—and, while supporting further research with the drug under "carefully controlled conditions," he expressed, "If a drug has been in research this long, how can it be good?"[92]

Despite Goddard's claim to support further LSD research, the FDA now clearly viewed LSD primarily as a dangerous drug of abuse and was suspicious or even dismissive of its potential benefits. It was natural that supporters of LSD research would suspect the FDA of moving to restrict research with the drug. However, the actions that the FDA took in regulating LSD research in these years suggests that it was in fact able to balance attempting to crack down on LSD's nonmedical use while still facilitating medical research. The controversy surrounding LSD had its most direct impact on the prospects of LSD research in April 1966, by influencing Sandoz to withdraw its IND for LSD research. As Sandoz had maintained itself as the drug's sole sponsor, all research was in jeopardy. The scale of LSD research in the United States would indeed drop significantly as a result. Nevertheless, a joint initiative of the FDA, NIMH, and VA prevented it from ending entirely.

By late 1965, the FDA and NIMH were already aware that Sandoz was planning to withdraw its sponsorship of LSD, as its patent for the drug had expired. At that time, the NIMH was supplying grants to approximately twenty investigations using LSD. Jonathan Cole, chief of the NIMH's Psychopharmacology Service Center, called a meeting of representatives of Sandoz, the NIMH, and the FDA, to discuss the future of LSD research on 7 December 1965. Cole asserted that there was "some evidence of benefit" with LSD therapy in the treatment of alcoholism, treatment-resistant neuroses, and "hardcore sociopathic personalities." He wished to ensure that Sandoz's withdrawal would not prevent NIMH grantees, and other legitimate investigators, from having access to the drug.[93]

The Sandoz representatives suggested that they could hand over their remaining supplies of LSD to the NIMH, which could act as the research sponsor itself. However, the NIMH was unable to take on this role. Three other prospects were discussed. First, the NIMH could find a new source for LSD and supply investigators who became their own sponsors by individually submitting INDs to the FDA. Second, the FDA could give LSD an effective NDA, approving it for commercial sale and routine use but "under very restrictive labeling." Seeming to support this possibility, Kelsey pointed out that research "could not go on indefinitely without some attempt at obtaining an approved NDA." Indeed, the regulations outlining the investigational IND phase of drug development stipulated that a drug's sponsor "shall not unduly prolong distribution of the drug for investigational use" but should submit an NDA "with reasonable promptness" after establishing its safety and efficacy."[94] However, Sandoz, although open to being a bulk supplier of LSD, was "not considering submitting an NDA." Cole suggested the final prospect: if some individual or organization, possibly Sandoz, would take on research sponsorship, the NIMH could cover all costs involved. The meeting ended with all parties agreeing that this last scenario was a possibility.[95]

Three months later, on 8 April 1966, Sandoz contacted the FDA to inform it that the company intended to withdraw its sponsorship of LSD and psilocybin without delay. Sandoz did not plan to take any measures to ensure continued legitimate research with the drugs. The company's American medical director, Craig Burrell, explained that the withdrawal was a result of the increased misuse of the drugs outside of medicine. Although Burrell was convinced that "no Sandoz produced LSD and Psilocybin reached black market channels," the increased publicity around the drugs and increasing black market production created a situation where "we can no longer bear the responsibility for the allocation and distribution of these substances."[96] Sandoz's cessation of LSD and psilocybin distribution was worldwide. The earlier plan of sharing the burdens of sponsorship between Sandoz and the NIMH was now off the table. Concerned by this prospect, officials from the FDA, NIMH, and VA discussed the matter with Sandoz. Together they decided that while most of the approximately seventy investigators would have their stocks of LSD recalled, twelve would be allowed to continue using the drug while they wrote up and submitted their own INDs to the FDA. On 11 April, Sandoz sent official notices to all LSD researchers, except the twelve, informing them of the cancellation of its sponsorship and recalling any stocks of the drug. Sandoz then replenished the twelve remaining investigators' supplies of LSD and delivered the rest of its stock, approximately twenty grams, to the NIMH, which would now take over the role of distributor.[97]

When Kennedy criticized the FDA at his May 1966 congressional hearings for the reduction in LSD research following Sandoz's withdrawal of its IND, he therefore failed to appreciate the nature of the IND regulations and to give the agencies fair credit for ensuring that research survived at all. Kennedy had called the hearings, entitled *Organization and Coordination of Federal Drug Research and Regulatory Programs: LSD*, to investigate the issue of interagency coordination in the regulation of LSD research and abuse. Although the growing abuse of LSD was of great concern to the Senate Subcommittee on Executive Organization, Kennedy stressed that the government's reaction should not hinder legitimate research, arguing that, "to some extent we have lost sight of the fact that [LSD] can be very, very helpful in society if used properly." With the number of LSD research projects dropping from seventy to just nine (with twelve investigators), he was concerned that the FDA had been "cutting down research."[98]

Defending their role, Commissioner Goddard, with NIMH director Stanley Yolles, explained to Kennedy that the regulations required that all investigators work under an IND. With Sandoz's withdrawal, investigators had to submit individual INDs if they wished to continue using LSD. The reason that some projects had not been terminated was that those researchers were using the drug on a daily basis, so any disruption caused by the approval process would have had a major detrimental effect on their research. These researchers still had to submit INDs, but the FDA had granted them a special exemption allowing them to continue using LSD in the interim. Goddard further explained that the reduction was also partly because some of the research projects were concluding at the time. Ultimately, while he invited the submission of INDs, Goddard explained that it was not the FDA's responsibility to stimulate research but simply to assess the adequacy of research proposals: as Goddard stated, "We certainly do not want to be in the position of thwarting research that is needed. . . . However, the responsibility for initiation does lie with the individual scientist."[99] Yolles stressed that the NIMH had accepted Sandoz's supplies of LSD precisely to ensure that valuable research continued. The NIMH had been under no obligation to become LSD's distributor and could have easily had the stocks destroyed. Yolles also confirmed that if they found research that needed to be performed but had not attracted scientists, the NIMH was willing to stimulate the research and carry it out.[100]

On 14 July 1966, the FDA published new regulations for the investigational use of hallucinogenic drugs. The regulations required an IND to be approved, rather than simply submitted, before drugs such as LSD could be sold or delivered to a researcher for clinical testing. FDA approval was also now required for researchers to receive the drugs for laboratory or animal research.[101] These regulations prevented dishonest persons, or unfit researchers, from gaining access to legal supplies of hallucinogenic drugs by abusing either the loose regulation of drug access for preclinical research or the period between IND submission and termination.

For bona fide researchers, these regulations could potentially delay the commencement of new clinical research. However, it is unlikely that these regulations would have had any real impact on such research. The NIMH was by this time the sole legal distributor of LSD, and it is unlikely that it would have distributed the drug to anyone before being thoroughly satisfied of their credentials and having consulted with the FDA. Indeed, the same expert committee advised the FDA on the adequacy of IND applications for research with psychedelics and the NIMH on requests for supplies of the drugs. Therefore, IND and drug supply applications were likely assessed simultaneously. The FDA had established this committee in 1964 on an ad hoc basis, and in 1967 it became an official joint FDA and NIMH public advisory committee, the FDA-PHS Psychotomimetics Advisory Committee.[102] It was one of twenty-six FDA public advisory committees, each of which advised on issues related to a different medical field, such as dentistry, oncology, or obstetrics.[103] The psychotomimetics committee was composed of twelve distinguished scientists, but none of its members had recent or extensive experience with the therapeutic use of psychedelic drugs.[104] In the first eighteen months after Sandoz's withdrawal, the NIMH received 114 requests for supplies of psychedelics. After review by the committee, all but six requests were approved. According to the committee's executive secretary, John Scigliano, those declined had mostly proposed to use the drug in therapy outside of a research framework.[105]

Conclusion

Had the FDA wished to curtail LSD research, in 1966 it had had the perfect opportunity. Rather than having to deny approval to researchers or cancel already approved projects, the FDA simply had to do nothing but let it die. With Sandoz's withdrawal, the only legal supply of LSD in the United States had disappeared, and every clinical research project had had its authority to conduct research automatically revoked. Had the FDA not acted, LSD research would have come to a complete halt. However, together with the NIMH and VA, the FDA acted voluntarily to ensure continued supplies of LSD were available to researchers. They even bent their own rules to allow certain clinical researchers to temporarily continue their use of the drug without an IND, in order not to disrupt their research.

Over the 1960s the field of LSD psychotherapy research transformed rather than died: from a large but loose collection of small, varied studies into a smaller number of major clinical trials working toward a common goal. While this can give the impression that research was in decline, the studies that remained were significantly more methodologically sophisticated than were previous studies. They therefore had the best chance of satisfying the second major requirement of the Drug Amendments of 1962: proof of drug effectiveness through "adequate and well-controlled trials."[106] Successfully doing so would prove more difficult than gaining approval to conduct the research.

Proof of Efficacy

LSD and the Randomized Controlled Trial

> There have been more than 2,000 papers in the scientific literature, but there is
> as yet no substantial evidence based on adequate and well controlled investiga-
> tions to support the use of this drug for any medical purpose.
>
> FDA commissioner James L. Goddard, 1966

In describing the state of LSD research before Representative Lawrence Fountain's *Drug Safety* congressional hearings in June 1966, FDA commissioner
James L. Goddard lifted the terms "substantial evidence" and "adequate and
well controlled investigations" directly from the text of the Drug Amendments of 1962. These were key terms in the legislation, used to outline the
new requirement for proof of drug effectiveness as part of the NDA process.
Goddard was not simply dismissing the value of the research that had so far
been conducted but also indicating that it was not up to the standard required
for drug approval under the new regulations. The previous month, at Senator
Thomas J. Dodd's hearings on LSD, Goddard had further described LSD research with alcoholics as "extremely preliminary" and, when asked why there
was no consensus on the drug's efficacy after ten years of research, explained
that difficulty in finding a placebo condition that would allow double-blind
testing was a "problem that has confounded much of the research up to now."[1]

While LSD research had survived the formalization of drug research and
development brought about by the amendments' investigational new drug
regulations, satisfying the efficacy provisions would be much harder. Although
proof of drug effectiveness was a seemingly simple, commonsense requirement, it raised the thorny issues of how effectiveness should be defined and
measured. Where the investigational new drug rules established clear gate-
keeping authority for the FDA, the efficacy provisions were written in broad,
subjective terms. Medical experts as well as the FDA had the responsibility
of interpreting them. In the years immediately following the legislation's pas-

sage, the FDA would provide nebulous understandings of research standards rather than clear guidelines.

Given this lack of clarity, and the centrality of research methodology in debates over the effectiveness of LSD psychotherapy, this chapter first explores the evolution of controlled clinical research methods over the mid-twentieth century, the theories behind them, and the role of the Drug Amendments of 1962 in changing research standards. Ultimately, the randomized double-blind placebo-controlled trial, which had been heavily promoted by research experts in the 1950s, rose in status to become the gold standard of research design in the eyes of both the FDA and research experts by 1962. Although this methodology was not strictly mandated by the amendments, anything less would provoke intense scrutiny. While the FDA and researchers alike advocated the randomized controlled trial as simply the most accurate and scientifically advanced research methodology, its focus on isolating drug effects from psychological influences reflected a "magic bullet" concept of drug efficacy. This chapter goes on to explore how this hidden assumption clashed, on both practical and theoretical grounds, with LSD psychotherapy's unique method of using a drug to catalyze a psychological treatment. These clashes would cause research difficulties that would plague LSD psychotherapy research until its demise in the 1970s.

Mandating Efficacy

The need to scrutinize how the efficacy requirements of the Drug Amendments of 1962 were interpreted arises from the broad and subjective nature of the provisions in the legislation. An NDA was required to provide "substantial evidence that the drug will have the effect it purports or is represented to have under the conditions of use prescribed, recommended, or suggested in the proposed labeling." "Substantial evidence" was defined as "evidence consisting of adequate and well-controlled investigations, including clinical investigations, by experts qualified by scientific training and experience to evaluate the effectiveness of the drug involved, on the basis of which it could fairly and responsibly be concluded by such experts that the drug will have the effect it purports or is represented to have under the conditions of use prescribed, recommended, or suggested in the labeling or proposed labeling thereof."[2] This definition did not greatly clarify the requirements, as "adequate and well-controlled investigations" was a term equally subjective as "substantial evidence." The FDA did not provide an elaboration of the requirements until 1969 and did not formalize the standards until 1970.[3] Between 1962 and 1970, drug researchers had to provide proof of drug efficacy in an NDA without official guidelines as to what form of proof would be considered "adequate and well-controlled."

The evolution of drug research methodology, increasing concern over drug effectiveness, and the passage and impact of the Drug Amendments of 1962 have all been topics of interest for a number of historians. However, these issues have largely been treated separately, with little analysis of their interplay and impact on drug research in the years immediately following the legislation. Just what the research standards became, and how much of a shift this represented to the standard of practice of drug research, has not been established.[4]

In the absence of official guidelines, what were considered "adequate and well-controlled investigations" can be deduced from two sources: comments on research standards from FDA officials and the opinions of medical experts. In the years immediately following the passage of the Drug Amendments of 1962, FDA officials addressed the research community on the changes brought about by the legislation. These discussions conveyed the FDA's general stance on appropriate research methods yet stopped far short of providing clear standards for research. In these statements, the agency showed a strong preference for double-blind placebo-controlled trials, while appreciating that these were not always possible.

In February 1963, the FDA held a conference in Washington, DC, to outline its planned implementation of the Drug Amendments of 1962. All interested parties were invited to the conference to hear papers from FDA officials detailing the new requirements of the legislation and how they would generally be applied. In an extended question and answer session, specific inquiries as to the FDA's interpretation of terms and requirements in the legislation were first voiced. Despite direct questions as to the standard of evidence required for proof of effectiveness, the answers of FDA officials remained vague. One audience member queried, "What standard will be used in determining effectiveness of a drug? What are the accepted characteristics of a controlled trial?" The acting director of the FDA's Division of New Drugs, Arthur Ruskin, replied simply, "We'll have to go to scientific authorities in the matter. . . . But I think all of us know, in general, what a controlled study is, and where double blind studies can be used."[5] When further questioned, "What will constitute adequate study, and subsequently adequate proof of efficacy?" in relation to tranquilizers, Ruskin elaborated somewhat: "It would include some sort of control investigation, with the use of a placebo and perhaps other tranquilizers that have known effectiveness, and possibly double blind studies." He did concede that "perhaps the most difficult area to have double blind studies is in the area of psychopharmacology."[6]

Over the next few years, FDA officials traveled the country giving talks to groups involved in pharmaceutical research and development, explaining the new requirements of the law. Regarding efficacy, FDA medical director Joseph Sadusk delivered the most notable of these addresses in 1964, before the American College of Physicians. As far as establishing standards of research methodology, the talk moved little past the view expressed by Ruskin. However, as political scientist Daniel Carpenter has argued, the speech powerfully asserted the FDA's new authority in this scientific matter precisely through its ambiguity.[7] Entitled "The Definition of the Efficacy of a Drug under the Law," the paper again set out the double-bind placebo-controlled trial as the ideal method of research. Nevertheless, Sadusk emphasized that "this is not the only type of study that can be called well-controlled" and cautioned that the method could not always be utilized because of ethical or practical concerns.[8] In such cases he did not suggest a clear alternative method but instead stated that the FDA would weigh the adequacy of a trial on factors such as its design, the expertise of the investigator, the methods used to record and assess results, and the nature of, and status of knowledge on, the disease being treated.

Ultimately, as Carpenter has argued, the term "adequate and well-controlled" became a descriptor given to a trial based on a subjective evaluation by the FDA, rather than a standard defined by protocols that a researcher could check off when designing a trial. As Sadusk stated, "What we want, and what the law requires, is data that would enable the appropriately qualified experts to say responsibly whether or not the drug may be expected to perform as it is represented. This kind of evidence is not hard for the qualified person to recognize when he sees it."[9] Researchers would not determine a drug's efficacy, with the FDA checking that they used appropriate methods; the FDA would determine efficacy based on experimental data furnished by the researcher. The double-blind placebo-controlled trial was the surest way of satisfying the FDA's standards, but every trial would be judged on a case-by-case basis, in the light of expert opinion on the adequacy of the research methods for the drug and disease in question. More thoroughly determining what could be considered an "adequate and well-controlled" trial therefore requires examining expert opinion on research methods. What did experts argue were the factors that could complicate the determination of a drug's efficacy? What were the best methods for overcoming those obstacles? Ultimately, expert opinion was much more insistent on the randomized double-blind placebo-controlled trial methodology.

Determining Efficacy—Medical Experts and the Evolution of Drug Research

Over the decades prior to the Drug Amendments of 1962, drug evaluation had become a topic of increasing interest for medical scientists. The field had evolved from entrusting the determination of efficacy to the opinion of experts to focusing on attaining objectivity through removing the biasing influences of the human participants in research. As the field of pharmacology expanded rapidly in the twentieth century, the need to quickly and accurately determine drugs' effectiveness became imperative to ensure increased drug production resulted in improved therapeutics. As researchers came to recognize how factors such as methods of patient selection, researcher or patient enthusiasm for a treatment, the placebo effect, variety in the natural course of disease, and methods of data evaluation could skew the results of research, techniques were developed to eliminate their influence. Randomization, blinding, standardized outcome measures, and statistical analysis became tools to control clinical trials to determine whether a drug was truly responsible for any apparent therapeutic effects. These elements were all combined to create the ideal objective drug assessment, the randomized double-blind placebo-controlled trial, which was well established, at least in theory, by the time of the Drug Amendments of 1962.

The randomized controlled trial was not an isolated invention of the mid-twentieth century but a coming together of various experimental techniques to address an increasing recognition of the factors that could compromise therapeutic evaluation. Historians have found antecedents of controlled assessment stretching back to the Old Testament and have pointed to several significant early cases: Scottish naval surgeon James Lind's 1747 comparative study of treatments for scurvy, the blind evaluation of mesmerism in eighteenth-century France, and the use of an inert placebo in a nineteenth-century French study on homeopathy.[10] These and other early studies showed an appreciation of fundamental issues in clinical evaluation, including the need to control for the natural course of illness, spontaneous remission, and the placebo effect. Starting in the 1930s, several drug trials advanced the theory and methods of controlled clinical trials significantly, which historians have pointed to as the chief influences on the growing formalization of the controlled trial methodology: Cornell University pharmacologist Harry Gold pioneered the use of placebo controls and double-blinding in a 1932 study of xanthines for the treatment of pain caused by angina pectoris, and British statistician and epidemiologist Austin Bradford Hill added initial random assignment of patients between treatment and control groups to a blind analysis of results, to further reduce bias, in a 1948 study of streptomycin in the treatment of tuberculosis.[11]

Hill soon became a leading figure in the promotion of the randomized controlled trial's theory and methods, which he outlined in articles published in the *British Medical Bulletin* and the *New England Journal of Medicine* in 1951 and 1952. Hill argued that controlled clinical trials were needed because of the rise in the number of drugs with similar effects being developed. Where penicillin's efficacy had been unquestionable given its dramatic and unparalleled effects, determining the comparative efficacy of the various antibiotics developed subsequently was much more complicated. The most common complaint against randomized controlled trials was that it was unethical to withhold a treatment believed to be effective in the name of research. Given this, Hill emphasized the need to start controlled trials with a drug immediately on discovery, before unsubstantiated claims of efficacy could be promoted, and countered that it was unethical to widely use a drug of unconfirmed efficacy.

Hill argued that to accurately evaluate drugs, clinical trials required patient samples of a size relative to the variability of the disease in question: where outcome was predictable, such as in leukemia, small samples could suffice, but where the natural course of the disease was unpredictable, a large sample was needed to distinguish the results of the treatment from chance. Patients then needed to be divided into treatment and control groups on a random basis to avoid any intentional or unintentional bias in allocation, such as mainly assigning patients who could be expected to favorably respond to treatment to the experimental group. If significant variables that could be expected to impact results (such as patient age) were present in the patient sample, then a method for ensuring an equal distribution from randomization was needed. Blinding both the patients and the researchers as to whether the patient was in the experimental or control group was then necessary to equalize the influence of their enthusiasm or skepticism over the treatment and avoid a skewed analysis of results. This blind was best achieved through the use of an inert placebo in the control group; however, practical issues or ethical concerns could require another technique to be devised.

Determining a clear treatment regimen and establishing objective measures for evaluating results prior to the trial's commencement further ensured the elimination of bias.[12]

The potential significance of the placebo effect in providing false impressions of efficacy was given additional weight in the 1950s by the research of Harvard anesthesiologist Henry K. Beecher and his colleagues. In a prominent 1955 article in the *Journal of the American Medical Association*—entitled "The Powerful Placebo"—Beecher summarized his findings, to the effect that failing to account for the placebo effect could be "devastating to experimental studies as well as to sound clinical judgement."[13] In extended studies of the treatment of severe postoperative pain, Beecher and his colleagues had consistently found that 30 percent or more of patients received satisfactory pain relief from placebos and that response to placebos varied significantly even within individual patients: of sixty-nine patients given two or more doses of a placebo, 14 percent consistently responded to it, 31 percent consistently did not respond, and the remaining 55 percent responded to some placebo doses but not to others. Surveying fifteen studies involving more than a thousand patients, Beecher found confirmation of his observations: placebos had a rate of effectiveness of approximately 35 percent in the treatment of a wide variety of subjective symptoms, including headache, anxiety, nausea, drug-induced mood changes, and the common cold. Further, placebos could mimic the unpleasant side effects of active drugs, producing many of the same subjective symptoms that they could also cure, such as headache, nausea, and drowsiness.[14] With the placebo effect frequently able to counter such severe and physiologically based symptoms as postoperative pain, Beecher's work clearly demonstrated the problematics of evaluating efficacy through simple clinical observation—particularly when subjective symptoms were involved—and he highlighted the critical need for double-blind placebo-controlled studies. Although he did not explicitly make the connection in his paper, given the focus on subjective symptoms Beecher's work would be particularly relevant to psychiatry.

By the early 1950s the theory and method of the randomized double-blind controlled trial were fully established and had been promoted in the United States. This, however, did not guarantee widespread support for the method among the medical community. Indeed, historians Harry Marks and Scott Podolsky have argued that the increasing promotion of the randomized controlled trial in the mid-twentieth century cannot be explained simply through epistemological developments—researchers by and large were not motivated to change their methods purely for the sake of scientific ideals. Indeed, prior to the 1950s, many researchers rejected the control techniques. They argued that, while ideal in theory, true control was never possible; thus, faith in control methods could give false authority to the results of a trial. They also argued that laboratory and well-conducted uncontrolled clinical research was sufficient.[15]

Such resistance to control methods was overcome primarily as a result of reformers, largely academic researchers, promoting the controlled trial as a defense against therapeutic claims for drugs that ranged from inaccurate to fraudulent. With the massive growth in the development of new drugs in the mid-twentieth century, the need for accurate methods of separating the wheat from the chaff gained a new imperative, especially in the face of intense marketing from pharmaceutical companies: successful promotion of ineffective, or less effective, new drugs threatened to undermine the achievements of medical science. This fear was based in a growing mistrust in the ability of any of the human participants in research to guard against the intentional or unintentional corruption of objectivity, which could creep in at any level. Reformers, therefore, promoted controlled trials as not only a way of increasing the accuracy of research but also for providing an easy way for physicians to judge the impartiality and reliability of the claims of manufacturers. As Marks argues, the evolution of clinical trial methodology was propelled less by the triumph of scientific theory than by "mistrust" in the industry to discern and promote the best medicines.[16]

The Randomized Controlled Trial in Psychiatry

If this was the case for medicine in general, what was the standard of research in psychiatry? In the 1950s, psychiatry was revolutionized by a wave of new drugs, beginning with the discovery of the first tranquilizer, chlorpromazine, in France in 1950. Over the decade, the discovery of the minor tranquilizer meprobamate and the antidepressants imipramine and iproniazid firmly established the field of psychopharmacology as a chief concern of psychiatry. The dramatic discovery of drugs to treat previously chronic, intractable mental illnesses in many ways paralleled the pharmacological revolution for infectious disease that had occurred over the previous twenty years with the discovery of antibiotics. However, there were some stark differences between the fields. Where the etiology of infectious disease and the therapeutic action of antibiotics were understood, the origins of mental illness and the mechanisms of action for the new drugs were largely mysterious. In fact, the effectiveness of the new drugs ran counter to the predominant etiological theory in the United States that mental illness was a result of psychological rather than biological factors.

This made rigorous clinical trials both more vital and more difficult. Without a firm understanding of the biological basis of mental illness and the mechanisms of action for the drugs, and without the ability to accurately evaluate them in the laboratory, the clinical trial was the only method for determining efficacy.[17] With mental illness being highly placebo responsive and both illness and treatment involving so many potentially significant, though little-understood, variables, clinical trials that would maximize objectivity and neutralize the impact of non-treatment-specific influences were needed for efficacy to be established at a reliable level. However, controlling the myriad variables in psychiatry presented a great challenge, as did the fact that all diagnoses and patient assessments were based on the interpretation of symptoms and their variation, which complicated attempts to establish objectivity and standardized methods for outcome evaluation.

The state of expert opinion on drug research in psychiatry in the mid-1950s was displayed at a major 1956 conference on drug evaluation organized by the NIMH and held in Washington, DC. Cosponsored by the National Research Council of the National Academy of Sciences and the American Psychiatric Association, the conference was called as a response to the inconsistent and largely inadequate quality of the reports on the efficacy of the tranquilizers chlorpromazine and reserpine. Through the conference, the organizers intended to examine the efficacy of these drugs through interrogating the problems involved in research in order to guide future studies.[18]

The meeting gathered together the nation's leading authorities on pharmacology and psychopharmacology, attracting a crowd of nearly one thousand. The proceedings show the level of consensus on appropriate research methods, the difficulties in their application, and the level and nature of dissent. For most of the participants, the basic elements of the randomized controlled trial—comparative controls, randomization, placebo use, double-blinding, and statistical analysis—were well understood and accepted as ideals in clinical research. As Johns Hopkins pharmacologists Louis Lasagna—who had collaborated with Beecher in his placebo research—and Victor Laties commented, "Placebo and double-blind controls are of proven value in experimental work, and the reasons for their use should not need to be discussed at length in the year 1956."[19] Instead of explaining and justifying the need for these basic elements in research, the conference was concerned with a more detailed analysis of the problems involved in trying to put the ideals into practice.

Performing valuable and accurate research required balancing the need for high levels of standardization and control with the practical realities of treatment. A precise research question needed to be established, and complex theoretical questions needed to be addressed: What level of difference between the results of the experimental treatment and control would be considered significant? What was an acceptable risk versus benefit ratio for the illness being tested? What constituted "improvement" in the illness? This last question was particularly pertinent for research in psychiatry, as results could not be easily determined through biological tests for the presence of disease. Were patients improved if they were simply quieter or more manageable, or did there need to be a significant reduction in symptomatology? The answer depended on the research question of the trial. If symptom reduction was the goal, which symptoms should be the focus, what constituted "significant" reduction, and how could this be reliably and objectively measured? The preferred method for evaluating results was with a clinical rating scale: a standardized test that usually consisted of interview questions, with a choice of predetermined answers that allowed scoring and quantification. However, the conference participants found that the available rating scales provided as many questions as answers, as their reliability, objectivity, accuracy, and comprehensiveness were poorly understood.[20]

Even seemingly simple practical issues in trial planning, such as what dosage of a drug to use, could on close analysis become complex. Using a fixed dose was the simplest way of establishing a standardized and objectively delivered treatment that allowed easy quantification and comparison. But the dosage might be too low or high, not frequent enough or too frequent, thus obscuring the drug's efficacy. Allowing flexible doses would better ensure the drug's potential was picked up, but as this relied on the skill of administering physicians to find the optimum dose for individual patients, an important variable was added to the trial that needed to be accounted for in its design.[21] Deciding on the duration of the experiment and the route of drug administration required considering and balancing similar factors.

The issue of control was of primary concern at the conference. The participants found a wide range of variables that needed to be controlled in addition to the natural course of illness and the placebo effect. These included changes in the patients' environment, routine, activities, and staff. Most considered historical controls—where the results of a treatment were compared to existing data on prognosis—unsatisfactory, given the inability to control many variables. Using patients as their own control, by switching them between a placebo and the experimental treatment, was only appropriate with certain conditions and drugs, where response to treatment could be expected to reliably "turn off and on like water from a tap."[22] Several participants highlighted the difficulty of establishing a secure double-blind with an inert placebo if the experimental treatment had conspicuous side effects. They therefore suggested that an "active placebo" could be used: a drug that produced side effects similar to those of the experimental drug but that would not interfere with the illness being treated. However, this could cause complications, as it was hard to guarantee that the drug would have no effect on the illness. Indeed, the drug could have a psychologically negative effect on treatment due to its unpleasant subjective effects, even if it had no biological effect on the illness.[23]

Given the complexities of designing clinical trials that put the ideals of the randomized double-blind controlled trial into practice, one of the major recommendations to come out of the conference was precise reporting of trial design in research publications. Reports should include all available data on patient selection, controls, variables considered, treatment schedules, statistical analysis, methods of evaluation, and any other aspects of research considered significant. Although designing a perfect trial was impossible, openly reporting these factors would allow the reader to make an informed assessment of the weight of the results and accurately compare them to other research.[24]

While the majority of the conference participants accepted the ideals of the randomized controlled trial, a significant minority of participants voiced concerns over the limitations of statistically driven research methods. In addition to the practical difficulties of implementing the randomized controlled trial model, these physicians argued that drug treatment was not a purely objective process but one that involved the "art of medicine." Consequently, they argued that the standardizing focus of the methodology was not well suited to capture the diversity of factors that contributed to a treatment's efficacy. These concerns foreshadow those that LSD psychotherapy researchers would voice in the 1960s as they faced pressure to incorporate controlled trial methods into their research.

Psychiatrist Lincoln Clark of the Salt Lake City Veterans Administration Hospital in Utah was particularly critical of the degradation of respect for clinical observation that accompanied efforts to increase objectivity in research. He argued that although "we like to think of ourselves as scientists and understandably feel more secure with reliable methods," clinical observation was the method that so far had provided most of the clinically useful information on the psychological effects of drugs. Indeed, he thought that "premature" use of rating scales and other standardized treatment and testing measures "because of anxiety about reliability" could be "very inefficient if not misleading."[25] This was because a drug might have effects or uses that a rating scale could not discern, as the questions it contained were based on a narrow or differing concept of treatment efficacy. He therefore argued that it was particularly critical that early stages of drug research be based on clinical observation. Audience member Dr. Kalinowsky also attacked the declining reputation of clinical observation by further highlighting the great achievements of uncontrolled research in psychiatry: "I would like to remind you of the fact that all of the treatments in psychiatry, drugs as well as the previous treatments, were all introduced through studies which were not well planned, which were not planned at all, but they were introduced on the bases of the observations of some clinicians in relatively small hospitals. . . . I might add that the large statistical studies which were done later added very little to the indications suggested by those small original studies."[26]

Clark extended his critique of the randomized controlled trial by challenging the validity of its ideal of isolating a "pure" drug effect from other influencing variables, which he argued could produce only a shallow understanding of a drug's efficacy. Indeed, learning how to manipulate these variables to draw the greatest efficacy from a treatment was a goal of research that was lost in the controlled trials.

> Psychopharmacological agents do not produce a constant effect under all circumstances but a variety of responses which depend upon non-drug factors.
> . . .
> In the artificial situation of an experiment these factors would be regarded as intervening variables which the investigator would seek to control in order to isolate the drug effect, but it is important to remember that such variables will not be controlled in the eventual clinical use of the drugs. . . . What we gain in reliability and validity by using, for example, formal, double-blind studies of groups of subjects under standard conditions, reliable rating scales, or other quantifiable methods, we lose in knowledge of the richness and depth of the psychological processes occurring in the drug response of the individual case. Yet such information may be the key to an effective use of the drug in the in-

dividual patient or lead to an understanding of why a drug benefits some cases in an experimental population and fails in others.[27]

Audience member Dr. Gardner also argued that extrapharmacological variables were not complicating factors to be neutralized but vital components of treatment. In his experience the new drugs were not especially effective when used "by themselves in a mechanical way." Instead their usefulness was as a "psychiatric catalyst between the patient and those trying to communicate with him and help him." By opening up communication, the drugs made patients amenable to psychological and environmental treatments, which would combine with the drug's effects to have an impact on the patient greater than that of the drug or other treatments alone. Studying the drug treatment in a "vacuum," Gardner argued, was akin to asking, "How strong must a hearing aid be for a person to be interested in what is being said[?]"—it was based on the incorrect assumption that the drug's biological action was the only relevant aspect of treatment.[28]

In response to these arguments, conference participants supporting the randomized controlled trial ideal asserted that there was nothing special about psychiatry that precluded the use of methodology, and that if there were non-drug variables deemed an important component of treatment, they could be incorporated into a trial's design. Lasagna, who perhaps significantly was not a psychiatrist, was particularly dismissive of claims that psychiatry provided insurmountably unique challenges to the researcher and that the art of medicine was lost in clinical trials. He argued that "any field which is in a disordered state prefers to believe that the reason for intellectual chaos is the overwhelmingly difficult problems confronting it" and commented, "I, myself, would prefer to see a little more science and a little less art in this field."[29] Jonathan Cole, one of the conference's primary organizers and chief of the NIMH's new Psychopharmacology Service Center, was also a strong supporter of the randomized controlled trial, having studied under pioneer Harry Gold during medical school in the mid-1940s.[30] He argued that extrapharmacological elements in a treatment need not be eliminated from research. Instead, their role in the treatment also needed objective evaluation, before being worked into an overall treatment efficacy trial design. That a drug was a catalyst for wider treatment was not a militating factor for a controlled trial but an additional hypothesis that also needed exploring—everything was "open to scientific test."[31] Conference chair Ralph Gerard, professor of neurophysiology at the University of Michigan, echoed this opinion, stating, "Obviously, if one feels that the effect of the drugs is primarily to make the patient accessible to other kinds of therapy, then the experiment must be designed to include that variable, which is perfectly possible."[32]

The conference proceedings suggest that in the mid-1950s psychopharmacology was at the cutting edge of clinical trial methodology. The majority of the participants supported the need for objective, standardized, and statistics-driven clinical trials to determine the efficacy of drugs and saw the methods of the randomized double-blind controlled trial as the best way of doing so. Those who expressed doubts regarding the superiority of randomized controlled trials were at least familiar with their theory and methods, and were more concerned that other forms of research retain respect in light of situations where the methodology might not be ideal, rather than objecting to its use outright. Given the organizing bodies of the conference and the fact that the participants were considered the leaders in their fields, the conference's proceedings can be seen not only as representative of expert opinion but also as a clear establishment of the orthodoxy of controlled trials.

Standard of Practice

Assessing the impact that the efficacy provisions of the 1962 amendments had on drug research and development depends on whether they introduced new research standards or merely reflected and formalized research standards as they evolved. From the perspective of clinical research experts, the latter certainly seems to be the case. Further supporting this view, the 1962 amendments were not the FDA's first attempt to regulate drug efficacy: under the Federal Food, Drug, and Cosmetic Act of 1938, the FDA considered efficacy when evaluating the proof of drug safety required in an NDA, as it considered the issues inextricably linked. This was especially important for drugs designed to treat life-threatening conditions, where risk had to be weighed against potential benefit, and the danger of wasting time with ineffective drugs had to be taken into account. For the evaluation of efficacy, FDA officials had expressed a preference for double-blind trials.[33]

However, further evidence strongly suggests the amendments did in fact represent a pivotal change in the regulation of efficacy and the conduct of clinical research: that, despite earlier efforts to promote sophisticated efficacy testing, adopting the complex and expensive techniques of the randomized controlled trial had remained ultimately voluntary. As Earl Meyers, chief of the Controls Evaluation Branch of the FDA's Division of New Drugs, observed in 1963, the FDA's prior powers to regulate efficacy had been limited: although

after 1938 it "invariably considered efficacy in connection with safety in clear-
ing new drugs when they were for a progressive or life-threatening condition
or when they had a significant toxic potential . . . the new drug provisions did
not authorize us to control exaggerated claims or to exclude from the market worthless but essentially innocuous products."[34] At the 1956 psychopharmacology conference, University of Utah pharmacologist Louis Goodman
described the reality of drug development before the amendments. Drugs
came to market on the back of "poor clinical publications," while "really
good, definitive, critical, convincing, and properly controlled clinical studies
are published only years after the drug has made the grade or has begun its
well-deserved disappearance from the therapeutic scene."[35] To evaluate the
impact of the efficacy provisions, it is necessary to examine the standard of
practice in drug research and development in the years before their passage.

Just as Goodman noted, the breakthrough psychiatric drugs of the 1950s
came to market on the back of very limited and poorly controlled clinical
studies, with methodologically sophisticated trials being reported only after
the drugs were already in widespread use. Indeed, in the case of the tranquilizer chlorpromazine, commonly considered the greatest therapeutic breakthrough in psychiatry's history, most of the premarket clinical testing did not
even concern its psychiatric potential.[36] In 1954, the FDA approved Smith,
Kline, and French Laboratories' NDA to market chlorpromazine for use in
countering nausea and vomiting, and in psychiatry. Although its psychiatric
use was approved in the NDA, and was considered throughout the development phase, the vast majority of effort in research and development was
centered on the drug's antiemetic properties. Research submitted to the FDA
included more than one thousand patients treated for nausea and vomiting,
compared to just 104 psychiatric patients. The research performed with psychiatric patients was also relatively conventional, testing its sedative, rather
than its remarkable antipsychotic, properties, although its unique nonhyp-
notic effects were noted. This was largely because Smith, Kline, and French
feared there was little market for a drug to treat psychosis, as this was such
an unprecedented concept. The company believed the drug would find its
quickest development path, and largest market, through its more conventional physiological effects.[37]

In 1954, reports of the first independent psychiatric clinical trials of chlorpromazine in North America began to be published. They consisted of impressions of efficacy garnered through researchers' clinical observations of
the effects of treatment in hospital patients with a variety of diagnoses. The

reports focused on closely monitoring the effects of the drug on patients' symptoms and their psychological effects. There were no indications of controls being used, and results were crudely tabulated with little information as to how they were evaluated. The studies all reported highly positive results.[38]

Over the next two years, a number of researchers published results from controlled trials of chlorpromazine. Although these trials all attempted a double-blind comparison with an inert placebo (and in some cases other sedatives), their designs varied significantly and fell short of controlled trial ideals: patients were not randomized into treatment and control groups, blinds were often imperfect, and patient groups were not standardized in term of diagnosis. Published results varied from strong to insignificant evidence of efficacy.[39] Interestingly, the most methodologically sophisticated trial reported negative results. Robert Hall and Dorothy Dunlap's 1955 trial at Agnews State Hospital in California randomly allocated 175 "semi-disturbed chronic schizophrenic" patients between chlorpromazine and an inert placebo in a double-blind fashion and used rating scales to evaluate results. The blind was partially broken because of revealing side effects and a flawed drug coding system. Results showed that although patients significantly improved during the trial, there was no significant difference in improvement between the experimental and placebo groups. The researchers concluded that chlorpromazine "has an action that is principally sedative, and . . . has little value for non-tense schizophrenics except possibly those with the paranoid subtype."[40]

In 1960, results from the first large-scale, multihospital study of the efficacy of chlorpromazine in the treatment of schizophrenia were published. The trial included 692 patients with "schizophrenic reactions," treated in thirty-seven Veterans Administration hospitals. Researchers divided the patients into four diagnostic subgroups, from which they were randomly allocated to receive chlorpromazine, promazine, phenobarbital, or an inert placebo. The trial was double-blind, with standardized doses and conditions of treatment, three rating scales used to evaluate results, and a detailed statistical analysis of the data. The results clearly demonstrated the superior efficacy of chlorpromazine over the other treatments.[41] However, by this time chlorpromazine was already well established as a treatment for psychosis: within eight months of being marketed as Thorazine in 1954, it had been given to two million patients.[42] Therefore, although clinical trials were improving in methodology in the decade before the Drug Amendments of 1962, their results seem to have had little influence on the popularity of chlorpromazine.

Controlled trials were not required for the drug to enter the market, and a negative report of efficacy from the most sophisticated trial of the mid-1950s appears to have had little impact on its uptake. By the time chlorpromazine's efficacy was conclusively established, clinical experience had already long cemented its place in psychiatry. Controlled clinical trials appear to have been conducted largely for the scientific interest of researchers and supported by pharmaceutical companies likely for their marketing use.[43]

The development path of iproniazid, the first monoamine oxidase inhibitor (MAOI) antidepressant, even more dramatically shows how unimportant research methodology was in determining a new drug's uptake in psychiatry prior to the Drug Amendments of 1962. Like chlorpromazine, iproniazid was approved for sale on the basis of a physiological effect. When its unique psychoactive effects were discovered, the fact that it was already on the market helped to ease its uptake in psychiatry. A derivative of the German V2 rocket fuel hydrazine, iproniazid was first synthesized in 1951 and found to be useful in the treatment of tuberculosis. It quickly passed to market, and soon side effects of mild euphoria and stimulation were noted, with a now-famous newspaper report of tuberculosis patients at Sea View Hospital in Staten Island dancing in the halls.[44]

Psychiatric research with iproniazid began in earnest in 1956 at Rockland State Hospital in New York, prompted by prominent psychiatrist Nathan Kline's search for a "psychic energizer" that could relieve depression.[45] Together with colleagues John Saunders and Harry Loomer, Kline began clinically investigating iproniazid with depressed outpatients, as well as with seventeen chronic hospital patients whom they described as "withdrawn, regressed, deteriorated, colorless and of flattened affect."[46] Results, published in 1957, showed that after five weeks 47 percent of the hospital patients had improved, which climbed to 70 percent after five months. These results were supported by case studies of individual patients who represented the various responses to treatment, such as a positive responder who went from being "mute and withdrawn" to "talkative and, at times, even a bit noisy," especially significant considering the patient had been hospitalized for twenty years.[47]

The trial was uncontrolled, and the results were based on clinical impressions. The researchers not only justified the absence of controls on the basis that it was a pilot study but also argued that the failure of the patients to respond to other prior treatments made them their own controls: a placebo effect caused by enthusiasm for a new treatment could not explain efficacy, as such enthusiasm would have been equally present in previous attempts to use new treatments. Furthermore, the chronic unresponsive nature of their illnesses argued against spontaneous remission or general fluctuations in the severity of their pathology. Significantly, this trial was methodologically almost identical to the first psychedelic therapy trial reported by Canadian Colin Smith in 1958, which tested twenty-four alcoholic patients, similarly chosen for the severity of their condition, included case studies to demonstrate the treatment's effects, and found half of the patients improved or much improved after an average follow-up period of one year.[48]

Given that Loomer, Saunders, and Kline's trial of iproniazid was designed as a pilot study, it is not surprising that it was uncontrolled. The researchers were looking to explore the drug's therapeutic potential, rather than provide definitive proof of efficacy for a well-defined treatment. More significant is that this level of research is what propelled iproniazid into widespread use. Between their first presentation of the research at a conference of the American Psychiatric Association, in April 1957, and February 1958, approximately 380,000 patients received the drug.[49] This ease and speed of uptake was possible as iproniazid was already FDA approved and therefore available to physicians. After hearing of its psychiatric use, physicians could immediately try it themselves. As LSD was not already available on the market, similar research results only promoted further studies, rather than widespread use. For iproniazid, the only difficulty that had arisen was convincing the drug's manufacturer, Hoffmann-LaRoche, to support its development as an antidepressant, because of side effects that had accompanied its high-dose use with tuberculosis. However, Kline's insistence convinced them, and his personal promotion of the drug in newspaper interviews and even before Congress did much to popularize the drug.[50] In 1964, Kline was awarded a prestigious Lasker Award for discovering the antidepressant effects of iproniazid.[51]

"Adequate and Well-Controlled Investigations"

Prior to the Drug Amendments of 1962 there was, therefore, a great division between the theoretical state of the art and the common practice of clinical drug research, particularly in psychiatry. The ideals of the randomized double-blind controlled trial were well established and actively promoted by research experts. Yet the methods were not common in the practice of drug development, as drugs could be approved by the FDA on the back of limited clinical trials and then find their place in medicine through widespread clinical use. What then could be considered an "adequate and well-controlled" trial? This would obviously depend who was being asked—an industry representative, a psychiatrist wishing to determine whether a drug was useful, or a scientist specifically interested in the issues of drug efficacy and research methodology. However, it is evident that, over the 1950s, not only did randomized controlled trials become firmly entrenched in the theory of experts but that the sophistication of clinical trials was increasing in practice, even if they were conducted primarily for academic purposes. Randomized controlled trials were also widely understood as a standard for rigorous research among those who did not use them—although the iproniazid researchers did not employ the methods in their study, they did feel the need to justify that decision. It is also perhaps unsurprising that many researchers and pharmaceutical companies would not perform complex and expensive randomized controlled trials unless required to. Accordingly, although uncontrolled research was common, this does not equate to it being widely considered "adequate."

Although regulators may not have been able to expect the randomized double-blind controlled trial to be fully realized in clinical research in the years before 1962, it was nonetheless the preeminent model on which to evaluate the quality of research. On this basis, it can reasonably be concluded that an "adequate and well-controlled" trial could be considered one that made a concerted attempt to address issues such as bias, the placebo effect, influencing variables, chance, and natural variation in disease through techniques such as comparative control; blinding; placebo comparison; randomization; standardized treatments, environments and measures; and statistical analysis. This interpretation is consistent with the FDA's publicly expressed preference for double-blind placebo-controlled trials where possible, with a weighing of various research factors when not. It is also consistent with the FDA's 1970 official description of the research requirements for efficacy testing, which similarly set out the components of randomized controlled trials as the necessary building blocks of a trial's design.[52]

The Drug Amendments of 1962 did not introduce the issue of drug efficacy or the methodology of the controlled trial to either drug researchers or the FDA. However, the amendments were significant in establishing a new regime for drug development that made those two previously subsidiary matters central requirements for research. The FDA and research experts, charged with interpreting and enforcing the requirement for "substantial evidence" of drug efficacy based on "adequate and well controlled investigations," were strongly convinced of the randomized controlled trial's supremacy. Deviating from the methodology would now invite intense scrutiny and suspicion.

LSD Psychotherapy and the Randomized Controlled Trial

The cementing of the randomized double-blind controlled trial as the model for pharmaceutical research posed a significant challenge to LSD psychotherapists. The lack of "adequate" controls in the large body of research amassed over the previous decade rendered the results insufficient to establish efficacy, despite their consistently impressive nature. New trials that would satisfy both the scientific community and the FDA were needed if any consensus on the effectiveness of any form of LSD psychotherapy were to be reached, let alone an NDA submitted and approved. However, performing controlled trials with LSD would not be a straightforward task, as the dramatic effects of the drug and LSD psychotherapy's complex therapeutic processes clashed with the randomized controlled trial methodology in both practical and conceptual ways.

Many researchers adamantly opposed the requirement for controlled trials, arguing that the prescribed research methodologies were neither appropriate nor possible. At the May 1965 Second International Conference on the Use of LSD in Psychotherapy and Alcoholism, held in Amityville, New York, the issue of controlled trials arose frequently as a topic of debate. Conference organizer Harold Abramson was particularly opposed to double-blind statistical methods of research. After pointing out that a double-blind was impossible to establish when administering LSD or an inert placebo because of the drug's dramatic subjective effects, Abramson argued that statistical methods were fundamentally inappropriate for the study of psychotherapy: "whenever the psyche is involved," he found it "difficult to understand" how studying patient averages could provide any meaningful insight into improving psychotherapy. Instead, close study of treatment effects in individual patients was needed. He also argued that the number of potentially important variables in a patient population rendered the prospect of true control unfeasible.[53] Dutch psychiatrist Cornelius Van Rhijn agreed that controlled trial methods were inappropriate for psychotherapy research, as psychiatry lacked the objective measures needed to allow fair comparison of cases: "In psychotherapy . . . there is no general agreement upon diagnosis, favorable or unfavorable cases, or the outcome of any form of treatment. So I think you are wasting your time and money on controlled experiments and double-blind studies on subjects, patients or cases, which cannot be divided into fixed classes with a fixed diagnosis of a fixed disease with a fixed or sure outcome with some sort of therapy. The only thing I can believe in is carefully controlled studies in which certain patients can act as their own controls."[54]

Canadian psychedelic therapy pioneer Abram Hoffer also featured among the staunch opponents of the double-blind placebo-controlled methodology. He argued that not only was the use of an inert placebo impractical but the logical alternative of an active placebo was conceptually problematic. To sustain a double-blind, an active placebo would have to mimic the symptoms of LSD intoxication, while lacking its therapeutic qualities. But it was these subjective effects—the psychedelic experience—that researchers considered to be the therapeutic component in treatment; thus, "any drug which produces a psychedelic experience should . . . be as effective as LSD." The use of an active placebo capable of adequately mimicking a psychedelic reaction would result in a trial where "one merely would have a comparison between two sets of psychedelic experiences."[55] The results of such a trial would misleadingly show a lack of efficacy for psychedelic therapy, as there would not be a significant difference between the results of the control and LSD groups. Hoffer also more generally attacked the double-blind method by turning around the call for proof of efficacy from treatments to the method itself: "I would like to state categorically that the double-blind is not scientific, has never been validated, and has been repudiated by mathematicians. It is a theoretical procedure which has never been proven, as far as I can tell, and I have challenged many people to give me evidence that the double-blind does what it is supposed to do."[56]

Delving deeper into the conceptual incompatibility of LSD psychotherapy and the randomized controlled trial reveals assumptions inherent in the methodology that conflicted with the therapy's theory and method. The randomized controlled trial rose in status in the postwar period on the grounds of its objectivity—its ability to neutralize the impact of influencing variables and thereby isolate a drug's true effects. Hidden in this notion of objectivity was a "magic bullet" concept of drug efficacy, whereby a treatment should work unconsciously, independent of potential nondrug influences, through a biological interaction between drug and disease or affliction. German medical scientist Paul Ehrlich first used the term "magic bullet" in the early twentieth century to describe the effect of antibodies in serum therapy: they selectively bound to and killed intruding disease cells, while leaving healthy tissues untouched. He hypothesized that drugs could work in the same way, a form of treatment he called "chemotherapy." Ehrlich's concept was influenced by both a growing understanding of bacteriology in the period and his research into the mechanism by which dyes could selectively stain certain tissues.[57] The development of the antibacterial sulfonamides in the 1930s and penicillin in the 1940s seemingly realized the magic bullet concept. These drugs revolutionized medicine, providing miraculous cures for infectious diseases that were leading causes of disability and mortality.[58]

Randomized controlled trials were ideal for testing magic bullet–type drugs, where treatment involved simply administering a medication. This form of treatment allowed the easy use of placebo controls; double-blinding; and standardized procedures, environments, and measures: if the biological activity of the drug was considered the only relevant factor in treatment efficacy, ignorance regarding the administration of an experimental or placebo treatment could not only be achieved but also posed no threat to the treatment's potential effect. The magic bullet antibiotics were not just ideal candidates for randomized controlled trial testing but also influenced the uptake of the methodology: the two rose in prominence together over the 1940s and 1950s through the pioneering research of Austin Bradford Hill and the need to accurately evaluate and differentiate the influx of new antibiotic drugs. Antibiotics were the most successful drugs ever developed, and the most advanced clinical research methods were best suited to test such drugs that worked through an objective biological action. Therefore, the magic bullet concept became not just an ideal form of drug efficacy but the dominant model. A drug's pharmacological activity increasingly came to be considered the only "specific" aspect of treatment, with all other "nonspecific," nonpharmacological influences merely clouding the accurate judgment of a treatment's efficacy.[59] The breakthrough psychiatric drugs of the 1950s largely conformed to this magic bullet theory of drug efficacy. While their method of action was unknown, the new antipsychotics, antidepressants, and anxiolytics seemed to most observers to work regardless of the treatment environment or the interpersonal skills of the physician. Pharmacotherapy became simply a matter of fitting a diagnosis to a medication.

LSD psychotherapy was completely at odds with the magic bullet theory of drug efficacy. Rather than a specific biological treatment, LSD was merely a tool in a psychotherapeutic process—a catalyst for attaining states of consciousness or experiences that could be used by a skilled therapist to therapeutic ends. The drug had no inherent beneficial effects. Instead, its efficacy lay in the psychological impact of the subjective drug experience, which was crafted through a unique relationship among the patient, therapist, and drug.

The controlled trial's alliance with the magic bullet form of drug efficacy would make providing proof of LSD psychotherapy's efficacy through the methodology problematic. The conceptual incompatibility of LSD psychotherapy and the standard randomized controlled trial was explored by psychologist Robert Mogar at the American Psychological Association's third Research in Psychotherapy conference, held in 1966. Mogar, who had conducted LSD research with the International Foundation for Advanced Study, argued that efforts to perform controlled research with LSD were flawed because of a fundamental misconception: "The major conceptual fallacy, usually implicit, is the assumption that only drug specific effects are real, valid, and lawful. Nonspecific variables that are difficult to define and measure rigorously are random, insignificant, and sources of error."[60]

Considered "extraneous," nondrug variables produced placebo effects, which, although often powerful, were judged to confound an accurate evaluation of the specific treatment because of their nonspecific nature. However, Mogar argued that if any form of psychotherapy was to be accepted as a legitimate form of treatment, attitudes toward the placebo effect needed reevaluating. Drawing attention to the "nonspecific-extraneous-placebo fallacy," he quoted psychiatrist Arthur Shapiro's statement that "the placebo is defined as the psychological elements in treatment; psychological elements constitute psychotherapy; therefore, psychotherapy is a placebo."[61] According to Mogar, research had shown that LSD produced no invariant effects aside from an "increased sensitivity to both internal and external stimuli . . . a markedly lowered threshold for arousal."[62] Thus, he argued, the notion of "drug specific effects" needed adjusting in the case of LSD, where nondrug variables powerfully shaped the patient's reaction to the drug. These variables could be categorized as those relating to the patient, therapist, therapist-patient interaction, and situation (set and setting). Before a valid assessment of the efficacy of a form of LSD psychotherapy could be performed, a more precise understanding of the role of these nondrug factors in creating a desired reaction was needed. Mogar suggested that research on this topic could involve inverting the standard form of controlled trial—where drug administration is the tested variable— by keeping drug administration as a constant, while varying the nature of nondrug factors. Once a specific LSD reaction was well defined and could be reliably produced, a study of treatment efficacy would need to be designed that would provide a comparative control for the treatment as a whole, rather than just one influencing variable.[63]

The common element underpinning these arguments was that LSD psychotherapy was not a drug treatment but a form of psychotherapy. However, because LSD psychotherapy utilized a drug, it came under the regulation of the FDA, and thus proof of its efficacy needed to be established in the same manner as required for a drug treatment. The randomized controlled trial was not designed to test the efficacy of psychotherapies, which was a much more complicated task than evaluating drug efficacy. While testers of drug treatments in psychiatry had to face the difficulties of establishing standardized diagnoses and outcome measures, and faced many potentially significant nonspecific variables, the specific element of their treatment—drug administration—was clearly defined and could easily be manipulated for the purpose of experiment. In contrast, there was little agreement among the numerous schools of psychotherapy—such as Freudian, Jungian, interpersonal, or humanistic—on any aspect of psychiatric illness or its treatment.

Psychotherapeutic schools offered different theories of the nature of the mind and the origins of mental illness and methods for treating it. Even within a school, the notion of specificity was complicated, as many conditions could be treated through the same methods. The goals of treatment also ranged from the reduction of specific symptoms to more difficult to define goals such as increased self-understanding and adjustment to life. Even if a form of psychotherapy was standardized for a particular patient population and for a specific goal, the fact that the treatment relied on active cooperation between two individuals meant that significant variables existed outside of the treatment framework. Summarizing the American Psychological Association's 1961 Research in Psychotherapy conference, proceedings editors Lester Lubrosky and Hans Strupp found that discussed variables fell into four major categories: the techniques of therapy, the therapist, the patient, and the match between therapist and patient.[64] Because of the critical nature of these personal and interpersonal variables, many psychiatrists regarded psychotherapy as an art as well as a treatment based in science. Randomized controlled trials required the manipulation of a hypothesized specific therapeutic element in treatment while all nonspecific variables remained constant. But with such a blurred boundary between the specific and nonspecific elements in psychotherapy, devising a method of evaluating any form of psychotherapy presented formidable challenges. As prominent psychotherapy researcher Jerome Frank commented in 1974, the complexity of psychotherapy had resulted in researchers either attempting to encompass all aspects of psychotherapy at the expense of accuracy or focusing on a manageably small element of treatment and "achieving rigor at the expense of significance."[65]

A major methodological issue in psychotherapy research was finding a control condition that would allow comparison between the outcome of psychotherapy and the natural course of illness. This need was particularly significant for psychotherapies that were conducted over long periods, where not only significant natural fluctuations in pathology could be expected but major changes in the patient's circumstances as well. Controlled trials accomplished this through the use of the double-blind placebo comparison, but this was not possible with psychotherapy: too little was known about the process of psychotherapy for a therapist to deliver a convincing but ineffective form of treatment to the patient. Even if this were possible, it would only be single-blind, as therapists could not be made ignorant of the fact they were delivering a sham treatment. In lieu of an adequate placebo treatment, researchers could compare the progress of treated patients with that of similar patients who were left untreated. A common method of attaining such a group was to enroll patients for treatment but then assign them to a long waiting list. Their changing pathology over time could then be compared with that of similar patients who entered treatment immediately. But experience proved the no-treatment waiting list problematic and hard to maintain: only patients with nonurgent problems could ethically be held back from treatment, refusal of immediate treatment could psychologically affect patients, and patients would inevitably drop off the list or find another form of formal or informal psychotherapy while they were waiting.[66] An alternative method was to compare two or more different forms of psychotherapy in the treatment of similar patients. This method had the benefit of theoretically equalizing nonspecific variables between treatments, as all patients would be receiving therapy from trained and committed practitioners. However, such studies struggled to find differential efficacy between treatments. This suggested that the nonspecific elements common to all psychotherapies were more significant than their specific theories and methods.[67]

In addition to these difficulties in designing controlled trials, psychotherapy research lagged behind drug research because of researchers' resistance to attempt outcome studies at all. In summarizing the American Psychological Association's first Research in Psychotherapy conference, held in 1958, Morris Parloff and Eli Rubinstein found that researchers avoided outcome studies partly because of the stigma that it was "applied" research, rather than more prestigious "basic" research, such as closely studying patients' personalities and psychopathologies or the process of psychotherapy to advance theory. The history of poor research methodology in outcome research exacerbated this stigma. Researchers also feared confirming that nonspecific factors were responsible for psychotherapy's effectiveness, as this could undermine their careers as trained and committed specialists.[68] Furthermore, as Mogar had argued, the placebo effect was a much more complex concept for psychotherapy than for psychopharmacology, as the need to control for psychological influences appeared to many psychiatrists and psychologists irrelevant in the context of a psychological treatment. The placebo effect, itself a form of psychological treatment, was a component of psychotherapy rather than a phenomenon that masked its true efficacy.[69] This argument as well as the efficacy of psychotherapy more generally did not go unchallenged in the 1950s and 1960s.[70] Nevertheless, in those decades psychotherapy carried enough prestige that these critiques could largely be ignored. Regardless, the reality was that all research was purely academic, as psychotherapies did not need to be of proven efficacy in order to be practiced: "talk therapies" did not involve any physically invasive procedures, making them of little interest to federal regulators and outside the jurisdiction of the FDA.

Like other psychotherapies, LSD psychotherapy was therefore a poor fit for the randomized controlled trial on both conceptual and practical grounds. Because of the treatment's lack of a clear division between specific and nonspecific impacting variables, the concept of a placebo effect was complicated, and an adequate control treatment was difficult to design. The drug's obvious effects and the required active participation of both therapist and patient in treatment rendered blinding practically problematic. These problems were significant for both psycholytic and psychedelic forms of LSD psychotherapy, but certain factors would make controlled research with psycholytic therapy even more difficult. Psycholytic therapy was simply the use of LSD to facilitate various forms of psychodynamic psychotherapy; thus, the treatment had no standardized theory, method, goals, treatment course, or outcome measures. Proving the efficacy of psycholytic therapy would require first standardizing such aspects of treatment. Psychedelic therapy at least had a standard method and goal in treating alcoholism, as well as a short course of treatment and an objective outcome measure in drinking behavior.

The specific challenges for research on psycholytic therapy were clearly shown at the first US conference to focus solely on research into LSD's therapeutic potential. Entitled "The Use of LSD in Psychotherapy," and held in Princeton, New Jersey, in 1959, the conference brought together twenty-six of the leading international LSD researchers. The verbatim proceedings of the conference, which was designed as a series of discussions rather than formal presentations, show that while there was little disagreement over LSD having therapeutic benefits, there was little agreement on exactly how to use and interpret the drugs effects. As participant Betty Eisner remembered, "There were 26 different ways of looking at psychotherapy as well as LSD: twenty-six different areas of expertise and experience, and 26 opinions on the drug."[71]

From the beginning of the conference's first discussion, led by Harold Abramson, it was evident that the lack of a common language regarding the specifics of psychotherapy, let alone LSD psychotherapy, was a major difficulty for therapists wanting to pool their experience: just three sentences into Abramson's description of his therapeutic method, the discussion turned to the definition of his framework of "psychoanalytically orientated psycho-therapy."[72] Despite host Frank Fremont-Smith's initial attempts to steer the discussion away from definitions—as "we certainly won't reach agreement today, tomorrow, or in 20 months on a common definition of any form of psychotherapy with a label attached"—the difficulties of overcoming the participants' different theoretical frameworks proved insurmountable: as he later stated, "The striking feature of the Conference so far is that we have not communicated. The verbal image that was good for one of us was not good for eight-tenths of the others."[73]

Terminology used to describe aspects of LSD treatment, such as "ego en-hancement," "reconstructive therapy," and even "subconscious" had far from universal understandings and often caused confusion among the partici-pants.[74] Similarly, even the common experiences of patients under LSD were interpreted differently, with the experience of being born or giving birth, for example, considered a memory by some and a fantasy by others.[75] Differences in interpretation were not the only difficulties that varying psychotherapeutic orientations caused. Beverly Hills psychiatrist Mortimer Hartman had found in his clinic that the orientation of the therapists fundamentally altered the experience of the patients and the material they brought forward. "In our group, for instance, which consists of two Freudians and two Jungians, the latter will get the transcendental experience in the patient much faster than the former. The two Freudians, on the other hand, will evoke the patient's childhood memories much more quickly than the two Jungians in the group. These results are due to the different orientations and different kinds of sug-gestion on the part of the therapists."[76]

In addition to researchers' differing theoretical frameworks making it dif-ficult to cement a clearly defined treatment paradigm for psycholytic therapy, with Ronald Sandison concluding that "every physician probably has to administer LSD in his own way," these difficulties highlighted further important questions for psychotherapy research with or without LSD.[77] With reactions under LSD highlighting the power of the therapist's conscious or unconscious suggestions, beliefs, and attitudes in shaping the therapeutic responses of the patient, it became clear that a greater understanding of the patient-therapist relationship was needed to understand the efficacy of any form of psychotherapy. The lack of understanding of LSD psychotherapy's efficacy was not a failing of the researchers but merely reflected the complexity of the task, as Fremont-Smith expressed in his concluding remarks:

> I would like just to touch on the fact that we have been dealing with the very essence of the nature of therapy of any kind, of the nature of the psychotherapeutic process, about which we certainly know too little. It involves the nature of human relationships, because psychotherapy involves both relationships within the person and between persons. . . .
>
> . . . [W]e should not feel too distressed because we cannot encompass all this; that would hardly be possible. . . .
>
> Added to these basic problems of human personality and human relationships, there is a drug, a pharmaceutical agent, and this both complicates and simplifies the situation. It brings it nearer to science, on the one hand, and throws into bolder relief the very complexity of the problem itself.[78]

Clearly defining the efficacy of psycholytic therapy would first require establishing the efficacy of the forms of psychotherapy that LSD was used to facilitate and then demonstrating that the addition of LSD improved results.

Psycholytic therapy research would fade in the United States more quickly than psychedelic therapy. In addition to the research difficulties, several factors likely influenced this: Sandoz's restriction of its IND sponsorship to hospital-based researchers, as psychodynamic psychiatrists were often in private practice or small clinics; the difficulties of submitting an independent IND, as we have seen earlier in the case of Harold Abramson; and the fact that most psycholytic therapists were not committed drug researchers but psychotherapists who would return to practicing the drug-free form of their treatment when faced with the challenges of continuing LSD research. Psychedelic therapy was better suited to large-scale, hospital-based clinical trials, and in many ways it had a greater medical significance. Nevertheless, as the rest of this book explores, despite the advantages that psychedelic therapy had over psycholytic for performing controlled research, the difficulties involved would still prove insurmountable.

The incompatibility between LSD psychotherapy and the randomized controlled trial highlights how the different regulation of psychopharmacology and psychotherapy would widen the divide between psychiatry's biological and psychological treatments. Psychopharmacology would become increasingly wedded to the magic bullet construct of drug efficacy, as drugs were required to be proven effective through a testing methodology that presumed a direct biological action. For psychiatrists interested in drug research and treatment, only a drug's objectively verifiable long-term effects on restoring normal psychological functioning fit the biological concept of treatment. These would become the only desirable drug effects. Immediate subjective psychological drug effects would increasingly be considered merely side effects because of their nonspecific nature. By treating mental illness in this fashion, the psychiatrists' role would increasingly mirror that of the physician treating infectious disease.

The efficacy requirements of the Drug Amendments of 1962 would unintentionally help to turn psychopharmacology into a purely biological form of treatment. While a theoretical divide had long existed between biological and psychodynamic psychiatrists, the former had not had a monopoly on drugs, as psychodynamic psychiatrists explored how their subjective effects could be used to explore and manipulate psychology. This would no longer be practically possible, as proving the efficacy of such use through controlled trials would present formidable challenges. Psychodynamic psychiatrists would therefore retreat from psychopharmacology to their mainstay of psychotherapy, which had a much greater tolerance for subjective and nonspecific influences in treatment. Each now having a monopoly on distinct forms of treatment, biological and psychodynamic psychiatry would become distinct specialties to a much greater extent than before the 1962 amendments.

As this chapter has established, the FDA and research experts would generally interpret the amendment's term "adequate and well-controlled investigations" as referring to the randomized controlled trial, and LSD psychotherapy was incompatible with that form of efficacy testing. However, the FDA's Joseph Sadusk had acknowledged that controlled trial methods were not always possible and stated that in such cases other forms of research could be judged adequate by the FDA. So it could be expected that the FDA would not have required LSD psychotherapists to utilize randomized controlled trials. Nevertheless, Goddard's 1966 statements that opened this chapter strongly suggest that the FDA would accept nothing less than evidence from sophisticated controlled trials to support LSD's efficacy. Further, at separate congressional hearings held that year, NIMH director Stanley Yolles stated that LSD use needed to be strictly constrained to "carefully controlled experiments until *incontrovertible* data are available documenting LSD's efficacy and safety."[79] That LSD psychotherapy researchers began attempting to employ controlled trials shortly after the passage of the Drug Amendments of 1962 also strongly suggests that the need to use the methodology had been made clear to them.

Conclusion

With the passage of the Drug Amendments of 1962, LSD psychotherapy researchers were placed in a unique and difficult position. They were the first researchers required to provide proof of efficacy for a form of psychotherapy, and at a time when there was no consensus on an accurate method for doing so. With LSD psychotherapy officially recognized as a drug therapy, researchers were required to adopt the techniques of the preeminent model of pharmaceutical research, despite that method's poor fit for evaluating LSD psychotherapy. Over the 1960s LSD researchers would nevertheless attempt to fit their research into the controlled trial model and thereby not only be able to continue their work but potentially convince the medical community as well as the FDA of the value of LSD in psychiatry. However, the difficulties of balancing scientific standards with the clinical demands of treatment would result in research moving sideways instead of forward, with more clinical trials resulting in more confusion, rather than a clearer picture of LSD psychotherapy's efficacy.

CHAPTER FOUR

Against the Tide

The Spring Grove Experiment

I have been doing LSD therapy for as long as I have been in analytic training. To date no good controlled study has come of either. Both are incapable of demonstration. Both have their metapsychology which is incapable of proof. It is my intention to change all that.

Charles Savage, c. 1962

In 1963, a study of the efficacy of psychedelic therapy was initiated at Spring Grove State Hospital, near Baltimore, Maryland. In many ways the timing of its inception was unfavorable, as this was the same year that Timothy Leary and Richard Alpert's antics at Harvard boiled over into the public sphere. Their dismissal from the university would come to represent a watershed moment in the transformation of LSD's reputation from a tool of medical research to a dangerous drug of abuse. Further, as the FDA gained oversight of LSD research through the Drug Amendments of 1962, research began declining in the formalized regulatory context. Yet, despite this, the psychedelic research program at Spring Grove would flourish over the 1960s, growing into the longest, largest, most sophisticated, and most successful such program ever undertaken in the United States, not coming to a close until 1976.

Psychiatrist Albert Kurland and psychologist Sanford Unger initiated the program to rigorously evaluate the effectiveness of psychedelic therapy in the treatment of alcoholism by submitting it to a randomized, double-blind controlled clinical trial. By bringing psychedelic research into line with the prevailing scientific standards and the FDA's expectations for drug evaluation under the Drug Amendments of 1962, Kurland and Unger aimed to provide convincing evidence for or against the efficacy of psychedelic therapy. Promising early results led the researchers to continuously expand the program. Over the decade they launched three further major clinical trials exploring psychedelic therapy for new indications: first neuroses; then anxiety, depression, and pain associated with terminal cancer; and finally narcotic addiction.

More experienced researchers also joined the team, leading Spring Grove to become a world center of expertise in psychedelic drugs.

By the end of the 1960s, all signs suggested that the Spring Grove clinical trials would confirm the efficacy of psychedelic therapy for a variety of indications. Yet, ultimately, their research would leave no lasting impact on psychiatry, and the program would fade into complete obscurity.[1] Chapter 5 explores why this eventuated, through an in-depth analysis of the designs of the Spring Grove clinical trials and the internal and external challenges that undermined the researchers' work. First, however, charting the constant growth and success of the program over the 1960s not only reveals that LSD psychotherapy was neither thwarted by the increasing regulation of that decade nor completely extinguished by the stigma of controversy, but also the conditions under which it thrived and the factors deemed critical for treatment success.

The Spring Grove LSD research program was hardly a fringe operation; it represented the cutting edge of experimental psychopharmacology. While their treatments may have been unorthodox, the researchers themselves were highly orthodox, many coming from Ivy League backgrounds and close association with the National Institute of Mental Health. Indeed, Kurland held several institutional leadership positions that made him a central, powerful individual in psychiatric research in Maryland. Rather than simply put psychedelic therapy to the controlled trial test, the Spring Grove researchers developed a large research program that worked to refine treatment methods and increase their understanding of the therapeutic process. Over the decade their clinical experience and preliminary results clearly convinced them of the effectiveness of their treatments, and they began planning to incorporate psychedelic therapy into the standard treatment program of Maryland's state hospitals. Despite the context of turmoil surrounding LSD in the 1960s, they still viewed LSD as potentially becoming a central tool of psychiatry, with wide implications for understanding and treating addiction and mental illness, and improving mental health. They would face little difficulty working toward their goals; convincing the wider medical community would be the greater challenge.

Inception and Expansion

Born in 1914 in Wilkes-Barre, Pennsylvania, Kurland served as a battalion surgeon during the Second World War, where he witnessed the effects of extreme stress on troops, including death by friendly fire and suicide. Influenced by these observations, Kurland undertook training in psychiatry on his return to the United States, including some training in psychoanalysis. In 1949, he joined the staff at Spring Grove State Hospital on the outskirts of Baltimore to complete his certification in psychiatry. Founded in 1797, at the time Spring Grove catered to a patient population of more than 2,700 with just twenty-three psychiatrists. Kurland was assigned to manage a sixty-five-bed unit for the criminally insane. Considering the hospital's extremely low staff-to-patient ratio, Kurland concluded that he would receive little supervision or training. He decided to further his education through research, despite having to conduct it on his own time and with no hospital funding.[2] His early publications included an evaluation of drama therapy and a study of "wife murderers."[3] In recognition of his work, in 1953 Kurland was appointed as the hospital's director of research, although initially his only staff was a secretary. The following year Kurland entered the field of psychopharmacology, investigating the emerging reports of the tranquilizing effects of chlorpromazine. He conducted an uncontrolled clinical trial with the drug and published positive results in 1955.[4]

As discussed in chapter 1, Kurland's first contact with LSD came in the mid-1950s, when he collaborated with Louis Cholden and Charles Savage (then of the National Institute of Mental Health) on research exploring the drug's effects in schizophrenic patients.[5] It was not until 1963 that LSD came back to Spring Grove. The impetus for research again came from the NIMH, this time from a young psychologist named Sanford Unger. Born in 1931 in New York City, Unger had received his PhD in human development from Cornell University in 1959 and joined the NIMH's Laboratory of Psychology as a research psychologist in 1960.[6] In 1962, reports making widely divergent claims for LSD's effects caught the interest of Unger's department. Unger volunteered to conduct an extensive review of the literature on the drug to try to bring some clarity to confusion over its effects.[7]

Unger's report, published in *Psychiatry* in 1963, considered how the variety of effects claimed for LSD, mescaline, and psilocybin related to extradrug variables and how personality change associated with the drugs related to specific types of experiences. Unger found that, through the reports of the drugs' variable effects, a few consistent elements could be ascertained: an " 'orgy' of vision" characterized by the experience of intense images, color, and light; a profound distortion in the subject's sense of self, a form of depersonalization or dissociation; the ability to clearly observe and report mental changes, a clarity of consciousness clearly distinguishing the drug state from delirium;

and, finally, a lasting impression that the experience was one of awesome power and significance, whether positive or negative.[8] The variable effects of the drugs were then largely dependent on the attitudes of those administering them, with experimenters expecting anxiety finding it, and psychotherapists finding experiences relevant to their theoretical framework. Unger concluded that by deliberately manipulating the expectations and attitudes of patients, their reaction to LSD-type drugs could be "systematically directed." Studying the increasingly frequent reports of rapid personality change following LSD use, particularly leading to sobriety in alcoholics, Unger found that such change was invariably associated with a transcendental, or mystical, drug reaction. Given the dramatic nature of these reports and the considerable public health implications if they were accurate, Unger concluded that this use of the drugs deserved "intensive investigation."[9]

Having discovered all he could from the literature on LSD, Unger's next step was to try the drug. A colleague who had had some clinical experience with LSD and who held a psychedelic view of its effects administered him 200 mcg. Unger's experience was profoundly psychedelic: he found his "awareness to be literally constituted by, or suffused with . . . bliss, awe, harmony."[10] His section chief and the director of clinical investigations at the NIMH also tried the drug, and they supported Unger's desire to further investigate its therapeutic potential. Subsequently, Unger traveled the country visiting LSD researchers to further explore the research that was already underway. Jonathan Cole, chief of the NIMH's Psychopharmacology Service Center, put Unger in touch with Kurland at Spring Grove.

By 1963, Kurland had built up considerable experience in the therapeutic evaluation of psychotropic agents. He had continued researching the efficacy of tranquilizers, progressing from uncontrolled studies to sophisticated randomized double-blind placebo-controlled trials.[11] In addition to his role as director of research at Spring Grove, in 1960 Kurland became director of research for the Maryland State Department of Mental Hygiene.[12] In this position he came under increasing pressure from the state commissioner of mental hygiene to find more effective methods for treating the growing population of alcoholics in the state's psychiatric hospitals. In response, Kurland oversaw research at Spring Grove testing the efficacy of the new antidepressant nialamide and the minor tranquilizer chlordiazepoxide in treating the addiction. Both trials returned largely negative results.[13] Kurland therefore read the emerging reports of the successful treatment of alcoholics with LSD with great interest. He noted, however, that controlled studies were needed to confirm its efficacy.[14]

Kurland and Unger decided to collaborate on a controlled evaluation of LSD in the treatment of alcoholism, and, with Cole's support, they applied to the NIMH for funding. Cole was skeptical of the uncontrolled research that backed the claims of LSD's therapeutic effectiveness and of the unconventional mystical descriptions of the therapeutic process. He was even skeptical of the value of the kinds of personality changes associated with the drug, commenting, "If a person becomes more relaxed and happy-go-lucky, more sensitive to poetry or music, but less concerned with success or competition, is this good?"[15] Nevertheless, he was concerned about the problem that alcoholism posed to the public health system, and he was not ready to disregard a treatment that could be useful. Cole also held Kurland's previous psychopharmacology research in high regard. The proposed study thus promised to bring better scientific standards to the unconventional field. Kurland and Unger's application was approved, and funding for the study began in 1964. Unger left the NIMH to work on the research full time at Spring Grove.[16]

The research began with a pilot study of sixty-nine male inpatients of the hospital's Alcoholic Rehabilitation Unit. The pilot phase was intended to build experience with the psychedelic procedure, establish its safety, and explore its therapeutic potential. From the start, the researchers' intention was to directly replicate the therapeutic method of the Canadian pioneers of psychedelic therapy. Like those researchers, Kurland and Unger focused on carefully manipulating the mind-set of the patient and the setting LSD was administered in, to produce a therapeutically useful psychedelic experience. They believed that the life of the alcoholic was one of severe alienation, which the psychedelic experience could alleviate by helping the patient to "foster the growth of new contact with himself and life," leading to "a major reorientation in the alcoholic patient's view of his own worth and his prospects."[17]

Prior to the administration of LSD, the patient spent an average of twelve to fifteen hours with the therapist, over two weeks, preparing for the experience. This intensive preparation included both psychotherapy—to bring the patient to a level of psychological readiness for change, as well as to build a strong rapport between the therapist and patient—and specific preparation for the LSD experience. Throughout the ten- to twelve-hour 450 mcg LSD session, the patient was accompanied by the therapist and a nurse. Rather than giving formal psychotherapy, their role during the session was to guide and shape the drug experience, provide support through challenging or frightening passages, and harness and integrate emotional reactions and psychodynamic material as it arose.[18] Music, eyeshades, and other items such as photographs and mirrors were used throughout the session to help the therapist guide the patient's experience. Further psychotherapy in the days following the LSD session was used to work through any unresolved conflicts that had emerged in the session and to cement positive insights and experiences into the patient's personality to help ensure they led to positive change.[19]

The effect of this treatment program was assessed with the Minnesota Multiphasic Personality Inventory (MMPI), which was administered prior to treatment and shortly afterward. The results, averaged from the data for all the patients, showed statistically significant improvements in all measures of psychopathology except hypomania. Particular improvements were found in ratings of depression and psychasthenia, a condition the researchers described as characterized by "rumination and preoccupation with negative, distraught thought content."[20] On a smaller series of patients, the researchers also administered the MMPI on the day before LSD administration, to judge whether the effects of the treatment were due primarily to the preparatory psychotherapy. Results suggested that this was not the case. A follow-up conducted six months after treatment found that one-third of the patients had remained abstinent. The experience with these sixty-nine patients also demonstrated that the psychedelic procedure of treatment was safe: both MMPI data and clinical evaluations confirmed that no patient was harmed by the drug experience.

In addition to this uncontrolled study, the pilot phase of research involved an attempt at a small controlled trial. The researchers studied the progress of twenty-five of the psychedelic therapy patients alongside another twenty-five similar alcoholic patients who were treated with only a limited amount of psychotherapy. However, the study fell apart because of a high dropout rate in the psychotherapy-only group. Both groups of patients had been housed in the same ward, and the researchers concluded that the dropouts were due to feelings of rivalry from the psychotherapy-only group toward the psychedelic patients and their disappointment at missing out on the exciting new treatment that they had volunteered for.[21] The difficulty in designing a control group that was both practicable and scientifically sound was a problem that would plague the researchers throughout their attempts to evaluate the therapeutic usefulness of LSD.

Over the decade, the Spring Grove researchers developed and refined their treatment method. The team placed particular emphasis on the importance of the preparatory psychotherapy, which increased in duration to an average of twenty hours. While it was the psychedelic experience that could rapidly transform patients' attitudes and behaviors, the researchers believed that this was only possible "after the achievement of psychodynamic resolution and self understanding during the preparatory psychotherapy."[22] They considered the drug session as "corrective and remedial" as opposed to uncovering: the goal was to change attitudes, values, and behavior rather than to uncover repressed memories or psychological conflicts. The procedure was designed to produce "meaningful catharsis, reciprocal inhibition of anxiety, conflict resolution, emotionally validated insight, attitude redirection, elevated self-esteem, and deepened philosophical perspective."[23]

In the second half of 1964, the psychedelic research program at Spring Grove began to grow, in both staff and ambitions. A major addition to the team was Charles Savage. Since his previous LSD research at Spring Grove, Savage had moved to California, where he had been among the first in the United States to explore the psychedelic therapy method developed in Canada: first at the Palo Alto Medical Research Foundation, then at the International Foundation for Advanced Study in Menlo Park. At Spring Grove he would take up the position of director of medical research, as well as appointments as assistant professor of psychiatry at Johns Hopkins Hospital and clinical assistant professor of psychiatry at the University of Maryland.[24] He would have a particular influence on the design of control treatments for the Spring Grove studies, bringing ideas that he had formulated at the International Foundation for Advanced Study but that had not been implemented.

As they moved on from the pilot phase in the alcoholic study, the researchers also launched into a new research direction: psychedelic therapy for the treatment of neuroses. They planned a new major clinical trial, which, like the alcoholic study, would be a sophisticated randomized, double-blind controlled trial. While psychedelic therapy had been developed and primarily studied in the treatment of alcoholics, several researchers had reported positive results with other categories of patients. Most notably, alongside their pioneering alcoholic work, Ross MacLean, Al Hubbard, and colleagues at Hollywood Hospital in Vancouver had reported treating thirty-nine non-alcoholic patients, twenty-six of whom were diagnosed with a form of neurosis. Of these patients, sixteen (61.5 percent) were considered "much improved" and seven (27 percent) "improved" after an average follow-up period of more than six months, leaving only three (11.5 percent) patients judged as unchanged.[25] Savage himself had also found positive results with a variety of nonalcoholic, nonpsychotic outpatients at the International Foundation for Advanced Study immediately prior to his arrival at Spring Grove.[26]

The Spring Grove researchers submitted a funding application for the neurotic study to the Department of Health, Education, and Welfare in August 1964, with Kurland as principal investigator and Savage as co–principal investigator. The study would begin in January 1965, and Savage would officially join the staff at Spring Grove in February.[27] The trial aimed to evaluate the efficacy of psychedelic therapy in hospitalized "chronically-ill psychoneurotic patients." The researchers recognized that this was a loose diagnostic category, representing a "heterogeneous group with a wide range of pathology pictures." However, the patients shared predominant symptoms of "incapacitating depression, or chronic, pervasive anxiety." Spring Grove admitted twenty to thirty such patients a month. They were considered poor candidates for treatment, and most had previously undergone hospital treatment. All newly admitted psychoneurotic patients would be screened for the study. Those with serious organic illness or "defective intelligence," those outside the ages of twenty-one to forty, those unwilling to undergo treatment, and those for whom follow-up would be difficult were excluded.[28]

By the start of 1966, with the controlled trials with alcoholic and neurotic patients underway, the Spring Grove researchers began planning to systematically explore a third indication for psychedelic therapy: pain and psychological distress associated with terminal illness. This followed their positive experience treating their terminally ill colleague Sarah in August 1965. In February 1966, Kurland submitted a grant application to the Department of Health, Education, and Welfare for a controlled trial. The application outlined the common experience of these patients that the researchers hoped to improve. They considered the modern "American Way of Death" to be highly problematic: while modern medicine had developed many methods to prolong life, the quality of life for dying patients was very poor, with prolonged life often equaling prolonged suffering. As society became increasingly secular, death had taken on a different meaning for many. Where in more religious times death had been understood as God's will and belief in an afterlife had provided comfort to both the dying and their loved ones, the secular perspective interpreted death as a "disease which ought to be eliminated . . . a consequence of personal neglect or failure . . . something to be shunned and not openly discussed." Denial was a common factor at the bedside, with all involved focusing on the hopes of a miraculous cure through herculean treatment instead of accepting death and preparing for it. This denial increased feelings of failure and defeat as the disease ultimately won out over treatment efforts. For the terminal cancer patient, the last stages of life were character-ized by "increasing pain, increasing anxiety, increasing morphine, increasing addiction, increasing demandingness, with the ultimate disintegration and degradation of the personality." With its focus on prolonging life at all costs, modern medicine left its patients "deprived of the opportunity to die with dignity."[29]

In addition to justifying the trial on the basis of their experience with Sarah, Kurland drew on the research of Eric Kast at the Chicago Medical School. Kast had been the first to treat cancer patients with LSD, and he pub-lished his initial results in 1963. His intention had been to study the potential analgesic effects of LSD, but he also found the drug to have a therapeutic effect on the patients' attitudes toward their condition. Kast theorized that LSD could have an analgesic effect due to its ability to produce profound distortions in an individual's body image and its effects on concentration. He believed that pathological pain was partly caused by an objective neuro-physiological process and partly by subjective psychological factors. The psy-chological element was primarily a conflict "between the desire to maintain bodily integrity and the wish to sequestrate the ailing part."[30] If LSD could lessen patients' need to psychologically hold onto the pain-producing parts of their body, they would become more dissociated from them and thereby experience less pain. LSD also decreased subjects' ability to maintain concen-tration on specific sensations: the focus of their attention shifted rapidly, and sensations that would usually dominate the mind, such as physical discom-fort, no longer took such a priority. Kast theorized that patients would be-come distracted from their pain, whether it was of physical or psychological origin, by the sensory and mental phenomena that the drug produced.

Kast tested his hypothesis by comparing LSD with two powerful opioid analgesics, meperidine and dihydromorphinone, in fifty patients who suf-fered from severe pain, thirty-nine of whom had a form of cancer. Kast found that although LSD took longer to have an effect, it had a significantly superior analgesic effect than either of the two opioids: patients experienced an aver-age of almost thirty-two hours of pain relief after receiving LSD, compared to less than three hours after the opioids. Beyond having an analgesic effect, Kast noticed that, after LSD, "patients displayed a peculiar disregard for the gravity of their situations, and talked freely about their impending death with an affect considered inappropriate in our western civilization, but most beneficial to their own psychic states." He interpreted patients' accepting attitude toward their condition as related to meaningful experiences of beauty produced by LSD. The changed perspectives lasted even longer than the drug's analgesic effects. Despite the positive effects of LSD, only twelve of the fifty patients wished for a repeat administration, which Kast believed was due to the experience being "hard work."[31]

The stated aim of the Spring Grove trial was to cross-validate Kast's research by testing two hypotheses: that LSD therapy could relieve pain and reduce the use of conventional analgesics in cancer patients, and that it could "reduce the depression and anxiety associated with impending death." All participants in the study were to be cancer patients from Sinai Hospital in Baltimore. They were to have exhausted all conventional treatments, be functional enough to cooperate, be expected to live for at least one month, and not be in remission.

Outside the Hospital

By the mid-1960s, the psychedelic research program at Spring Grove State Hospital had developed into the largest such program in the country. The researchers were conducting two significant controlled clinical trials and were planning for a third. Designed with both clinical needs and scientific rigor in mind, the trials promised to provide conclusive evidence of the efficacy of psychedelic therapy in treating alcoholism, neurosis, and pain and psychological distress associated with terminal cancer. At the same time, however, the sociopolitical climate surrounding LSD was worsening. As discussed in chapter 2, nonmedical use of LSD was increasing, and the drug's partial criminalization under the Drug Abuse Control Amendments of 1965 did little to deter this. Indeed, controversy and concern over the drug increased considerably the next year: historian Erika Dyck has found that reports on LSD in the *New York Times* jump from five in 1965 to more than five hundred in 1966.[32] Typical stories from the period contained sensationalized accounts of LSD use provoking prolonged psychotic breakdowns and violent behavior, often leading to death.

Perhaps representative of LSD's media coverage was a prominent, and since widely cited, *Life* magazine cover story from March 1966. Published under the cover headline "The Exploding Threat of the Mind Drug That Got Out of Control: LSD," the series of short articles painted a picture of a drug with dramatic, unpredictable effects that was overtaking and threatening America: the "large underground cult" of LSD users was spreading, with an estimated one million doses likely to be consumed that year. The authors warned starkly of the dangers of "bad trips," quoting one user's experience: "It was horrible. . . . I saw my face. It was very large and it had scars running down it. I experienced the desire to die, but not actual death, the desire to rip my skin off and pull my hair out and my face off, things like that. . . . I definitely won't take acid again."[33] *Life*'s science editor Albert Rosenfeld further warned that the "bizarre psychic effects" of the drug could lead to not only psychiatric casualties but also death: "People on LSD sometimes believe they have the power to fly, or to walk on water. One young Californian walked in front of a speeding car, convinced it could not harm him—and was killed. A woman in Europe, into whose drink a prankster dropped some LSD, thought she was going crazy and committed suicide. For these people and others like them, LSD was not merely dangerous—it was lethal."[34] Driving the point home, he concluded, "What the LSD user may be buying is a one-way ticket to an asylum, a prison or a grave."

Yet Rosenfeld also conceded that—although it remained to be proven—LSD might be "extremely useful" in psychotherapy, where it could help give patients "astonishing insight into themselves, thereby accelerating their recovery."[35] Further, another section of the coverage quoted religious scholar Walter Clark suggesting that psychedelic drugs allowed scholars to study "religious experience in the laboratory" and that "no psychologist of religion can afford to be ignorant of them." It also quoted a retired navy captain, who claimed that LSD had helped him to solve a difficult technical problem while designing intelligence equipment, by releasing "the normal limiting mechanisms of the brain." Tempering this enthusiasm, the section cited LSD researcher Sidney Cohen as being worried that "indiscriminate" LSD users would suffer brain damage. The section concluded by lamenting that legitimate research was now restricted to the clinical domain, as "there is no reason to suppose that doctors are the only men serious enough to approach the drug," and warned that further criminalizing the drug was futile and could result in "driving away people with prudence and intelligence while scarcely inconveniencing the really reckless, dangerous" users.[36]

While the *Life* articles attempted to provide some balance to its portrayal of LSD as a wildly dangerous drug—acknowledging that it had potential benefits when used responsibly—other articles did not. One particularly scathing article, published two months earlier in January 1966 in *This Week* magazine, took aim at not just the dangers of LSD's nonmedical use but at the safety and effectiveness of its supervised medical use as well. *This Week*, a Sunday magazine nationally syndicated to thirty-nine prominent newspapers such as the *Los Angeles Times*, and—of greatest relevance to the Spring Grove researchers—the *Baltimore Sun*, had a total circulation of almost ten million.[37] The article had the potential to do serious damage to LSD psychotherapy's reputation. Entitled "The Nightmare Drug," it characterized LSD as *"a menace, a deadly chemical brainwash that can, in the wrong hands, wreck a mind and shatter a life."* The authors went beyond this, arguing that *"LSD is dangerous even under medical supervision"* and that disturbing visions experienced by patients undergoing LSD psychotherapy had resulted in severe depression and suicide. Further, they reported that research into LSD's therapeutic potential had "established this bitter and alarming fact: *LSD seems to be a monumental bust."* They supported this claim with quotes from several psychiatrists—including Roy Grinker, who had pioneered drug-assisted psychotherapy in developing narcosynthesis during the Second World War and who now edited the prestigious journal *Archives of General Psychiatry*—that attested to LSD psychotherapy failing to live up to its hype. The reporters did acknowledge that studies out of Canada had reported great success with alcoholic patients, as well as patients with other psychiatric disorders. Yet they emphasized the perspective of critics of these studies—that they were unreliable, as they were neither randomized nor double-blind.[38]

There is some evidence that the public and political controversy over LSD was having a negative effect on the conduct of some studies. In 1966, LSD researcher Charles Dahlberg and his colleagues conducted a survey of twenty-nine other researchers, inquiring whether the recent adverse publicity had hindered their work. Many confirmed they were experiencing difficulties: volunteers were increasingly drug seekers considered to be inappropriate research subjects, patients and their families were more anxious about the drug, researchers and their colleagues were increasingly ambivalent and cautious in their attitudes toward LSD, and some projects had even been terminated.[39]

Despite this, Savage's June response to Dahlberg was that while the adverse publicity had had some effect, "I can't say that this has been a major source of interference in our studies." He explained that while pressure from anxious family members did lead to "occasional dropouts," patient attitudes toward the drug were not easily influenced by the publicity: "The state hospital is a closed community and although patients do watch television and read the newspapers, they seem to be more susceptible to the propaganda from other patients who have been successfully treated." More problematic were the normal difficulties of treatment and research, such as keeping alcoholics in the hospital long enough to complete their course of therapy. Ultimately, he believed that "if we don't complete the program, it will be the fault within us and not the publicity."[40] He did, however, recognize that this situation could change if the controversy continued to increase.

Although the controversy in itself did not have a major impact on the Spring Grove researchers, it did threaten their work by influencing Sandoz Pharmaceuticals to withdraw its sponsorship of LSD research in April 1966, as discussed in chapter 2. Since the passage of the Drug Amendments of 1962, the Spring Grove LSD research program had operated under Sandoz's IND.[41] The FDA required that all premarket clinical drug research be conducted under an IND, and Sandoz had maintained itself as the sole IND sponsor for LSD research, as well as the drug's sole manufacturer and distributor. The withdrawal of Sandoz's IND meant that the Spring Grove researchers could no longer legally continue their LSD research and would have no access to further supplies of the drug. However, this hurdle also ultimately had little impact on the progress of the researchers' work.

On 14 April, Kurland wrote to Frances Kelsey at the IND Branch of the FDA in search of help in his predicament. He outlined the research underway at Spring Grove, which he reported as delivering very promising early results, and requested permission to submit an IND to continue this work. Kurland was particularly concerned about how to obtain additional supplies of LSD. He had enough stock of the drug to cover the present trials, but if these studies led to further research avenues (which he believed they would), he would require extra supplies. In a follow-up letter the next day, Kurland confirmed that Sandoz had given him permission to use the data contained in its IND to complete his own.[42]

Another option for ensuring the continuation of the Spring Grove research was discussed by Savage in a May 1966 letter to Canadian LSD researcher Ross MacLean. Savage stated that it had been suggested to him that the Spring Grove researchers should file a New Drug Application for LSD, thus applying to make it an approved prescription drug, though closely controlled "presumably somewhat on a par with morphine." He wondered, on the one hand, whether this would increase the availability and misuse of the drug. On the other hand, he thought that fear of malpractice suits and other "legal and social sanctions" would restrict its use to experienced practitioners. A perhaps more crucial problem was that putting together an NDA would apparently cost in the region of half a million dollars.[43] Where this suggestion came from, and whether it was feasible, is not clear. The idea of giving LSD an effective NDA for restricted usage had been floated when representatives of Sandoz, the NIMH, and the FDA had met to discuss Sandoz's potential withdrawal from LSD sponsorship in December 1965. Kelsey had seemed to support the idea; therefore, from the perspective of the FDA it appeared that an NDA was not out of the question.[44]

Even an effective NDA, however, would not have ensured a continued supply of LSD without a manufacturer or distributor. Ultimately, as previously discussed, this situation was resolved with the NIMH's negotiation with Sandoz to take on its significant remaining stocks of LSD and act as the drug's distributor. The FDA then helped to smooth the transition to independently sponsored research by allowing researchers who were using LSD on a regular basis to temporarily continue doing so while they put together and submitted their own INDs.[45] Whether as a result of cost or other factors, Kurland and colleagues went through with their submission of an IND rather than an NDA. Because of the assistance of the NIMH and FDA, LSD research at Spring Grove was not notably disrupted by Sandoz's withdrawal from the field of LSD research.[46]

In the face of the controversy surrounding LSD, the Spring Grove researchers not only survived but actively pushed back and thrived. Over late 1965 and early 1966, the researchers collaborated with CBS News to create a television documentary that demonstrated their therapeutic use of LSD and the results it could have. Entitled "LSD: The Spring Grove Experiment," the program was produced by the series *CBS Reports* in light of the national concern over LSD, as the public was frequently exposed to conflicting reports of the drug's effects and dangers. By demonstrating their use of the drug, the Spring Grove researchers hoped to help educate the public not only on LSD's therapeutic potential but also how carefully it needed to be handled: it was a powerful drug that required expert preparation and supervision to administer safely.[47] By the time the documentary aired on 17 May 1966, this message was particularly pertinent: five days earlier Senator Thomas J. Dodd's subcommittee had begun hearings on LSD that starkly characterized it as a dangerous drug of abuse, and the hearings were widely reported in the media. LSD was an issue of major national and local concern, and, on the same night that the CBS broadcast aired, Baltimore television station WBAL aired the first of a four-part series of investigations on LSD as part of its news programming. The drug had also been a topic of focus for three newscasts on ABC-TV the previous week.[48] Into this milieu, the Spring Grove documentary gave a bal-

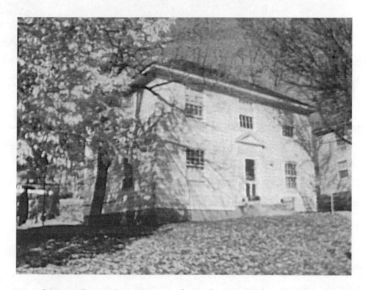

Cottage 13 at Spring Grove State Hospital, as shown in the *CBS Reports* documentary "LSD: The Spring Grove Experiment." Originally built as employee accommodation, the cottage housed the psychedelic research team and featured two specially furnished treatment rooms. "LSD: The Spring Grove Experiment," *CBS Reports*, produced by John Sharnik and Harry Morgan, aired 17 May 1966 (New York: CBS News Archives, 2016), DVD.

anced and detailed exploration of LSD's therapeutic effects and offered a rare view of psychedelic therapy from the patients' perspective.

Narrated by Charles Kuralt, the documentary followed alcoholic patient Arthur King and neurotic patient Peg Meginnis, from their intake interview through to six months after discharge. It showed them individually going through the psychedelic therapy procedure with Unger and explored how it impacted their lives and how they interpreted its effects. After intake interviews, where King and Meginnis outlined the problems that had led to their hospitalization, the documentary showed the two patients in preparatory psychotherapy, where they delved into their problematic attitudes and relationships with their families and Unger told them how to react to potentially frightening drug experiences. Their LSD sessions then took place in a dedicated room, made up as a pleasantly furnished living room. The patients were often reclining on a comfortable couch, wearing eyeshades and headphones, listening to emotive instrumental music. At other times they sat with Unger looking at family photographs, a rose, or a mirror. Unger directed them to observe how the objects or images changed as they thought about their problems: King saw the rose change from radiant to shriveled and black when Unger suggested that they go to a bar to have a drink. As they discovered insights into their behaviors and attitudes, the patients became overwhelmed with emotion, crying or laughing. King described one such profoundly emotional part of his experience:

> There was at one time a laughter that broke through and I think it was the best laugh I ever had in my life. It was just tremendous emotional release and I really felt wonderful at that time. It was just terrific just to laugh. At the end I felt a great weight had been taken off of me, instead of feeling it was the end of something, I felt like it was the beginning. Like it was something had opened up, and things could be seen in a different light.[49]

Unger maintained supportive and comforting physical contact with the patients throughout the session—holding their hands or cradling them while they broke down.

At the six-month follow-up interview, both patients reported dramatic improvements in their lives. Thirty-three-year-old King was now employed as an insurance examiner and was taking evening classes in accounting. He had completely abstained from alcohol and reported no desire to drink. He attributed this to the resolution of internal conflicts that he had previously used alcohol to repress. These conflicts had concerned his inability to feel close to other people, despite his desire to. After treatment, King felt much less distant from his family and community. He also reported a significant rise in his self-esteem, optimism, and motivation. Instead of viewing his future pessimistically, only hoping that his children would do better than he had, King now believed he had a future ahead of him and the right to make the most of it, asking himself, "What's wrong with my becoming something? What's wrong with my doing things? I feel that I'm a person too, that I got a life to lead and a long way to go yet."[50]

Meginnis, a housewife in her late forties, spoke even more dramatically of the changes in her attitudes and behaviors after LSD therapy. Her husband had committed her to the hospital after she had suffered a mental breakdown. Over the previous years, Meginnis's feelings of emptiness and estrangement from her somewhat distant husband had developed into increasingly paranoid beliefs about him: that he was having an affair, was a criminal, was severely ill, and was trying to murder her. Her fears escalated to the extent that she believed her husband was behind a local bank robbery. She reported him to the Federal Bureau of Investigation, which subsequently interrogated

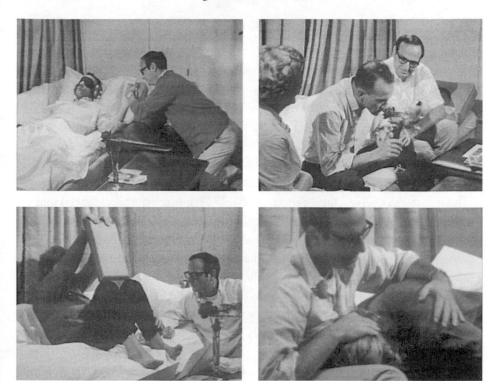

The CBS documentary highlighted the intimate support Sanford Unger provided to patients Arthur King and Peg Meginnis as they underwent their LSD sessions and the intense range and depth of emotions they experienced. "LSD: The Spring Grove Experiment," *CBS Reports*, produced by John Sharnik and Harry Morgan, aired 17 May 1966 (New York: CBS News Archives, 2016), DVD.

and released him. She later took him to a psychiatrist after seeing disturbing images in family photos that she believed he was responsible for. Much to her surprise, the psychiatrist recommended that she, not her husband, be committed. After her LSD treatment, Meginnis not only recovered from her delusional thinking but also reconnected with her husband and led a transformed life:

> Before I went to the hospital I hadn't slept inside my house a whole night. I slept outside on the lawn or in the car, because I thought I would be murdered if I slept inside. I spent every waking moment trying to solve this terrible agony. And I cut off all connections with humanity. And what is it compared to that now? Now I enjoy life the way I should. And life is, it's so much fuller. I never dreamed . . . I didn't have the conception, of what it was like to . . . receive love,

and to give love, and to still be myself, and to not have to earn it. Life is fine now.[51]

When Kuralt asked whether conventional psychotherapy could have delivered the same results, Meginnis described how the drug experience transformed the power of psychotherapy: "Well, I was given the words before, and psychotherapy is verbal, understand? I was given the words, 'you are a scared kid, you are really frightened inside, but you have taken a lifetime to build a wall around it.' I listened to the words, see. Now with LSD, I experienced the words. I experienced it. All the fear that was trapped in me was released. It was hell, see, but I experienced it."[52] Meginnis's husband agreed that the value of the LSD experience was that insights actually led to change: "I think that somewhere along the line, before she even took LSD, she knew that she was sick. But this didn't change what was going on in her mind about me, until after she took the LSD." Psychedelic therapy did not simply lead to new insights; it transformed insights from theoretical knowledge to experiences. Experiencing insights meant that they were emotionally, rather than merely intellectually, validated. These insights were therefore more easily integrated into the patient's personality.

Kurland also appeared in the documentary. He described how, in all his years of research, the rapid effects of LSD on behavior, thinking, and emotion, had "been one of the most dramatic experiences that I have ever observed." Yet, in assessing its therapeutic potential, he remained a cautious scientist. He recognized that his enthusiasm for the drug could skew his impression of its efficacy, so he would remain "somewhat suspicious" until he had amassed much more data. Unger, however, hinted at the difficulties researchers faced in obtaining data that would satisfy the scientific community: "It's one thing to be a scientist, to be objective, detached. It's another thing to be a therapist. Psychotherapy is a human enterprise—it's in contact between humans. This is an intimate situation, one is exposed in a way that otherwise would never occur. There can't be distance, or so-called objectivity. The commitment to patient is perhaps the prerequisite ingredient."[53] Here Unger touched on one of the central conflicts of LSD psychotherapy research: while objective data on LSD psychotherapy's efficacy was needed, psychedelic therapy could not be an objectively administered treatment. Indeed, it required the active utilization of many of the subjective, nonspecific factors that controlled trials were designed to eliminate: primarily, suggestion, empathic support, and enthusiasm. These nonspecific variables were used to craft and direct the

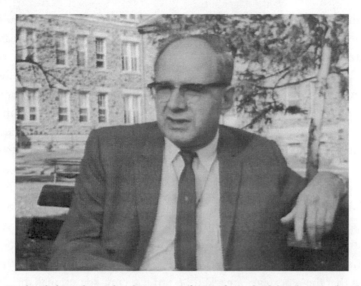

Albert Kurland describing the dramatic effects of psychedelic therapy for the CBS documentary. "LSD: The Spring Grove Experiment," *CBS Reports*, produced by John Sharnik and Harry Morgan, aired 17 May 1966 (New York: CBS News Archives, 2016), DVD.

psychedelic experience, yet they were also the basis of the placebo effect. Therefore, researchers faced the difficult task of turning psychedelic therapy into a procedure that was standardized enough to allow the use of controls and quantitative assessment yet that maintained its personalized, subjective, intimate, and variable nature enough to retain its therapeutic potential. This difficulty in balancing of scientific rigor with therapeutic method would be a defining issue in LSD psychotherapy research as it moved through the 1960s and early 1970s, and indeed it would be the major factor to limit the success and influence of the Spring Grove research. At this stage, however, the documentary presented an optimistic picture of the future of LSD psychotherapy: that careful, sustained scientific research would ultimately reveal how to control and harness the drug's effects for the good of humankind.

The broadcast received rave reviews. United Press International's Rick Du Brow described it as a "mind-opening documentary" that avoided sensationalistic coverage and praised its "gentle and skeptical—yet openminded" approach. Cynthia Lowry of the Associated Press described the two treatment cases in the documentary as "dramatically successful," concluding that while LSD was dangerous when "young people use it for kicks . . . it may—and the word 'may' is stressed—be a godsend in the treatment of some mental and emotional disorders." Passing on one of the key messages that the researchers had intended for the program, she also stressed that the "long careful 'preparation'" that patients received was "as important as LSD's amazing effect on the mind." These two reviews were widely published in newspapers around the country.[54] More locally, Donald Kirkley of the *Baltimore Sun* similarly praised the documentary as a "helpful antidote to the sensational stories" surrounding LSD and for showing the care that needed to be exercised to safely administer the drug—perhaps hyperbolically describing the researchers as handling the drug "with the extreme caution of a demolition squad defusing a bomb." He concluded that although the drug was dangerous outside of medical supervision and more research was needed, "there is hope that investigation ultimately will confirm its beneficial nature, under proper control." One dissenting review came from Harry Harris of the *Philadelphia Inquirer*, who claimed that the reportage "smacked of 'miracle cure' sensationalism." Rather than praising the researchers for stressing that careful preparation was needed to safely administer the drug, he cast this in a negative light—the drug was dangerous and had the potential to make patients worse. Further, perhaps revealing more about himself than the documentary, Harris balked at the "embarrassingly intimate closeups" of the patients in their LSD sessions as well as the details provided on Meginnis's backstory, concluding that the program was "excessively prying—good drama, but bad manners."[55] Overall, the documentary appears to have achieved what the Spring Grove researchers hoped. It brought balance to the media coverage on LSD, reminded the public that the drug had great psychiatric potential and was still actively being researched, and stressed that safe and successful treatment required far more than simply administering the drug.

As the Spring Grove researchers attempted to balance public perceptions of LSD, they remained engaged with the still large and dynamic field of LSD research in the mid-1960s. Indeed, these years saw several significant conferences in the United States that focused attention on LSD research. Largest was the May 1965 Second International Conference on the Use of LSD in Psychotherapy and Alcoholism, organized by Harold Abramson and held at South Oaks Psychiatric Hospital in Amityville, New York. The conference featured thirty-six papers from LSD researchers from across North America and Europe. In March 1966, the Fifth International Congress of the Collegium Internationale Neuro-Psycho-Pharmacologicum, held in Washington, DC, featured a panel on "psychotomimetics as treatments in psychiatry" with eleven papers presented. In May and June of that year, Savage cochaired the American Psychological Association's third Research in Psychotherapy conference. The NIMH-funded conference featured papers grouped around three themes, one of which was LSD.[56] LSD psychotherapy was clearly still of significant interest to mainstream mental health professionals, rather than an obscure, niche field. The conferences each featured papers with a variety of focuses, from theoretical considerations to clinical trials, covering all forms of LSD psychotherapy. The general tone of the conferences was positive for the effectiveness of the various LSD therapies and optimistic about their future. The Spring Grove researchers featured prominently in each meeting, reporting details on their treatment method, trial designs, and positive preliminary results.[57]

Outside of these conferences, the Spring Grove researchers maintained close relations with other LSD researchers, as well as others interested in the field. By 1966 Unger had not only visited all of the LSD researchers in the United States but had twice toured Europe, visiting LSD psychotherapists in Norway, Denmark, Germany, Holland, and Czechoslovakia. Sandoz funded at least one of these trips, where Unger helped European psycholytic therapists to set up psychedelic therapy programs. He had also traveled to Basel, Switzerland, to visit LSD's discoverer, Albert Hofmann.[58] During the mid- to late 1960s, Spring Grove also hosted a constant stream of visitors interested in its psychedelic research. The visitors included numerous officials from the FDA, NIMH, and Maryland state government, and even an official from the World Health Organization. Many visitors were physicians from hospitals and universities from across the country, as well as overseas. Among these were other LSD researchers, including prominent German psycholytic therapist Hanscarl Leuner, Kenneth Godfrey from the Topeka, Kansas, Veterans Administration Hospital, and John Lilly of the Communication Research Institute in Florida. Other visitors came from a background in religion, seeking to explore the religious implications of the psychedelic experience. These visitors included philosopher and popularizer of Zen Buddhism Alan Watts; Walter Houston Clark, professor of psychology of religion at Andover Newton Theological School, Massachusetts; and Huston Smith, professor of comparative religion at Massachusetts Institute of Technology.[59]

In June 1966, the Spring Grove researchers again entered the public and political fray: reflecting their status as the leading psychedelic researchers in the country, Kurland, Savage, and Unger were brought to testify before Representative Lawrence Fountain's *Drug Safety* congressional hearings investigating the regulation of LSD. Although Fountain's subcommittee was primarily concerned with the drug's increasingly widespread nonmedical use, the members were also concerned that the government's focus on LSD's dangers and its regulation could hamper research and recognition of its legitimate uses. Therefore, the three researchers were asked to testify as to how research was progressing under the new regulations. The subcommittee questioned the researchers respectfully as experts on the drug. They inquired about their work and their opinions on various aspects of LSD's use and misuse, without expressing disdain or skepticism. Overall, the researchers said nothing to suggest that their work had so far been hampered. Savage, however, was concerned that the potential future criminalization of personal possession could deter patients from volunteering for treatment, because of the increased stigma attached to the drug.[60]

The subcommittee members questioned the researchers in great detail over the nature of their treatment and their results to date. Kurland, Savage, and Unger stressed that LSD's medical use was very different from that of other drugs: it did not have any "inherent beneficial effects" and was therefore not a chemotherapeutic agent but a tool in a psychotherapeutic process. This characteristic, and the drug's dramatic subjective effects, had made it particularly challenging to design controlled studies, due to the difficulty in finding an adequate placebo treatment. Despite this, they were confident that their research efforts would provide a rigorous examination of the efficacy of psychedelic therapy. The Spring Grove researchers reported their impressive preliminary results with both alcoholic and neurotic patients. Indeed, Unger described the results to date from the controlled alcoholic study as "so good that I nearly don't like to report it. I mean that. My feeling is that the present rate won't, can't continue."[61]

Questioned on the issue of the safety of LSD psychotherapy, the researchers testified to a remarkable absence of negative outcomes, which they believed was due to their rigorous preparation and screening. Indeed, Kurland remarked that lack of "attempted suicides or psychotic reactions" was "puzzling," as the severely alcoholic population they were treating frequently had other underlying psychiatric pathology and traditionally had a high mortality rate after hospital discharge. In the psychoneurotic study there had been two adverse events. The first was a psychotic episode in a patient not long after her LSD treatment. The patient had a history of these episodes, and she recovered after conventional treatment. The second was an attempted suicide after discharge. The attempt was considered minor. Neither of these events could be conclusively tied to the LSD treatment, but the researchers recognized that this was a possibility. While attesting to LSD's safety under their conditions, the researchers stressed that uncontrolled use was dangerous. The drug produced a period of intense emotionality, and there was no guarantee that these emotions would be positive. Without guidance, negative emotions could spiral out of control, leaving the user traumatized. In the worst-case scenario, this kind of reaction could lead to suicide.[62]

The subcommittee also questioned the researchers regarding the control of nonmedical use of LSD. While they had little experience with nonmedical use of LSD, the researchers expressed doubt over whether further criminal sanctions would be effective. Unger was also concerned with the social ramifications of criminalizing users, who he believed were mostly college students who were by and large "not irresponsible people nor . . . particularly psychiatrically disturbed."[63] He suggested that the dangers associated with nonmedical use of LSD could be minimized through the establishment of centers where interested individuals could experience LSD under appropriate supervision. Representative John Dow expressed support for Unger's idea in theory, although he doubted that such centers would be effective in preventing uncontrolled use. However, Unger argued that the drug was not addictive and that it was unlikely to be heavily abused except among a minority of already disturbed individuals. He believed that education was the only way to combat irresponsible use of LSD and that further criminalization would merely fuel the public's curiosity about the drug. The subcommittee members did not openly endorse or oppose this view, although they did add that further criminal sanctions could make LSD more attractive to black marketeers, as increased risk raised prices.[64]

After successfully weathering 1966, the following year the Spring Grove researchers faced a new controversy that again threatened to destroy their work: the possibility that LSD caused chromosomal damage. In March 1967, Maimon Cohen and colleagues from the State University of New York, Buffalo, published in *Science* the results of a small in vitro study that found that the addition of LSD to cultures of human leukocytes significantly increased the rate of chromosomal abnormalities compared to control cultures. The researchers also found similar abnormalities in the chromosomes of a patient suffering from paranoid schizophrenia who had undergone fifteen sessions of LSD psychotherapy.[65] The news media jumped on the findings, with the *New York Times* publishing a report on the study the same day it was released, citing Cohen as saying that the chromosomal changes "could lead to mental retardation and physical abnormalities in the offspring of LSD users," al-though conceding that such possibilities were yet to be proven.[66] Coming just five years after thalidomide had dramatically demonstrated the dangers that drugs could present to an undeveloped fetus, these claims were particularly alarming and suggested that LSD was not safe even in the hands of medical experts.

The Spring Grove researchers responded to this threat to the safety of their treatment and the future of their research by conducting their own study, which they published in 1969. Other attempts to investigate Cohen's findings through in vivo studies had provided contradictory results, with some con-firming high rates of chromosomal abnormalities in (primarily illicit) LSD users, while others did not. These studies also had serious methodological flaws: they lacked comparative analysis of chromosome aberrations in sub-jects before LSD ingestion and often failed to control for other factors that could impact chromosomes, such as other drugs, viral illnesses, and impu-rities in black-market LSD. The Spring Grove clinical trials provided the op-portunity to study the effects of pharmaceutically pure LSD on chromosomes in LSD psychotherapy patients under controlled conditions. For the study, conducted in collaboration with Joe-Hin Tjio from the National Institute of Arthritis and Metabolic Disease, the researchers took blood samples from thirty-two patients from the alcoholic and neurotic studies, both before and after LSD ingestion. They found no significant differences in the aberration rates between the samples.[67] These results were confirmed in 1971, when *Science* published a review of sixty-eight studies that concluded that in moderate doses pure LSD "does not damage chromosomes in vivo, does not cause detectable genetic damage, and is not a teratogen or a carcinogen in man," and that outside of pregnancy (as a routine precaution) "there is no present contraindication to the continued controlled experimental use of pure LSD."[68]

The actual impact that fear over chromosomal damage had on LSD re-search in the late 1960s is difficult to assess. The reports of genetic danger were widely reported on in the media, along with cases of babies born with deformities purportedly caused by LSD, although there was in fact little sci-entific basis for determining this.[69] In the shadow of thalidomide, the claims undoubtedly did damage to LSD's public and medical reputation, and it took time to amass studies to thoroughly examine and refute these claims. Un-surprisingly, the later studies confirming LSD's safety received far less press attention than the earlier claims of its dangers. Yet, ultimately, the FDA made no moves to restrict research in these years, and by 1967 the number of approved psychedelic research programs was already fairly limited. As the next chapter explores, these studies were mostly concluding in the years 1967–1971, and their results would be far more significant in shaping the future of LSD research than fear over the drug's safety. For the Spring Grove researchers at least, as we will see below, the chromosome controversy appears to have had little effect on research progress over the late 1960s.

Further Expansion

Aside from seeing the beginning of the chromosomal scare, for the Spring Grove researchers 1967 continued the research momentum established over the previous years. Despite the surrounding controversy, so far its actual impact at Spring Grove had been minimal—the research program was stable and well regarded. The researchers were not only managing to withstand the controversy but had taken a role in combating it, by educating the public about the drug and conducting a rigorous study of its safety. They were active in the international research community, and their experience and expertise was respected by political leaders who were wary of the drug. From this position, the Spring Grove LSD program would continue to expand in scale, scope, and expertise.

By the start of 1967, the Spring Grove researchers had developed enough confidence and support for their psychedelic therapy procedure with alcoholics to begin planning for its eventual integration into the standard treatment procedure of the state's hospitals. The first site for expansion was to be Crownsville State Hospital, near Annapolis. Their plan was not to simply establish a psychedelic therapy unit at Crownsville but to conduct a "demonstration project"—a sophisticated study of the implementation of psychedelic therapy in a new environment—that would act as a test and model for further expansion. Crownsville had the highest number of alcoholic admissions in the state, so it was a logical site to conduct the project. The researchers were careful not to represent their treatment program as a miracle cure, emphasizing that they conceived the introduction of psychedelic therapy to a hospital as neither "capable of 'transforming,' nor even of *radically* affecting the rate of enduring treatment success." Nevertheless, they believed that a "substantial number" of patients who improved little from standard treatments would be "materially benefitted."[70] In addition to its large alcoholic population, Crownsville did not have a strong tradition in research, so the site offered a good opportunity to test whether the positive atmosphere toward research in general at Spring Grove had influenced the success of its LSD treatment.

Should the treatment be successfully adopted at Crownsville, the study would then aid other institutions in implementing their own psychedelic programs by helping them to anticipate the difficulties they might encounter.

The researchers planned to commence this demonstration project after the completion of the controlled Spring Grove alcoholic study in 1969, dependent on positive final results. Nevertheless, experience so far led the researchers to expect these positive results, and the plan had already met the approval of the Maryland commissioner of mental hygiene and the superintendent of Crownsville. State support for the project reflected not only the Spring Grove researchers' positive preliminary results but also the gravity of the problem of alcoholism and Kurland's place in Maryland's psychiatric administration. Alcoholism was the leading cause of psychiatric hospital admissions in the state, amounting to two-fifths of male admissions and one-eighth of female admissions. The prognosis for these patients was poor, with a Spring Grove study finding less than 10 percent maintaining sobriety one year after discharge following standard treatment.[71] Kurland, as director of research for the state's Department of Mental Hygiene, was responsible for finding new treatments to alleviate this situation. He had initiated the Spring Grove LSD studies for this reason. It was therefore the department's responsibility to use the results of his research endeavors to better the situation of its psychiatric patients. The department's commissioner, Isadore Tuerk, had been the superintendent of Spring Grove in the 1950s when Kurland had joined the staff and began his research career. Tuerk was most likely responsible for installing Kurland as director of research for the Department of Mental Hygiene, just as he had installed him in the same position at Spring Grove.[72] While Tuerk's personal opinion of LSD therapy is not clear, his long and close relationship with Kurland strongly suggests that he had great faith in his integrity, abilities, and ambitions. Therefore, he supported, or at least did not thwart, Kurland's plans to expand LSD research in the state.

Ultimately, the demonstration project did not go ahead, and the Spring Grove research never expanded to a second site. The reason for this is unclear. The expansion was contingent upon the final results of the alcoholism study. As the next chapter explores, these results would be somewhat ambiguous, but at the very least they suggested more research. Therefore, poor results in the study seems an unconvincing explanation. The increasing controversies surrounding LSD could have led either the state or Crownsville to withdraw its support. This is certainly a possibility; however, there are many alternative—or contributing—more mundane possible explanations, including a lack of funding, staff time, or other logistical difficulties. Nevertheless, regardless of the reason that it failed to come to fruition, the plan for expansion in early 1967 demonstrates that, at a time of increasing controversy around LSD and a shrinking national scale of research, in Maryland psychedelic research remained a state-supported endeavor that promised to provide treatments to meet the needs of the state's psychiatric hospitals.

In addition to making plans to expand their research to other sites, in 1967 the Spring Grove research team expanded its ranks with the addition of two significant new members: psychiatrists Stanislav Grof and Walter Pahnke. These researchers came from diverse backgrounds, in terms of qualifications and experience, and their academic and clinical interests would help further expand the scope and sophistication of the Spring Grove research. Grof, from Czechoslovakia, was one of Europe's most prominent and experienced LSD psychotherapists. His research had begun in 1956, when he ingested LSD as a student volunteer in the psychiatry department of the Charles University School of Medicine in Prague. The profound experience that ensued left Grof in no doubt that the drug had great implications for psychiatry. After completing his medical degree that same year, Grof joined a research team at the city's Psychiatric Research Institute to further investigate the drug. There he spent several years employing LSD and similar drugs as psychotomimetics, to study the possible biochemical origins of psychoses. At the same time Grof had been training in psychoanalysis, which led him to conclude that his LSD subjects' experiences were revealing psychodynamic processes, rather than representing model psychoses. He therefore began exploring psycholytic therapy. Grof first traveled to the United States in 1965 to present his research at the Second International Conference on the Use of LSD in Psychotherapy. He was subsequently offered a fellowship from the Foundations' Fund for Research in Psychiatry, of New Haven, Connecticut. He used this to take up a position of clinical and research fellow in the Department of Psychiatry and Behavioral Sciences at Johns Hopkins University in 1967. At the time, this department had a close relationship with the LSD researchers at Spring Grove, so Grof began collaborating with them.[73] Adopting the psychedelic method, Grof would become a senior member of the Spring Grove team, taking leading roles in both the conduct of the clinical trials and the administration of the research program. He would later publish numerous monographs from his experiences in LSD research, cementing his place as an international authority on psychedelics.[74]

Pahnke made a significant and immediate contribution to the sophistication of the research program at Spring Grove. Pahnke came from a background in both medicine and religion. His prior research had focused on the religious implications of psychedelic drugs, particularly on the relationship between the psychedelic experience and the spontaneously occurring mystical states of consciousness considered divine in many religions. Based on this research, Pahnke categorized the typical elements of mystical experiences, developing a model that could be applied to psychedelic experiences. When brought to Spring Grove, this model helped the researchers to better conceptualize the therapeutic experiences of their patients. While the team had long considered the mystical LSD experience the most beneficial, Pahnke's research helped it to better define and understand this reaction, improving the precision of its therapy and research. Given the importance of this understanding, it is worthwhile considering Pahnke's past research in detail.

Born in 1931 in Harvey, Illinois, Pahnke undertook his initial research with psychedelics for his PhD in Religion and Society at Harvard University, awarded in 1964. This research followed his completion of doctor of medicine and bachelor of divinity degrees at the university.[75] Pahnke's PhD centered on a study often referred to as the "Good Friday Experiment," or the "Miracle at Marsh Chapel." The experiment compared the experiences of volunteers who had been administered psilocybin or a placebo, in a double-blind fashion, against a typology of mystical experience. Pahnke's aim was to examine the similarities and differences between the psychedelic experience and naturally occurring mystical states, while controlling for the role of extrapharmacological factors in producing the experimental mystical state. His interest in the topic had been stimulated by both the increasing reports of mystical states resulting from psychedelic drugs and the traditional use of psychoactive plants, such as the peyote cactus, in many of the world's religions, particularly among indigenous cultures of the Americas. Timothy Leary, who was still at Harvard in 1962 when the experiment took place, both advised on the design of the study and participated in it, acting as a guide for the research subjects.[76]

The first stage in Pahnke's research was to develop a typology of the "genuine" mystical experience. This typology presupposed that mystical experiences had certain core characteristics that were universal, irrespective of a person's religion and culture or the setting or historical period in which they occurred. Where mystical states gained their significance to a specific religion was in their interpretation, rather than in the basic types of experiences that they were composed of. For this argument, and the categorization of the elements of the mystical experience, Pahnke drew on the work of scholars of

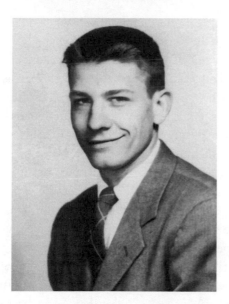

Walter Pahnke, circa 1955. William Richards Collection of Walter Pahnke Papers, courtesy of Purdue University Libraries, Karnes Archives & Special Collections.

mysticism such as William James, James B. Pratt, Richard M. Bucke, Walter H. Clark, and Walter T. Stace.[77] As the research would confirm the high degree of similarity between psychedelic and mystical states, Pahnke's typology gives insight into the kinds of experiences that patients commonly encountered in their psychedelic therapy sessions.

The first and most important of nine universal characteristics of mystical experiences Pahnke named "unity." This was then further divided into "internal unity" and "external unity." Internal unity was the experience of an "undifferentiated unity," characterized by the loss of the usual sense of self, or ego—a "fading or melting away into pure awareness." In this state, awareness no longer revolved around the senses. Despite the dissolution of the ego and loss of sense impressions, consciousness and the ability to experience these phenomena were retained: the subject perceived "no empirical distinctions or particular content except the awareness of the unity itself." External unity saw retention of the senses but instead a powerful feeling of "oneness" with all animate and inanimate objects in the external world: "The subject feels a sense of oneness with these objects, because he 'sees' that at the most basic level all are part of a single unity." This feeling of "all is one," nevertheless, did not override all normal understanding of the separation between subject and object but instead operated on a different level of consciousness: "The essences of objects are experienced intuitively while their outward forms are experienced through the senses."[78]

The second universal characteristic of mystical experiences was a "transcendence of time and space." This was often described as a feeling of "eternity" or "infinity," where not only the experience's relation to clock time was lost but also "one's personal sense of his past, present and future." The third characteristic was a "deeply felt positive mood." Subjects often described these intense, overwhelming feelings of "joy, blessedness, and peace" with terms such as "ecstasy," "beatitude," "bliss," and "rapture." The fourth characteristic was a "sense of sacredness" regarding the experience—feelings of "awe and wonder" and "profound humility before the overpowering majesty of what is felt to be holy." The fifth characteristic, "objectivity and reality," encompassed the experience of intuitive, insightful knowledge. This knowledge was not factual but had the quality of illumination, or a profound sense of understanding, achieved through transcendence into an "ultimate reality" that existed at a higher level of consciousness than "ordinary reality." To subjects, this knowledge was inherently authoritative, as it was directly experienced rather than conveyed to them.[79]

The sixth characteristic of "paradoxicality" referred to the tendency for mystics to describe many of their experiences in paradoxical terms. For example, internal unity was often described by the same mystic as feeling both "empty" and "full," and subjects' awareness of their ego dissolution was dependent on the retention of a self that experiences it. Mystics also typically claimed that words were inadequate to describe their experiences. While they obviously did write impressive accounts of their experiences, this seventh characteristic—"alleged ineffability"—can be seen in the difficulty of effectively communicating elements that seem paradoxical, as well as in the experience of profound intuitive knowledge that is not, and cannot be, conveyed. The eighth characteristic was that the mystical experience was by its nature transitory. Whatever lasting effects they had, experiences such as unitary consciousness could not be indefinitely maintained. The final characteristic was that the mystical experience resulted in "persisting positive change in attitude and/or behavior" in the subject. These positive changes could be in the mystic's personality structure or outlook toward, and relation to, others, life in general, or mysticism itself. These changes often constituted a profound transformation of the mystic's outlook on life, toward greater love, tolerance, understanding, optimism, and appreciation of life in general.[80]

Having constructed this typology, Pahnke set out to use it to assess psychedelic experiences as mystical states of consciousness. The experiment saw twenty Christian theological students attend a two-and-a-half-hour Good Friday service in a private chapel. Prior to the service, Pahnke administered psilocybin to half of the students and niacin as an active placebo to the other half, in a randomized double-blind fashion. Theological students, and the stirring religious setting, were chosen to help "maximize the possibility that mystical phenomena would occur." The placebo, which produced a tingling sensation and relaxation, controlled for whether any mystical phenomena were a result of this suggestive set and setting alone. The students were given preparation for the experience, but neither they nor the experimenter had prior personal experience with psychedelic drugs. Guides who were familiar with psilocybin supervised the students during the experiment, and half of the guides also received the drug during the experiment. These guides were "supportive but non-directive," helping to create an atmosphere conducive to mystical experiences, while letting the students' experiences unfold by themselves. The guides were not familiar with Pahnke's typology.[81]

Pahnke then used independent judges, who were ignorant of the nature of the experiment, to rate the correlation between the subjects' written accounts of their experiences and the typology of mystical experience. Analyzing these ratings—as well as data from additional questionnaires and interviews with the subjects—revealed that the experiences of the psilocybin subjects correlated more closely with the mystical typology than did those of the placebo subjects, to a statistically significant degree.[82] The results led Pahnke to conclude that psilocybin could "induce states of consciousness which are apparently indistinguishable from, if not identical with, those experienced by mystics."[83]

While completing his PhD, Pahnke was awarded the Sheldon Travelling Fellowship from Harvard, which allowed him to travel Europe to observe and participate in LSD research being undertaken there. During the trip he received training in LSD psychotherapy from Hanscarl Leuner, at Georg-August University in Göttingen, Germany. On his return to the United States in 1964, Pahnke undertook his psychiatric residency at the Massachusetts Mental Health Center in Boston, where he continued to explore using psilocybin with nonpsychiatric volunteers. In 1966 he began training in psychedelic therapy at Spring Grove State Hospital and joined the team there as a research psychiatrist upon completing his residency in 1967.[84]

Once at Spring Grove, Pahnke took over directorship of the study of psychedelic therapy in the treatment of terminal cancer patients.[85] He simplified his typology of the mystical experience and used it to define and evaluate the "psychedelic peak experience" in order to study the relationship between the "completeness" of patients' psychedelic reactions and treatment outcome using the following criteria: "(1) Sense of unity and oneness (positive ego transcendence, loss of usual sense of self without loss of consciousness). (2) Transcendence of time and space. (3) Deeply felt positive mood (joy, peace, and love). (4) Sense of awesomeness and reverence. (5) Meaningfulness of psychological and/or philosophical insight. (6) Ineffability (sense of difficulty in communicating the experience by verbal expression)."[86] By this stage the Spring Grove researchers had renamed their therapeutic method "psychedelic peak therapy." This name reemphasized that their treatment was defined by the kind of experience it utilized, rather than simply the category of drug involved. While this kind of LSD reaction had been the central characteristic of psychedelic therapy since its development, increasingly the term "psychedelic" had become more generalized: other researchers had been conducting high-dose treatments without the mystical framework, and many recreational users of LSD had adopted the term.[87]

Besides expanding in staff and scope, the Spring Grove research program also upgraded its facilities in the late 1960s. Until late 1968, the psychedelic research had been conducted in a modest, two-story cottage—cottage 13—on the hospital's grounds.[88] Since 1959, Kurland had been in negotiations with the state and federal governments to establish a dedicated psychiatric research facility for Maryland. After delays due to budgetary and planning issues, the Maryland Psychiatric Research Center (MPRC) opened in late 1968. The MPRC was designed as an interdisciplinary facility for clinical, psychological, biological, chemical, and psychosocial research focusing on the causes, manifestations, and treatment of mental illnesses.[89] Located on the Spring Grove grounds, the three-story, forty-thousand-square-foot, air-conditioned building housed extensive laboratory, data processing, and clinical facilities. For psychedelic research, the MPRC included two purpose-built treatment suites that included homey furnishings, overnight facilities, private bathrooms and kitchens, and closed-circuit television monitoring from a nearby conference room.[90]

The Spring Grove LSD researchers took leading roles in the MPRC's administration, with Kurland appointed as superintendent, and Savage directly below him as associate director. In the Clinical Sciences Division, which housed the psychedelic program, Pahnke was appointed chief of psychiatric research, and Unger chief of psychological research. In 1969 Pahnke was

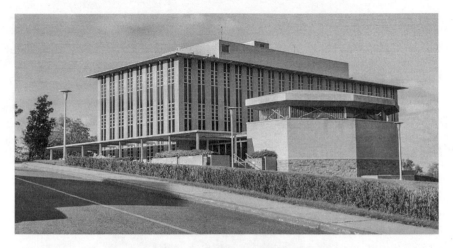

The Maryland Psychiatric Research Center on the grounds of Spring Grove State Hospital, circa 1972. The psychedelic research program operated out of the center after it opened in 1968. Photo by Richard Yensen.

promoted to director of clinical sciences research, and Grof took his place as chief of psychiatric research.[91] The important role of the Spring Grove psychedelic research staff—and their work—in the establishment and administration of the MPRC reflected the respect that they had garnered at both the state and federal level. Rather than fringe workers in a controversial field, they were government-funded scientists at the forefront of psychiatric research in Maryland.

In addition to the new premises, 1968 also saw the Spring Grove researchers initiate their fourth psychedelic research program: the treatment of narcotic (heroin) addiction.[92] This was the final clinical indication into which the team would expand its research. The trial was a natural progression from the alcoholic study, based on the assumption that if psychedelic therapy could help treat addiction to one drug, it would most likely help those addicted to others. Narcotic addiction was generally considered to be even more highly resistant to treatment than alcoholism: the researchers cited one study from the Public Health Service Hospital at Lexington, Kentucky, which specialized in treating narcotic addicts, that found a 94–97 percent relapse rate for its patients. Yet they noted that another Lexington study, conducted by Arnold Ludwig and Jerome Levine, had found success treating narcotic addicts with a unique treatment combining LSD with hypnosis and psychotherapy. This study, however, had been on patients who remained hospitalized throughout the posttreatment evaluation period; it had tested not for long-term absti-

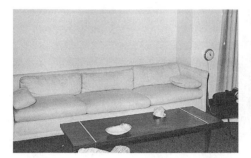
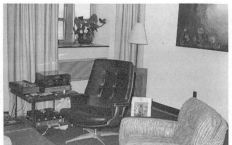
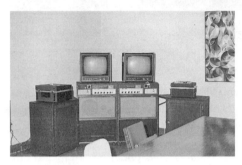

One of the two psychedelic therapy treatment rooms at the Maryland Psychiatric Research Center, circa 1972. Audiovisual monitoring was available from the center's staff meeting room, which provided remote-controlled zoom and positioning of the black and white video cameras located in each room. Photos by Richard Yensen.

nence or social adjustment but for changes in ratings of psychopathology. Therefore, at Spring Grove the researchers planned to expand on this work by evaluating LSD's effectiveness in promoting long-term narcotic abstinence by conducting a controlled trial with the psychedelic peak therapy method that they were finding successful with alcoholics.[93]

As their fourth clinical trial was getting underway, the Spring Grove researchers began to present preliminary results from their other three trials. While it was still too early to draw firm conclusions, results to date suggested that psychedelic peak therapy was significantly benefiting their patients. In November 1968, the researchers presented results for the neurotic and cancer studies at a psychedelic drugs symposium hosted by the Department of Psychiatry of Hahnemann Medical College, Philadelphia. For the neurotic study, the researchers reported that psychedelic therapy showed significantly greater patient improvement than conventional psychotherapy on measures of depression, obsessive-compulsive syndrome, introversion, neuroticism, and anxiety. Patients also showed greater improvements in measures of positive mental health, such as ego strength, spontaneity, self-regard, and "self-actualized values."[94]

Data from the pilot phase of the cancer study found that, of twenty-two patients who had undergone treatment, 27 percent showed "dramatic" positive change, while another 36 percent showed "meaningful" change. The positive changes were in ratings of "depression, anxiety, emotional tension, psychological isolation, fear of death, and the amount of pain medication required."[95] The researchers' hypothesis that the peak experience was most conducive to positive change was supported by the observation that, of the six patients who had the most intense peak experience, five were also considered to have experienced the greatest posttreatment improvement. They also observed that patients who were in the earlier stages of their illness improved the most.

More detailed data was available for the preliminary results of the alcoholic study. In July 1969, the Spring Grove researchers presented results from the six-month follow-up point to a symposium on psychedelic drugs at the annual convention of the American Medical Association in New York. They found a statistically significant advantage for psychedelic therapy over the control condition, with 53 percent compared to 33 percent of patients considered "essentially rehabilitated" in terms of drinking behavior and 44 percent compared to 25 percent in terms of "global adjustment," which included factors such as employment and interpersonal relationships. These results prompted the researchers to put forward a modest claim of efficacy: "In practical terms, we can say that a given alcoholic patient receiving a single high dose of LSD in the context of psychedelic-peak psychotherapy and experiencing a profound psychedelic-peak reaction has the best likelihood for improvement six months later."[96]

Buoyed by their positive preliminary results and reflecting their expertise in LSD administration, in 1969 the Spring Grove researchers amended their IND with the FDA to allow them to administer LSD to mental health professionals and scientists for training purposes. The researchers had long allowed their own staff to have a personal LSD session to familiarize them with the treatment process.[97] The new program would make Spring Grove a national center for such training. The program was a response to frequent requests from mental health professionals for an LSD session to aid them in their own work, which the researchers were usually forced to decline. They proposed that acceptable reasons for requesting a session would include training for independent psychedelic research, a desire to better understand the symptoms of schizophrenia or the problems of youth drug abuse, or to develop psychotherapy skills by increasing self-understanding and insight. Candidates would go through similar screening, preparation, and session and aftercare procedures as did patients. The researchers designed the training program as a study, with forty candidates receiving LSD over two years and data collected to assess how the LSD session impacted them both professionally and personally.[98] The program continued beyond this plan, and, by 1976, 203 mental health professionals had received a training session with LSD. However, no published research resulted from the study.[99]

Besides expanding the scope of their LSD research program, the Spring Grove researchers continued to work to improve their psychedelic peak therapy treatment method. Since the inception of the Spring Grove psychedelic research program, music had been used extensively in LSD sessions to help guide patients' experiences. In 1969, music therapist Helen Bonny joined the team to perform research that would deepen its understanding of the role of music in psychedelic therapy.[100] In 1972 she published a paper with Pahnke in the *Journal of Music Therapy* discussing in detail how music was of benefit in LSD sessions. They summarized five ways that music facilitated therapy: "1) By helping the patient relinquish usual controls and enter more fully into his inner world of experience; 2) by facilitating the release of intense emotionality; 3) by contributing toward a peak experience; 4) by providing continuity in an experience of timelessness; 5) by directing and structuring the experience."[101] They then outlined how specific kinds of music were used during the different phases of LSD's effects to direct patients' reactions. During the onset of the drug's effects, pleasant, calm music was played to relax and reassure the patient. As the effects intensified, more rhythmic and dynamic music was used to provide "an undercurrent of support and forward movement," helping to draw the patient into the drug experience.[102] During the height of the drug's effects, powerful, inspiring music was used to help bring the patient to the peak experience. As the drug's effects diminished, the music would return to a quieter, calming tone. During the early and later periods of the session, music of various genres was played, including the patients' own selections. In the periods of greater drug intensity, the music was either instrumental or included vocals in languages the patient could not understand. This was to prevent patients from engaging intellectually with the lyrics, which would prevent them from "letting go" to achieve the higher peak experience.

Conclusion

By all appearances, at the close of the 1960s the Spring Grove LSD researchers had every reason to be optimistic. Over the decade, despite the increasing controversy surrounding LSD, their research program had continuously expanded in size and scope, and they continued to enjoy good relations with regulators and medical authorities inside and outside of Maryland. With extremely promising early results, all signs suggested that they would soon confirm the efficacy of psychedelic therapy, and—at least in Maryland—it appeared that the process of integrating the treatment into the standard treatment procedure of state hospitals could soon begin.

Yet, ultimately, in the 1970s no consensus would emerge on the efficacy of any form of LSD psychotherapy for any indication. Over the decade LSD psychotherapy research would slowly diminish until it came to a complete halt. The studies that had been conducted would have little impact on mainstream psychiatric theory or practice, despite the continued absence of effective treatments for alcoholism, narcotic addiction, or end-of-life anxiety. The Spring Grove LSD research would be largely forgotten. The failure of the early promise of the Spring Grove program to lead to a consensus on psychedelic therapy's efficacy reveals problematic difficulties involved in submitting psychedelic therapy to standard drug research methods and the complexity of the notion of "objectivity" in clinical research.

CHAPTER FIVE

Elusive Efficacy

The Trials of Psychedelic Therapy

LSD seems to be a facilitator and in the present study it seems to have facilitated mediocrity, however brilliantly reported and adumbrated by elegant statistical techniques.

Charles Savage, 1971,
review of Ludwig, Levine, and Stark, *LSD and Alcoholism*

By the late 1960s, the time was approaching for a final determination on the usefulness of LSD in psychiatric treatment. For more than fifteen years, researchers had been reporting dramatic effects for the drug, but methodological limitations had prevented a scientific consensus from forming. Now a series of controlled studies was coming to a conclusion, which promised to provide objective evidence to a psychiatric field divided between believers and skeptics. The Spring Grove psychedelic research program had grown to become the largest in the nation, with sophisticated studies evaluating the efficacy of LSD in four clinical areas. Yet, rather than leading the psychedelic field to scientific legitimacy, the group faced internal and external challenges that undermined its work.

Internally, as final results for the Spring Grove clinical trials took shape between 1971 and 1973, problems emerged in their design. While the researchers had gone to great lengths to design trials that balanced clinical needs with scientific rigor, they could not always be fully implemented as planned, and elements such as control groups and random patient assignment did not always work as intended. These and other problems influenced often lackluster and inconclusive results. They also left the researchers open to critiques that could undermine positive elements in their results.

An even greater challenge came from other researchers. The Spring Grove researchers were far from alone in continuing LSD research in the late 1960s. Between 1967 and 1970, six other research teams also reported results from controlled studies that purported to submit the claims for psychedelic therapy's effectiveness in treating alcoholism to the rigorous controlled trial test. Final reports from these studies arrived before those from Spring Grove and reported uniformly negative results. They therefore overshadowed the underwhelming Spring Grove results and appeared to deliver a scientific consensus: LSD therapy was an ineffective treatment for alcoholism. However, the uniformity in both the intent and outcome of these clinical trials hid a great variation in the most fundamental element of a clinical trial's design: the treatment being evaluated. While the original claims for LSD's effectiveness in treating alcoholism had been made for its use in a specific treatment method—psychedelic therapy—only the Spring Grove researchers actually utilized this method.

The internal and external challenges that the Spring Grove researchers faced shed light not only on the fate of LSD psychotherapy but on the problematic complexity of controlled clinical trials. Each research group claimed that the randomized controlled trial methodology would provide objective data on the efficacy of psychedelic therapy. Yet they designed their therapeutic methods and control groups in widely divergent ways based on their own biases and assumptions, which their final results ultimately reflected. Their use of the randomized controlled trial methodology therefore obscured rather than clarified the efficacy of psychedelic therapy. Rather than neutralizing bias, the method hid it behind a veil of objectivity.

Internal Challenges

Faced with the challenge of designing a randomized controlled trial evaluating psychedelic therapy in the treatment of chronic alcoholism, the Spring Grove researchers attempted to devise a method that would render feasible double-blind treatment administration, without compromising their intensive psychotherapeutic treatment procedure. Maintaining a double-blind would require a control treatment that mimicked the subjective effects of LSD, for both the patient and therapist, yet lacked its therapeutic properties. This was a complex proposition, as the researchers considered these subjective effects—specifically the mystical psychedelic experience—to be the drug's therapeutic property. When Charles Savage joined the team in 1965, he brought with him an idea he had developed at the International Foundation for Advanced Study. Psychedelic researchers generally considered that a high dose of LSD, as well as the right "set and setting," was necessary for a subject to attain the full psychedelic experience. Savage theorized that the best active placebo for the psychedelic experience would be a nonpsychedelic LSD experience, produced by a small dose of the drug. The low dose would leave patients and therapists in no doubt that they had taken LSD but would not have the same therapeutic effects as a high dose. This double-blind design would allow researchers to control for the therapeutic influence of the nondrug, specific elements of psychedelic therapy—preparatory psychotherapy and a prolonged session with a therapist—as well as a placebo effect produced by the nonspecific factors involved in all drug treatments, such as expectation, suggestion, and enthusiasm.[1]

Initially, the researchers also planned a second control group. On being accepted into the study, patients would be randomly assigned either to immediately proceed through the LSD treatment procedure or to a waiting list. Patients on the waiting list would initially go through the same preparation for psychedelic therapy as those in the experimental group but would then be discharged to wait six months for their LSD session. After being readmitted to undergo their LSD session, the researchers would follow the progress of these patients for a further six months. Such waiting list control groups were common in psychotherapy research. Here it would provide comparative data on the effects of the preparatory psychotherapy alone over the first six months. Further, by ultimately not denying the patients treatment and by keeping waiting list patients separate from those who received their LSD session immediately, the design would avoid the damaging effects to staff and patient morale that the researchers had experienced when they attempted to implement a no-treatment control group in the pilot phase of their research.[2] Despite the benefits that this second control condition would provide, for unknown reasons it was ultimately not implemented in the study.

For the NIMH-funded double-blind study, patients were randomly assigned, on a two-to-one basis, to receive either a high 450 mcg dose of LSD, or a low 50 mcg active placebo dose, in the identical context of their technique of psychedelic peak therapy. The researchers also allowed an optional repeat LSD session after six months for patients who needed it. This was done for the sake of the therapists, who felt great pressure at only having one shot to deliver a therapeutic experience to their patients. Savage also believed that, for some alcoholics, a single session was simply insufficient to produce lasting change.[3]

The Spring Grove researchers published final results for the alcoholic study in 1971. One hundred and thirty-five male alcoholic patients had undergone treatment. Although the study's design had allowed for up to three LSD sessions, only eighteen patients ultimately received more than one session.

Therefore, the researchers chose to exclude these patients from their analysis of results. The patients had received on average approximately twenty hours of therapy (excluding the LSD session) over a seven-week treatment period. An independent team of social workers assessed the results through a battery of psychological tests administered prior to treatment, prior to discharge, and then at six, twelve, and eighteen months after discharge.[4]

After the significant results in favor of the high-dose group at the six-month follow-up point (discussed in chapter 4), at the twelve- and eighteen-month points there were no statistically significant differences between the results of the high- and low-dose groups. The positive results for the high-dose group had not been lost; in fact, they had either remained steady or improved: for drinking behavior the results had shifted little, with 53 percent of patients rehabilitated at six months, and 54 percent at eighteen months, while for global adjustment the rate had risen from 44 to 53 percent. However, the rate of treatment success in the low-dose group had risen significantly, from 33 to 47 percent for drinking behavior and from 25 to 41 percent for global adjustment.[5] Additionally, removing the double-blind revealed that random assignment of patients between the low- and high-dose groups had failed to provide an even distribution of demographic factors that could influence treatment success: the high-dose group had a significantly greater number of patients who were married and who had completed high school, while the low-dose group had more patients with five or more hospital admissions. These factors had the potential to bias the high-dose group in favor of positive results.

These results were obviously disappointing, as clinical impressions as well as early results had suggested that the treatment was very effective. The final results, however, suggested that any advantages of high-dose psychedelic therapy were short lived, and the uneven demographic factors in the treatment and control groups called into question the validity of even this short-term advantage. While on the surface these results appear to demonstrate that psychedelic therapy was at best of only limited efficacy, in later years Savage reflected on flaws in the design and conduct of the trial that undermined the significance of the results.

Initially, Savage had been "not unhappy with the results." He had been disappointed that the positive results at six months had been only at a $p < 0.05$ level of statistical significance (results would be produced by chance alone less than five times out of one hundred)—despite this being the standard level for determining significance in clinical trials—and that this advantage had not been maintained beyond six months.[6] Nevertheless, he had considered that "a 54% recovery rate seemed hardly nugatory." Furthermore, he had assumed that the level of statistical significance would increase as more patients took part in the study. This had not eventuated, as the study had been "abruptly" concluded, "for no very good reason" other than the therapists' fatigue at working within the study design and their preference to begin working with a new, shorter-acting, psychedelic compound, dipropyltryptamine (DPT).[7]

That the trial stopped because of therapist fatigue provides two important insights into LSD research at Spring Grove. First, it shows how taxing the psychedelic therapy procedure was for the therapists. The procedure was inherently demanding, as it involved a marathon ten- to twelve-hour therapy session, during which the therapists had to provide effective support and guidance to a patient undergoing a dramatic and variable emotional experience. Performing this, as well as the intensive preparation, was made even more taxing by knowing that one-third of the patients—those in the low-dose group—were not expected to benefit greatly from their efforts. While ideal from a scientific point of view, the double-blind controlled trial form of research was a disheartening prospect for therapists whose main goal was to deliver an effective treatment to each patient.

Following this perspective, the second insight is that the researchers designed and conducted the study with more than simply scientific rigor in mind—as Savage wrote to Jonathan Cole at the NIMH in 1965, the intent of the study was to "develop an effective program for the treatment of alcoholics *while at the same time* retaining sufficient control so that the role of LSD can be assessed."[8] Controlled efficacy assessment was a secondary, if not subordinate, goal to treating patients. Reflecting this, Savage explained that the assignment of patients between high- and low-dose on a two-to-one rather than equal basis was done to "placate the therapists."[9]

Further reflecting on the disappointing results of the study, Savage realized that the sample size had not been the major factor limiting the potential significance of results: he now believed that "prolongation of the studies would have made no difference, because *every one* got LSD."[10] Although designed as an active placebo treatment, the efficacy of low-dose psychedelic therapy had not previously been tested. Instead, its use was based on the theory that the low dose would be insufficient to produce a psychedelic experience and that this reaction was necessary for treatment effectiveness. The researchers had evaluated the second half of this hypothesis at the six-month follow-up point, by analyzing the results in relation to what they called "psychedelic reactivity"—the intensity of the patients' subjective drug experiences, regardless of dose. The results were statistically significant in favor of the more profound reactions for global adjustment. Drinking behavior results displayed a similar trend although they were not statistically significant.[11] The researchers did not, however, provide an analysis of the relationship between dose and psychedelic reactivity.[12] So, while they found some evidence that the more profound psychedelic experiences were most beneficial to patients, the exact links among dose, subjective response, and therapeutic effects were still far from clear.

This became particularly problematic, as results for low-dose psychedelic therapy suggested that it was a more effective treatment than they had expected. Indeed, the researchers concluded that, for many patients, the "considerable abreaction and catharsis of psychodynamically charged material" that occurred frequently in low-dose sessions was "quite helpful."[13] Thus, it appeared that low-dose psychedelic therapy was not a true placebo condition but rather a somewhat effective treatment in its own right. As Savage commented, the study was therefore "not a controlled study but a dose response curve study": rather than providing data on the efficacy of psychedelic therapy, it provided data on the comparative efficacy of two forms of psychedelic therapy.[14]

The planned second waiting-list control group would have provided some clarity to this situation. Savage commented only that it was "unaccountably ... eliminated from the study."[15] Considering that that the design and conduct of the study had been strongly influenced by therapeutic demands, the therapists may have protested against discharging patients to fend for themselves for six months before treatment. Although the researchers designed the waiting list control to avoid the damaging effects on morale experienced with a no-treatment group, it is still possible that the therapists' belief in psychedelic therapy's effectiveness left them unwilling to knowingly delay treatment to patients in need. Although with the low-dose treatment the therapists were also delivering a treatment that they did not expect to be effective, in this case the double-blind psychologically shielded both therapists and patients from this knowledge, making the design easier to implement. Other possible explanations include simply insufficient funding, staff, or time to treat and follow a third group of patients.

Despite the difficulties and disappointments in their alcoholic study, the Spring Grove researchers still found some significance in their results. While the unexpectedly positive results for the low-dose group made the evaluation of the efficacy of the high-dose treatment problematic, these results also suggested that the uneven demographic factors between the treatment groups had not significantly skewed favor toward the high dose. The researchers recognized that the inclusion of a nondrug control group would have provided a much clearer picture of overall treatment efficacy. Nevertheless, the positive results for both groups compared to existing data for the hospital's standard treatment routine suggested that psychedelic therapy was effective: a previous study at Spring Grove, with comparable alcoholics, found a 12 percent recovery rate at eighteen months, compared to 54 percent at the same point for high-dose patients in the LSD study. As significant as this was, since it was not part of the same study, it could not be formally considered in determining proof of efficacy. Overall, the researchers concluded that the "clinical achievements of only one psychedelic peak experience and its maintenance for a period of several months in these types of patients is an observation that cannot be discounted."[16] They proposed further research to learn how to "sustain and maximize" these positive results.

For their NIMH-funded clinical trial of psychedelic peak therapy in the treatment of neuroses, commenced in 1965, the Spring Grove researchers did implement a non-LSD control group. However, again random assignment of patients between treatment groups failed to evenly distribute significant patient variables. Here, the researchers found evidence suggesting that this undermined their results.

For the neurotic trial, patients accepted into the study were randomly assigned to one of three treatment groups. Group 1 was the baseline control group: patients underwent the hospital's standard treatments for their condition. These treatments included tailored use of drug therapy, electroconvulsive therapy, group and individual psychotherapy, and participation in milieu programs. This control group provided data on the efficacy of the hospital's standard treatment procedure, against which the experimental treatments could be compared. Groups 2 and 3 were then given psychedelic therapy with a low or high dose of LSD: group 2 patients would receive 50 mcg of LSD, and group 3 patients would receive 350 mcg. Assignment to these two groups was double-blind. The psychedelic therapy procedure and all assessment and follow-up evaluations were performed in a similar manner as in the alcoholic study.[17]

The researchers published the final results for the study in 1973, in the *Journal of Altered States of Consciousness*. Despite the inclusion of the non-LSD control group, the results were even more disappointing than those of the alcoholic study. Ninety-six patients took part in the experiment. Initially, a comparison of psychological tests performed prior to treatment and shortly afterward showed a statistically significant superior efficacy for both high-dose and (to a somewhat lesser extent) low-dose psychedelic therapy over conventional therapy. Statistical analysis showed little significant difference between the high- and low-dose treatments. Despite these positive early results, at the six-month follow-up point, tests failed to find any significant difference among the three groups. At the twelve-month follow-up there was some indication of superior efficacy for high-dose psychedelic therapy, but a high dropout rate had left the patient sample unrepresentative of the original population. Therefore, the results could not be considered accurate. At eighteen months there were again no significant differences among the three groups.[18]

The inclusion of the non-LSD control group in this trial suggests that the negative results attained were due simply to the lack of efficacy for psychedelic therapy in the treatment of patients suffering from chronic, severe psycho-neuroses. Yet, despite the superiority of the neurotic trial's design compared to the alcoholic trial, the Spring Grove researchers still questioned whether flaws in the study diminished the significance of results. Where the alcoholic study had included only male patients, the neurotic study included both male and female. Random allocation of patients had resulted in a disproportionately high number of women in the high-dose LSD group. This was significant, as an analysis of results in terms of gender suggested that female patients improved most with the low-dose treatment, while male patients improved most with the high-dose.[19]

The researchers theorized that differences in dose response between men and women could be due to both differences in their illnesses and in the support they received at home and in the community after discharge. Since the study's inception the researchers had acknowledged that the psychoneurotic diagnosis encompassed patients with wide variations in pathology, even if their chief complaints were consistently depression and anxiety. The researchers found that women in the study typically suffered from "anxiety reactions" or were "hysterical depressives" and struggled to "cope with marital and/or home problems." These patients often found the high-dose LSD session too confronting, and any improvements were frequently undone on their return home: instead of finding any "rewards for becoming less depressed . . . her husband and children may increase their demands on her." Men were more often suffering from "character problems" and had psychological defenses that impeded engagement with standard therapeutic techniques.[20] For these patients the intense high-dose LSD session was particularly useful, as it could break through these defenses. They also found that, with men, improvement often met with great community support, such as new employment opportunities.

The researchers' considered this analysis as only speculative, because of its post hoc nature. Nevertheless, if accurate, then the failure of randomization had undermined the efficacy of high-dose psychedelic therapy, as the patient population in that treatment group was biased in favor of nonresponders. Ultimately, the results of the Spring Grove neurotic trial were discouraging if not conclusive. Nevertheless, they were not damning to the Spring Grove psychedelic research program as whole. While there had been some history of claims of efficacy for psychedelic therapy for patients with neurotic illnesses, alcoholism had always been its primary indication. Alcoholism, or more generally addiction, was a distinctly different illness from psychoneurosis, so the results of this trial could not indicate a lack of efficacy for psychedelic therapy in the treatment of alcoholism or other addictions.

Significant challenges also faced the Spring Grove study of psychedelic therapy in the treatment of emotional distress and physical pain associated with terminal cancer. While in 1966 the researchers had planned a controlled study for this indication—similar in design to the alcoholic and neurotic studies—a lack of funding left them unable to implement it. Despite early indications of the effectiveness of the treatment, funding applications to the Public Health Service (PHS) and National Cancer Institute were unsuccessful. Research did continue, using limited funds from the Maryland State Department of Health and Mental Hygiene, the Mary Reynolds Babcock Foundation, and an all-purpose grant from the PHS.[21] However, this funding was not adequate to launch the controlled trial, so research stayed in the uncontrolled pilot phase. Why the PHS did not award specific funding for this trial, when it did for the other three Spring Grove LSD clinical trials, is not clear. It was most likely not due to any significant flaw in its design or a more fundamental opposition to the research but simply to a lack of funds to cover all worthy research applications.

Nevertheless, the Spring Grove researchers continued to publish positive results from their uncontrolled pilot research. Their final report, published in 1973 in *International Pharmacopsychiatry*, assessed the treatment's effects in thirty-one patients. The researchers compared pre- and posttreatment ratings of patients' degree of depression, anxiety, experience of pain, fear of death, psychological isolation, and difficulty of management. They found a statistically significant improvement for all categories, to the high level of $p < 0.001$. The researchers reported that 29 percent of the patients were "dramatically improved," while 41.9 percent were "moderately improved." Only two patients (6.4 percent) worsened over the treatment period, even though the degenerative nature of the patients' illnesses would have predisposed all of them to a worsening disposition. Despite the significant reduction in patients' experience of pain, narcotic use did not decrease to a statistically significant degree. The researchers suggested that LSD treatment made many patients more comfortable on their standard regimen of narcotic pain relief but did not go so far as to remove the need for narcotics. Other patients may have continued their narcotic use out of habituation or addiction.[22] Despite the highly positive results and the careful manner in which they had been collated and analyzed, without a control group they could not provide convincing evidence of efficacy.

The Spring Grove researchers found their most clearly positive results for the efficacy of psychedelic therapy in their NIMH-funded study of the treatment of heroin addicts, published in 1973 in *Archives of General Psychiatry*. Seventy-four volunteer male narcotic-addicted inmates from Maryland correctional institutions had been paroled early to participate in the study, initiated in 1968. The inmates were randomly assigned to either the treatment or control group. Members of the control group were enrolled as outpatients at the Narcotic Clinic in Baltimore, also known as Coleridge House. There they underwent an existing outpatient program for paroled narcotic addicts that involved daily monitoring of urine for drug use, weekly group psychotherapy sessions, and close parole supervision. Patients in the treatment group were admitted to this same clinic as inpatients for four to six weeks while they underwent psychedelic therapy. After treatment, they were discharged to the same outpatient care the control group received. Participation in the program was a condition of the patients' parole; repeated drug use or failure to attend the clinic, as well other parole violations, would result in reimprisonment.[23]

In this trial, random allocation successfully ensured an even distribution of significant demographic variables between the treatment and control groups. The researchers analyzed results in terms of abstinence from narcotics and global adjustment for the first twelve months of the patients' participation in the outpatient program. Abstinence could be evaluated accurately through the clinic's daily monitoring of patients' urine for opiates. These results revealed that 25 percent of the psychedelic therapy patients maintained complete abstinence over this period, compared to just 5 percent of the control group. This result was statistically significant to the level of $p < 0.05$. A further three LSD patients maintained complete abstinence for more than a year following a brief relapse on their entry into the outpatient program. Including these patients raised the abstinence rate up to one-third.[24]

Global adjustment scores trended in favor of psychedelic therapy at twelve months, but there was no statistically significant difference between the average scores of the two groups. Comparing individual scores, however, revealed that four times more LSD patients received the top global adjustment score than did control patients. While the treatment seemed to have had little impact on the global adjustment scores of the majority of patients, those patients who did react to treatment seemed to benefit maximally. Twelve of the thirteen LSD patients who received the maximum adjustment score were also among those judged to have the achieved the "psychedelic peak experience" in their LSD session. Thus, the researchers concluded that "the peak experience is a facilitative, but hardly an essential or sufficient ingredient for behavior change."[25]

Although the majority of narcotic-addicted patients did not remain abstinent following psychedelic therapy, the treatment was significantly more successful than the standard outpatient treatment. Heroin addicts were notoriously difficult to treat. The researchers highlighted the patients' lack of motivation for treatment, with all admitting that they had volunteered solely in the hope of obtaining early prison release. In an unpublished report, the researchers further described that "a tremendous socio-cultural gulf between the patients and the therapists" made establishing rapport and trust difficult: "The modal therapist was white, Anglo-Saxon, Protestant, and from the upper middle class; the typical addict was a ghetto-raised Negro with an 8th grade education. One therapist, attempting to assert his legitimacy, pointed out that he had once actively done physical labor but literally brought down the house when under cross examination he admitted that he had been the manager of a supermarket. The addict's view was, 'Doc, if you haven't lived in the street, you don't know what it's like.'" The researchers thought that they generally did manage to adequately overcome this gulf and that "even the racial problem was contained either out of mutual denial or respect."[26] Nevertheless, they suggested that black therapists could be more effective.

Given these difficulties, even the modest abstinence rates achieved could be considered significant. As the control condition was not a placebo treatment, the researchers conceded that the trial did not delineate whether it was the LSD session or other components of the overall psychedelic therapy procedure that was behind any treatment effects. The researchers had intended to clarify the role of the psychedelic experience in psychedelic therapy in the alcoholic and neurotic trials (through the low-dose LSD control treatment), allowing them to simply compare psychedelic therapy to an alternative treatment here. Nevertheless, as the low dose had not functioned as a true placebo condition in those studies, this question remained unanswered. Countering this potential critique, the researchers pointed out that it was unlikely that nondrug elements in the treatment condition were solely responsible for treatment effectiveness, as "no consistently positive claims have ever been associated with individual psychotherapy and/or brief residential treatment for chronic heroin abusers."[27]

For the Spring Grove researchers, clear and convincing scientific evidence demonstrating the efficacy of their psychedelic peak therapy procedure remained largely elusive. The randomized controlled trail method of evaluation had proven highly problematic, with control conditions and random assignment often not working as intended. Ultimately, the researchers believed, but could not prove, that these issues undermined their results, making psychedelic therapy appear less effective than it was. The researchers found their best success in the narcotic trial when they focused on providing a clear comparison between two distinct treatments, rather than on achieving a double-blind condition. Yet, without this, the findings still lacked the weight of evidence expected in modern clinical science. Overall the results of the Spring Grove studies were underwhelming and inconclusive, but not disastrous. Despite the disappointments in the alcoholic trial, there were still clear indications of effectiveness. Further research with a different control condition was fully justified. Psychedelic therapy for terminally ill cancer patients remained a treatment deserving controlled research. Yet developments in the wider field of LSD therapy research overshadowed any positive reading of Spring Grove's results.

External Challenges

Before the Spring Grove researchers had a chance to release their final results, their potential impact had already been greatly diminished by a wave of negative reports from six other studies. Like the Spring Grove researchers, these other researchers had also initiated their studies after reading the reports of dramatic recovery among alcoholics following psychedelic therapy. While intrigued by these results, the researchers were all highly critical of the uncontrolled research that had produced them and decided to put the treatment under scientific examination. The clinical trials that followed were all conducted in hospital settings and were funded by the federal or state government. With varying degrees of sophistication and success, they all designed their studies with substantial numbers of patients, control groups, blinding procedures, long follow-up periods, and statistical evaluations of the significance of results. The trials all broadly conformed to the formalized mode of pharmaceutical research required under the Drug Amendments of 1962.

But, instead of replicating the psychedelic therapy method as developed in Canada, each of the six non–Spring Grove research teams devised its own treatment that resembled it but also differed from it in critical ways. The only constant characteristic of the tested treatments was that they involved no more than three LSD sessions. Otherwise, each study evaluated the efficacy of a unique treatment that incorporated only selected aspects of psychedelic therapy. None of the treatments involved extensive preparatory psychotherapy or intensive session guidance. In fact, several involved no psychotherapy at all, and nursing staff or research assistants were often responsible for supervising drug sessions, rather than trained therapists. These changes to the treatment technique undermined any intentions to provide a fair and rigorous evaluation of psychedelic therapy in the treatment of alcoholism.

The foremost challenge to the significance of the Spring Grove research came from a clinical trial of LSD in the treatment of alcoholism led by Arnold Ludwig and Jerome Levine at Mendota State Hospital in Wisconsin. This trial was particularly important for several reasons: it was the only trial to expressly use psychotherapy as part of the tested treatment, it had the most sophisticated design and the largest number of patients, results were extensively analyzed and published in a significant monograph, and it received a major award from the American Psychiatric Association. But perhaps of greatest significance was the fact that, since 1964, Levine, when not conducting his own research, had been employed by the NIMH's Psychopharmacology Service Center to oversee LSD research in the nation. By the time of the publication of Ludwig and Levine's final results in 1970, Levine had taken over as chief of the unit, now renamed the Psychopharmacology Research Branch.[28] Therefore, the attitudes toward LSD therapy and research expressed by Levine reflected the outlook of the NIMH.

Ludwig and Levine were highly skeptical of the positive reports of psychedelic therapy's efficacy from uncontrolled studies, so they attempted to evaluate the claims in a scientifically rigorous manner. However, although their therapeutic method involved psychotherapy, it still differed significantly from the psychedelic therapy method. The researchers invented a new and unique LSD therapy, which under scrutiny showed negative results. That the NIMH official responsible for LSD research could not appreciate the importance of exactly replicating the therapeutic method of psychedelic therapy for an accurate evaluation of its efficacy strongly suggests that the Spring Grove researchers had little hope in distinguishing their studies from those with different methods.

Ludwig and Levine had first begun working with LSD in 1962, at the US Public Health Service Hospital for narcotic drug addicts in Lexington, Kentucky. There they developed a treatment combining LSD with hypnosis —"hypnodelic therapy"—to treat narcotics addicts and, later, alcoholics. Their impetus for investigating LSD came through frustration at the ineffectiveness of the hospital's normal psychotherapeutic treatment and anecdotal reports from colleagues that a few patients who had been given the drug in a non-therapeutic experiment had claimed the experience changed their outlook on life and values in a positive direction, away from drugs. A literature review confirmed that many researchers had claimed this kind of therapeutic effect for LSD. Ludwig and Levine decided to systematically investigate whether the drug could benefit their patients. However, instead of modeling their treatment on that for which success had been reported with alcoholics, they developed their therapy based on their own conceptions of how addiction could be treated. Indeed, they founded their method on a dismissal of the role of the psychedelic experience in therapy, stating that they "could not see much therapeutic benefit being derived from the illusions, hallucinations, or nirvana-like feelings which frequently accompany administration of the drug." Instead, the researchers believed that for a treatment to be effective, "it would be necessary to control the LSD experience and divert or channel whatever therapeutic potential it might possess toward the more conventional notions of psychological therapy, such as directing the patient's attention to his present problems and trying to get him to understand them in terms of his previous conflicts."[29] Ludwig had been experimenting with hypnosis, and he considered it a potentially good tool for directing the LSD experience in such a way.

Hypnodelic therapy involved hypnotizing the patient in the period between LSD administration and the onset of its effects thirty to forty-five minutes later. During this stage the therapist established a stronger than usual bond with the patient and gave suggestions that the treatment provided a new chance for insight and improvement. Once the patient was under the effects of the drug, the therapist conducted a two-hour psychotherapy session along the lines of conventional psychodynamic therapy but with increased depth, suggestibility, and intensity. Emphasis was placed on recalling and reliving past traumatic events and comprehending negative dynamic processes. After the session the therapist lifted the hypnotic trance and transferred the patient to an overnight room. The patient remained there alone, except for periodic checks by a nurse, for the rest of the drug's period of action (another eight to ten hours). The therapist encouraged the patient to use this time to further think through the issues discussed during the session and possibly write up the experience.[30]

In 1965 Ludwig and Levine published the results of a controlled pilot study of hypnodelic therapy in the treatment of narcotic addiction. The trial was not double-blind but randomly assigned seventy patients among five treatment groups: brief psychotherapy, hypnotherapy, hypnodelic therapy, LSD administration plus psychotherapy, and LSD administration without psychotherapy.[31] Results revealed that hypnodelic therapy was significantly more successful than the other treatments. But, as the follow-up tests were performed while the patients were still hospitalized, they did not test abstinence from drugs or life adjustment but therapeutic effect on measures of psychopathology.[32] This trial provided the formula for the later alcoholic trial: a controlled comparison of various combinations of LSD, hypnosis, and psychotherapy. The major changes lay in the population, follow-up period, and sophistication in evaluation.

Ludwig and Levine had both been working at the Lexington Public Health Service Hospital as a condition of their draft deferment, which committed them to two years of service to the PHS on the conclusion of their medical residencies. At the end of Levine's service in 1964, Jonathan Cole, chief of the NIMH Psychopharmacology Service Center, hired him for the task of "stimulating, supporting and consulting" on studies to evaluate the therapeutic usefulness of LSD and similar drugs in psychiatry.[33] Cole had been under increasing pressure to assess whether there was any truth to the claims from various researchers that LSD was therapeutically useful. Levine had long-held interests in both chemistry and psychology, and years earlier had contacted Cole in the hopes of fulfilling his PHS service at the Psychopharmacology Service Center. Cole had tried but been unable to arrange this. When Levine came out of his service with clinical experience with LSD, he appeared an ideal candidate to oversee psychedelic research for the NIMH.

In addition to consulting with LSD researchers such as those at Spring Grove, Levine fulfilled his role by continuing his collaboration with Ludwig, who had moved to Mendota State Hospital. There they had the opportunity to more thoroughly explore the efficacy of their therapeutic techniques with alcoholic patients.[34]

Ludwig and Levine, joined by research analyst Louis Stark, approached the task of assessing the efficacy of LSD psychotherapy with great skepticism of all the research that had gone before them. Besides critiquing prior studies for being uncontrolled and having small patient samples, the Mendota researchers expressed suspicion over the objectivity of those researchers, commenting that "therapeutic claims for this drug have been more of the nature of religious testimonials or statements of clinical conviction than cautious scientific observations and interpretations."[35] But they also claimed to maintain a balanced perspective, recognizing that a poorly designed study did not equate to a poor treatment: while a "skeptical attitude was justified," "given the impotency of current treatment procedures for alcoholics and the magnitude of the problem, it seemed wise to pursue and investigate any treatment approach which might offer help, even though the approach be viewed as radical, unconventional or untested."[36] The researchers set out to right the wrongs of previous studies. The stakes were high, because "if the glowing claims for LSD could be substantiated, the drug would indeed revolutionize psychiatric treatment," but the proof would "only be forthcoming through an impartial arbiter, known as *scientific method*, which makes no compromise with bias, regardless of its source."[37]

The NIMH-funded study took place in the Alcoholic Treatment Center of the Mendota State Hospital over four years, with results published in 1970. The experimental treatments were given against a background of the center's normal procedure: after recovering from withdrawal at the hospital, patients were admitted to the center for thirty days, where they underwent "milieu therapy," consisting of industrial therapy, group counseling, community therapy, Alcoholics Anonymous meetings, lectures, films, and "opportunities for individual counselling."[38] A total of 176 male patients took part in the study. The researchers reasonably concluded that a double-blind trial was impractical with LSD, so again decided on a controlled comparison method. Patients were randomly assigned to one of four treatments, with an equal number of patients in each treatment group. Half of each treatment group was also randomly assigned to receive Antabuse on discharge, a drug that causes severe nausea when alcohol is consumed. Thirteen psychiatrists administered the treatments, seven of whom were second- or third-year psychiatric residents. All were volunteers who were trained in hypnosis and LSD administration by Ludwig through "extensive reading material" and "demonstration sessions."[39]

In lieu of the double-blind, the researchers attempted to minimize a bias toward the experimental treatments by withholding information regarding the nature of the trial. They told patients that they would receive one of four treatments involving, either alone or in combination, LSD, hypnosis, a "contemplative session," or Antabuse. But they were not told that it was an experimental comparison but instead that the most appropriate treatment for their condition would be chosen. The researchers provided the patients with only basic information regarding LSD, and neither the patient nor psychiatrist knew which treatment was going to be used until just prior to the session. To control for therapist skill, psychiatrists were given an equal number of patients from each treatment group.[40]

The four tested treatments were hypnodelic therapy, psychedelic therapy, drug therapy, and milieu therapy. The Wisconsin researchers' form of psychedelic therapy was the same as hypnodelic therapy, but without hypnosis: LSD plus conventional psychotherapy focusing on the patients' major problems. The other two treatments were different forms of control treatments. Drug therapy was the administration of LSD without psychotherapy. This controlled for the role that psychotherapy played in the effectiveness of either of the two LSD psychotherapy treatments. Milieu therapy involved no drugs or psychotherapy, but a period of "contemplation and meditation" alone, where patients were told to think hard about their problems and make plans for the future. This gave a baseline assessment of the efficacy of the hospital's standard treatment procedure, against which the results of the experimental treatments could be compared.

Prior to all treatments, patients went through a two-hour psychiatric interview with their assigned therapist to gather personal information on which to base any psychotherapy. All treatments then took place in an "ordinary clinical office setting" and lasted approximately three hours, after which the patient was placed in an observation room overnight. The dose of LSD for the three drug treatments was 3 mcg/kg of body weight, somewhat lower than other studies (i.e., 225 mcg for a 75 kg patient).[41] Thus, although two of the tested treatments involved LSD and psychotherapy, they had little in common with the psychedelic therapy method established in the 1950s, which often featured extensive preparatory psychotherapy and focused on attaining the psychedelic experience through the manipulation of the patient's "set and setting" by the therapist, who acted as a supportive guide throughout the entirety of the drug's period of action

Social workers blind to the patients' treatments performed the patient evaluations. They employed a battery of tests prior to the first therapist meeting and prior to discharge, and then at three, six, nine, and twelve months after discharge. The tests rated patients on aspects of personality, psychological health, drinking behavior, and social adjustment. They also interviewed a relative of each patient prior to treatment and at six and twelve months. The successful follow-up rate was remarkably high for this category of patients— ranging between 88 and 96 percent, with the highest rate achieved at twelve months.[42]

Ludwig, Levine, and Stark extensively analyzed the data from the follow-up assessments to determine any statistical significance in the improvement rates of the four treatments. They found that although all four groups showed significant improvement in most areas of assessment, none of the LSD treatments produced significantly different results from the control treatment. They also analyzed the influence of thirty-six different variables on the success of treatment. These variables included the patients' marital status, age, whether their therapist had finished residency, motivation for improvement, pretreatment personality assessment, and number of hospital admissions. The variables seemed to have no significant impact on results. They also found Antabuse to be ineffective.[43] Lastly, the researchers took into account how treatment success related to patients' subjective experience of their LSD session. Reports showed that, among other measures, 65.6 percent enjoyed the experience, 8.4 percent had a "mystico-religious" experience, and 47.3 percent reported positive benefits. No statistically significant variation was found in the distribution of these factors among the treatments, and they appeared to have no significant influence on treatment outcome.[44] The researchers were confident enough in their methodology and the comprehensiveness of their study to state that their negative results produced such "inescapable conclusions about the purported efficacy of LSD for the treatment of alcoholism as to preclude any further investigation, at least as far as evaluating the usefulness of the particular techniques used in this study."[45]

The five other research groups evaluated treatments that on the surface appeared more similar to psychedelic therapy, with the treatment taking place in a more typical psychedelic setting. However, closer examination reveals that they were largely stripped of psychedelic therapy's therapeutic elements. Leo Hollister and colleagues at the Palo Alto Veterans Administration Hospital in California utilized a therapeutic method that most starkly contrasted to that of psychedelic therapy. The tested treatment not only involved no psychotherapy but also provided minimal preparation and session guidance. In fact, the method equated to little more than the administration of a high dose of LSD. By the mid-1960s, Hollister was a prominent psychopharmacologist who had been at the forefront of research methodology for more than a decade. His prior research had mostly been biologically oriented, and this likely influenced how he approached LSD therapy. The influence of Hollister's research background on his clinical trial illustrates how mainstream psychopharmacologists struggled to appreciate the fundamental difference between psychedelic therapy and their established "magic bullet" mode of drug treatment.

Hollister had not entered the fields of psychiatry and psychopharmacology deliberately. After training in internal medicine, in the early 1950s Hollister took up a position at the Veterans Administration Hospital in Menlo Park, California, which mainly treated psychiatric patients. In his medical role there, in 1953 he began researching reserpine as a treatment for hypertension. Soon afterward a representative of the drug's manufacturer informed him that the drug might also be useful for psychiatric patients. Therefore, Hollister began collaborating with some of his psychiatrist colleagues to test reserpine's effectiveness in treating schizophrenia. Having had some experience with the placebo-controlled double-blind method of drug evaluation, he conducted the research in this manner. According to Hollister, this was the first time that a parallel-group double-blind placebo-controlled trial had been conducted with schizophrenic patients.[46] Finding the treatment successful, Hollister expanded his research to controlled studies of chlorpromazine in 1954, after finding research suggesting that it had similar antipsychotic effects. He then collaborated on the most sophisticated clinical trial to have yet been undertaken in the field of psychopharmacology: a large-scale, multi-hospital, randomized, double-blind placebo-controlled study of the efficacy of chlorpromazine in schizophrenia. The trial, reported in 1960, confirmed the drug's efficacy.[47] By the start of the 1960s, despite having no formal training in psychiatry, Hollister found himself at the forefront of psychopharmacology.

In 1962, Hollister published two reports on his initial research with psychedelics. The first was a comparison of the states produced by various psychedelic drugs to the schizophrenic state, which found distinct differences.[48] This finding undermined the value of using the drugs to study the origins and manifestations of psychotic illnesses. His second report concerned a small-

scale attempt to evaluate the effect of psychedelics on conventional psychotherapeutic interviews. Hollister and his colleagues found that the drugs
did produce some improvement in their psychotherapy sessions, but they
stressed that the small sample, as well as limitations in their research design,
precluded them from reaching any convincing conclusions.[49]

Hollister was highly skeptical regarding the claims of effectiveness for the
various forms of LSD psychotherapy that had been reported since the early
1950s. This was primarily due to the uncontrolled nature of previous studies.
However, his criticism also went beyond the role of LSD in therapy to the
lack of evidence for the efficacy of the forms of psychotherapy that LSD was
supposed to facilitate, such as abreactive or group therapy. Hollister conceded
that controlled trials, particularly double-blind trials, were difficult to perform with LSD. Nevertheless, he argued that methodologically sound studies
were possible. He also drew attention to the "curious" situation where few
LSD psychotherapy researchers had experience evaluating conventional psychopharmacological treatments, commenting, "One might be more inclined
to believe claims made by anyone of demonstrated reliability in other areas
of clinical psychopharmacology."[50] In this judgment, he overlooked the fact
that, as LSD psychotherapy was indeed a form of psychotherapy, many researchers came to the field from backgrounds in psychodynamic, rather than
biological, psychiatry. For this reason it is not surprising that they had not
conducted prior drug research.

Hollister and his colleagues set out to bring scientific rigor to the evaluation of LSD in the treatment of alcoholism. In doing so they adopted a
medical form of treatment—one that apparently assumed that any beneficial
effects of LSD were inherent in the drug's action. Seventy-two male alcoholics were treated in the NIMH-funded randomized double-blind trial, which
compared a large 600 mcg dose of LSD against the stimulant dextroamphetamine as an active placebo. They published their results in 1969. Rather than
undergoing preparatory psychotherapy, prior to the treatment patients simply had a discussion with their psychiatrist regarding their drinking problem
designed to minimize guilt over their condition: they were told that their
alcoholism was not the result of any "psychological weakness" but simply that
they had "been hooked by an addicting drug." Following this perspective, the
treatment was not conceived as an attempt to address personality problems
but was to be used simply as an "introspective experience." The researchers
did not give a rationale for how this experience could aid alcoholic patients.
Specific preparation for receiving LSD was also almost nonexistent: as the

researchers wrote, "Within the bounds of medical ethics, patients were given as little concrete information as possible about the drugs to be tested." In fact, they were not even named.[51]

The treatment then consisted of merely administering the drugs in a comfortable room, with brief reassurance provided by an attending research assistant when needed. Music was available, but the research assistant made no attempt to guide the session, other than to emphasize that it was for self-examination. At no point—neither in the experiment's preparation or treatment nor as part of the general ward procedure—was any psychotherapy given. The whole treatment program was remarkably brief, lasting less than one and one-half weeks from hospital admission to discharge. This time included all necessary medical detoxification as well as the experimental treatment.[52] By comparison, the treatment period in the Spring Grove alcoholism study lasted an average of seven weeks.[53] At the two-month follow-up, the LSD patients had a significantly greater rate of improvement than did the dextroamphetamine patients, but by the six-month follow-up there was no significant difference between the two groups. A high dropout rate prevented a fair analysis of results at the twelve-month follow-up point. With the lack of any active form of therapy in the treatment, it is unsurprising that negative results were found. The researchers interpreted the results as demonstrating the lack of efficacy of this form of treatment.[54]

Hollister and his colleagues did place a caveat on the significance of their findings: they emphasized that the results were relevant only to the treatment method that they tested. Indeed, they acknowledged that the concurrent research at Spring Grove involved preparatory psychotherapy and a "therapeutic intervention" during the drug session, which could have an impact on treatment effectiveness. However, they defended their therapeutic method by claiming that they were testing the "original contention" that LSD administration with "little or no specific psychotherapy" could benefit alcoholics.[55] This was misleading, as Hollister cited Saskatchewan researcher Colin Smith's 1958 report, in which patients received two to four weeks of preparatory psychotherapy, and Smith explicitly stated that the drug "would almost certainly be valueless without psychotherapy and rehabilitative measures." The other cited studies, while varying in technique and featuring less-extensive preparation, still described both preparatory psychotherapy and intensive session guidance.[56] In fact, Hollister even gave passing mention to the inclusion of psychotherapy in these studies when initially citing them. Whether or not Hollister intentionally ignored these aspects of the treatment techniques he claimed to test, it appears that, rather than improving his objectivity, his prior experience evaluating conventional psychiatric drugs biased him toward viewing drugs as magic bullet treatments.

Although Hollister's therapeutic method seems an obvious departure from the established method of psychedelic therapy, treating LSD as a magic bullet treatment was not uncommon: two other clinical trials of LSD in the treatment of alcoholism conducted in the second half of the 1960s also involved no psychotherapy. Like Hollister, these researchers appear to have made no real efforts to treat their patients outside of administering the drug.

Keith Ditman, of UCLA, had been researching LSD since the mid-1950s. His earliest study was a comparison of the effects of LSD with the experience of delirium tremens, which found significant differences.[57] Despite no therapeutic intent in the study, many of the subjects given LSD reported beneficial effects.[58] In addition to this research, throughout the 1960s Ditman published critiques of LSD psychotherapy research—highlighting the lack of controlled trials—and studied the harmful effects of the nonmedical use of LSD.[59] Ditman and colleagues' NIMH-funded LSD and alcoholism trial, published in 1969, paid some attention to set and setting, with the experiment taking place in an "LSD setting," although the researchers did not explain exactly what this meant. In the double-blind experiment, ninety-nine male patients were expecting to receive LSD but were instead randomly assigned to receive either LSD, the stimulant methylphenidate, or the minor tranquilizer chlordiazepoxide. Neither the patients nor those involved in their treatment were informed that drugs other than LSD were administered. Results were measured not in terms of the treatments' effects on long-term drinking behavior but on an analysis of patients' drug sessions for the prevalence of experiences usually deemed therapeutic, such as increased self-understanding. The study found LSD to be no more therapeutic than the two control drugs.[60]

At the Topeka Veterans Administration Hospital in Kansas, Kenneth Godfrey had been conducting research with LSD and alcoholics since 1963. Over the mid-1960s Godfrey's method of administering the drug had evolved considerably, as he attempted to find a way to reliably produce a psychedelic reaction. Originally, he administered LSD in a highly clinical fashion: alone, except for a technician, patients were observed through one-way glass while being subjected to psychological tests. This method mostly resulted in psychotomimetic reactions. In light of this, Godfrey began to administer the drug in a more comfortable environment, with more supportive company and some music. On the advice of Abram Hoffer, he visited both Sanford

Unger at Spring Grove and Humphry Osmond at the New Jersey Neuro-psychiatric Institute to learn more about their psychedelic therapy method. Following this he gradually adopted the psychedelic method of LSD administration, with patients undergoing their session in a private home-like room, with constant supervision from a supportive nursing assistant, and with music as well as flowers, pictures, and mirrors used to manifest emotive and symbolic experiences. With this method patients consistently achieved the psychedelic experience.[61]

Despite Godfrey's clearly psychedelic framework and his consultation with Unger, Hoffer, and Osmond, it is not clear whether he always employed psychotherapy as part of his treatment, and when he did it varied from the psychedelic therapy model. In 1965 he reported only that he had found that classical psychoanalytical interpretations given to patients during their sessions "fell on deaf ears" but that more broadly symbolic interpretations could be helpful.[62] By 1967, his technique involved significant group therapy, a 50 mcg preparatory group LSD session—which helped to reveal individual psychodynamics—and a high-dose session led by a therapist. Godfrey reported promising results, with follow-up finding 25 percent of patients abstinent and maintaining a positive life adjustment and another 25 percent rated as somewhat improved, after a period of up to three and a half years.[63] From his enthusiastic descriptions of the insights and changes in patients produced by LSD, Godfrey was clearly convinced of the effectiveness of psychedelic therapy. While recognizing that more research was necessary, he showed an appreciation for the need to balance rigor with therapeutic method, stating, "The design for such research must be as scientifically precise as possible, but at the same time clinically tenable."[64]

Over the 1960s, Godfrey planned several formal clinical studies with LSD that evaluated both psychedelic and psycholytic forms of LSD therapy. In 1967, with his colleagues Robert Soskin and Harold Voth, the latter a psychoanalyst from the nearby Menninger Foundation, Godfrey drafted an ambitious research program that would evaluate treatment with six different patient groups: psychedelic therapy with alcoholics, psychedelic therapy with the wives of alcoholics (based on their belief that inadequate support or hostile attitudes at home often undermined alcoholics' recovery), psycholytic therapy with psychosomatic patients, psycholytic therapy with patients with neuroses and character disorders, psycholytic therapy with chronic psychotic patients, and psychedelic therapy to treat anxiety and depression associated with chronic physical illness. All were to be controlled to some degree. An internal review committee assessed the funding proposal and broadly supported it but suggested that the studies be separated into individual grant applications, lest the NIMH reject the whole program on the basis of one of the studies.[65] In 1969 Godfrey submitted a funding application to the Department of Health, Education, and Welfare for a controlled study comparing the efficacy of psycholytic therapy with two control conditions: psychotherapy alone and periodic LSD administration without accompanying psychotherapy. Patients in the study were to be typical psychotherapy candidates, predominantly suffering from neuroses.[66] This proposal appears not to have received funding.

Results from a controlled evaluation of psychedelic therapy at the Topeka Veterans Administration Hospital were published in 1970. Although Godfrey had led the LSD research program there, he was not the architect of the study. In fact, Godfrey's name appeared nowhere on the paper. Instead, William Bowen was listed as the lead author. In a 1969 letter to Hoffer, Godfrey claimed that he had nothing to do with the study per se: the authors, who had not been involved in treating the patients, had used patient records and conducted some further patient follow-up to put together the study and published it without his consultation. Godfrey described the authors as having an "axe to grind."[67]

The report featured two studies. In the first, forty-one male alcoholic subjects treated with high-dose (500 mcg) LSD therapy were compared with forty patients who underwent only the hospital's standard alcoholic treatment program, which the LSD subjects had also undergone. These were not concurrent treatment groups, but rather represented a comparison of patients admitted in 1965–1966, when LSD was offered as part of the hospital's routine treatment procedure, to patients admitted the subsequent year, when it was not. Patients were therefore not randomly assigned between the groups. The second trial was similar in design to the Spring Grove studies, with forty-four patients randomly assigned in a double-blind fashion to receive either the high or a low 25 mcg dose of LSD. A further fifteen patients who either refused LSD treatment or were rejected because of physical or psychiatric contraindications were also followed as an additional control group.[68] The studies were thus less methodologically sound than standard randomized controlled trials, as changes to the treatment milieu over time could impact results when using a nonconcurrent control group. Furthermore, using patients who refused or were refused treatment as a control group meant that those patients differed in significant ways from patients in the treatment groups, providing a flawed comparison.

The therapeutic method for both trials was the same. Patients were prepared for their LSD session through group lectures, where they were instructed to "go along" with the drug's effects and positive expectations for the treatment were emphasized. A nursing assistant trained for the task supervised the drug sessions, primarily to give intensive support to the patients and to provide encouragement that they could use the experience to improve their lives. This form of guidance, while more involved than that employed in Hollister's research, still appears to be much less directive than the method employed at Spring Grove, where a qualified therapist more actively worked to shape and harness the patient's experience. The background ward treatment was composed of lectures, exercises, and other activities designed primarily to improve interpersonal problem-solving skills. Although Godfrey at times employed group psychotherapy as part of his LSD treatment, no form of psychotherapy was given to the patients in these studies, apparently because of "limitations on staff time."[69] No significant differences were found between the results for the experimental or control groups in either study at the one-year follow-up point. Combining the data from the two studies did not reveal any significant differences between the high-dose patients and the control groups.

Discussing their poor results, Bowen and colleagues recognized that in LSD studies the attitudes of the researchers could have a profound influence on the nature of patients' drug experiences. But they considered it unlikely that researcher attitudes had negatively affected their results, as the treatment team was not only experienced with LSD but also had held a "favorable view" of its effectiveness.[70] They now believed that past impressions of effectiveness were due to dramatic personality changes that frequently did appear in patients but that ultimately could not be maintained after discharge when patients were exposed to the stresses of life. They suggested that providing greater aftercare to patients could improve long-term results, and an attempt to implement and evaluate such a program was currently underway at the hospital. This was probably a fair analysis of the experience of many patients who did not experience long-term benefits from LSD treatment and their expanded program had a sound rationale. Nevertheless, the study still failed to provide a fair evaluation of psychedelic therapy as it did not incorporate psychotherapy or intensive session guidance into the tested treatment.

Further, it had significant methodological limitations, and—although their balanced analysis suggests that the researchers were not opposed to LSD's use in psychiatry—the apparently underhand way in which the study was conducted, and the researchers' unknown motives for this, calls into question whether other unknown factors may have influenced its outcome.

The clinical trials of LSD therapy for alcoholism led by Milan Tomsovic and Wilson Van Dusen may have involved some level of psychotherapy. Nevertheless, from the limited discussions of this aspect of treatment in their reports, it appears that the researchers did not consider psychotherapy an integral part of treatment. They also employed only minimal session guidance. Tomsovic's study at the Sheridan Veterans Administration Hospital in Wyoming was the only non–Spring Grove trial to return a somewhat ambiguous result. Patients in the study were prepared for LSD treatment through a lecture and readings designed to reduce apprehension. The treatment then consisted of a single 500 mcg LSD session, administered in a comfortable room with music and visual stimuli available. A nurse was present during the session; however, the nurse did not attempt to direct the patient's experience but instead simply provided support when needed. The day after their treatment patients spent one hour discussing their experience in their "regular therapy group."[71] The study compared the results for 52 male volunteers for LSD therapy from the hospital's Alcoholic Rehabilitation Program against the results from two control groups: a further 45 patients who also volunteered for LSD but were later randomly assigned to undergo only the unit's standard treatment program, and 123 patients from a separate ongoing follow-up study of the success of the Alcoholic Rehabilitation Program. Despite the mention of patients having a regular therapy group, it is not clear to what extent any patients in the study received psychotherapy.[72]

The researchers conducted follow-up evaluations at three, six, and twelve months after discharge. At each point, results trended in favor of LSD therapy in terms of patients' drinking behavior but were statistically significant only at twelve months, and then only between the LSD treatment group and the LSD volunteer control group. This result was significant at the high $p < 0.01$ level of significance. However, as the results for patients who underwent only the hospital's standard alcoholic treatment program after volunteering for LSD were significantly worse than those for patients who routinely went through that same program, the researchers concluded that being offered and then denied LSD had a detrimental effect. On this basis, patients denied LSD after volunteering did not represent a fair control group, and the results of treatment were best compared with the study of the program's normal effectiveness. Here the results were not statistically significant. The researchers did propose an alternative interpretation: those who volunteered for LSD may have been patients who were best suited for drug treatment. The volunteers were observed as engaging poorly with the routine treatment program, as they were holding out for LSD. Therefore, the significant difference between the results for the LSD patients and volunteer controls may have shown efficacy within a specific subgroup of patients, with the background treatment program having little influence on their rates of improvement. Nevertheless, the researchers appeared to favor the former analysis.[73]

Psychologist Wilson Van Dusen and colleagues at Mendocino State Hospital in California conducted a clinical trial that tested a treatment method that most closely resembled the psychedelic therapy method of the Spring Grove and original Canadian researchers. The California Department of Mental Hygiene funded the trial, and results were published in 1967. Van Dusen was intimately familiar with the psychedelic experience. In 1961 he had published an account of his exploratory research with LSD in *Psychologia*, entitled "LSD and the Enlightenment of Zen," in which he compared the experiences of some LSD subjects to the state of satori in Zen Buddhism. He described this state as a "central human experience" that could forever alter the subject's life, as it deepened the "very root of human identity." Van Dusen had experienced this state himself under LSD, where he soared "into paradise" and saw the "structure of the whole of things . . . beyond time and space to the eternal unchanging One who was at the same time the whole of changing creation." He had found that it normally took several LSD sessions for a subject to reach satori and that it usually emerged after the "individual finds the core of his identity and finds he can afford to give it up in psychological death."[74]

Van Dusen's clinical trial with alcoholics was an attempt to confirm the positive results of Canadian researchers Ross MacLean and Colin Smith. As well as criticizing the lack of controls in their research, Van Dusen and his colleagues expressed skepticism over the role of the LSD session in the impressive results of MacLean's study: those patients had apparently been chosen for their good motivation and support networks, and had been given extensive social and vocational support outside of the reported treatment framework. Van Dusen and colleagues had learned this from personal communication with MacLean's colleague Al Hubbard. The Mendocino researchers originally designed their trial as double-blind, with scopolamine as an active placebo. But the blind had proved impossible to maintain, so they abandoned this design. Instead, results for the LSD patients were compared with those for patients who had undergone the hospital's standard alcoholic treatment program just prior to the beginning of the experiment. All patients were female. The average dose of LSD was 400 mcg. Before treatment, patients were rated as to their prognosis, based on factors such as marital status, motivation, and economic resources, and assigned to one, two, or three LSD sessions, with a poorer prognosis resulting in more sessions.[75] A total of seventy-one patients went through the LSD treatment.

Few details of the therapeutic framework surrounding the LSD sessions appear in Van Dusen's report. The patients resided in the hospital's alcoholic unit, described as a "small therapeutic-community-like setting" with "various social activities" and work assignment. Patients were also assigned, or often chose, a staff member who "worked with them before, during and after the experience." These staff members were male psychotherapists and female psychiatric technicians. The nature and extent of the "work" that these staff members did with the patients was not described, so it is not entirely clear whether the patients received psychotherapy. The lack of discussion of this aspect of treatment strongly suggests that if there was any psychotherapy, it was not extensive, and the researchers did not consider it critical to the LSD treatment process. Preparation for the LSD session was both informal and formal: patients learned what to expect from other patients who had already undergone treatment, as well as from the investigators. They were "vigorously counselled to cooperate with the experience," rather than try to resist the drug's effects. The researchers recognized that set and setting were a "critical factor in outcome" and claimed to use the drug "as a facilitating agent in a therapeutic setting."[76] Therefore, it seems that the researchers understood some of the unique aspects of psychedelic therapy. Yet their treatment would still vary significantly from the established methods.

The LSD sessions were conducted with groups of up to four patients. The researchers chose this format for pragmatic reasons: Mendocino State Hospital admitted 1,600 alcoholic patients annually; time-consuming individual treatment was not practical. Although more than one patient was present in the treatment room, each patient had an individual therapist, and some privacy was provided by cloth room dividers. The setting was typical of psychedelic therapy: a comfortable, dedicated room, with visual and auditory stimuli. Where the treatment session varied most from psychedelic therapy was in its conduct: rather than the experience being carefully guided by the therapists, "the day belonged to the subjects," who were free to spend their time how they wished. The therapists interacted with the patients only when requested to. Although music was played during the session, from the report it appears that it was merely in the background, rather than carefully and individually tailored to heighten and direct the experience. The researchers reported that the subjects spent most of their time in quiet contemplation. Some dwelled on issues such as relationships and the meaning of life, but "rarely did they examine drinking." In the days following the session, the patients "worked through" their experience with their therapist.[77]

Van Dusen did not provide a therapeutic rationale for the conduct of the LSD sessions in his clinical trial. However, in his previous report of using the drug with experimental subjects, he had expressed his opinion that the LSD reaction was best left to guide itself, stating that there "is an inner wisdom to the LSD reaction that is better without my intervention. . . . [T]his way subjects learn along their own lines at their own pace."[78] It would seem that he carried this view over into the drug's therapeutic use, still viewing it as effectively a magic bullet treatment: with some preparation and a comfortable setting, the drug could produce an experience that was intrinsically therapeutic.

At the eighteen-month follow-up point, the researchers reported that there were no significant differences between the LSD and control groups on ratings of drinking behavior or social adjustment. Pretreatment ratings of prognosis, the number of LSD sessions administered, measured demographic factors (such as age and duration of alcoholism), and ratings of the nature of the patients' drug experiences also appeared to have had no influence on results.[79] However, further considerations must be taken into account. Controlled trials assess the likelihood of whether the apparent effects of a treatment are indeed due to the treatment or are simply a product of chance or a placebo effect. The level of statistical significance found for the results of a study reveals not how effective a treatment is but simply the level of confidence in the validity of the results. Therefore, it is important to consider not only the comparative efficacy of the treatment and control conditions but the degree to which patients were actually benefiting from treatment, regardless of what caused this benefit.

Average improvement rates for the LSD group in Van Dusen's study appear to have been low. At each follow-up point, patients were rated as to changes in their drinking behavior on a four-point scale, where a score of 2 indicated that the patient had worsened, 3 indicated no change, 4 indicated improvement, and 5 indicated much improved. These scores were then averaged for the group. The score for the LSD group reached its highest level at the eighteen-month follow-up, but it was still only 3.97—bordering on improved but on average insufficient to be classified as such.[80] While it is difficult to accurately compare these results to those from other studies, given the different rating systems, a superficial comparison with the average improvement rates from the Spring Grove alcoholic study suggests that the Spring Grove patients benefited much more significantly: on a drinking behavior rating scale from 1 to 10, with a score of 1 signaling daily drinking and 10 signaling total abstinence, high-dose LSD patients had improved an average of 3.82 points at the eighteen-month follow-up.[81] Van Dusen's averaged results do not mean that no patients improved: such a middling score could result from individual scores ranging widely, from 2 to 5. Yet the fact that the researchers expressed their results only as averages suggests that they saw no significance in the variation of individual scores or the totals for each category of results.

Van Dusen and his colleagues recognized that their treatment results were not as positive as those of the original Canadian researchers. They suggested that the high rate of success they routinely had with their patients could have left "no room for improvement."[82] This does not seem a convincing explanation: at eighteen months the control group was only just rated as improved, with an averaged score of 4.03. Furthermore, the reason that psychedelic therapy had seemed remarkable to researchers was that there was no particularly effective treatment for alcoholism. If the Mendocino researchers had developed a successful milieu treatment for alcoholism, it surely would have seemed unfair to use this not only as a control treatment but also as the backdrop to the experimental treatment.

Ultimately, whether the poor results were due to the lesser emphasis on preparatory psychotherapy, the lack of guidance during the LSD session, or some unknown factor in the backdrop or conduct of the study is not clear. One significant difference in Van Dusen's study was that it treated female patients, where the other alcoholism trials had all treated male patients. Results from the Spring Grove neurotic study suggested that women were less responsive than men to high-dose psychedelic therapy. While this gendered response may have been specific to the neurotic patient population, gender was certainly a significant variable between Van Dusen's and the other researchers' studies that could have influenced results and that deserved further scrutiny.[83] Regardless, Van Dusen's results suggest that some factor in the study had a significant impact on uncontrolled ratings of treatment effectiveness compared to the studies of Kurland and the original Canadian researchers. Van Dusen and his colleagues seem to have used a controlled trial to demonstrate that an apparently ineffective treatment was indeed ineffective.

Debating Design: Scientific Rigor and Therapeutic Method

When the Spring Grove researchers reported the results of their alcoholic study in 1971, they emphasized the critical significance of treatment methods to results. The researchers dismissively categorized Hollister's treatment as "psychedelic chemotherapy," a method with minimal psychotherapy where "the major emphasis was on the administration of the drug itself."[84] While they did not mention Ditman's or Bowen's work, their methods could easily have been included under the same rubric. The Spring Grove researchers described their treatment as "distinctly different" from these methods, implying that the negative results of psychedelic chemotherapy had no implications for their own work. In the report they made only passing mention of Ludwig, Levine, and Stark's research, discounting it as simply a modification of psychedelic chemotherapy. While this appears to be the Spring Grove researchers only published critique of the other clinical trials, in an unpublished review from 1971, Charles Savage gave a detailed, scathing account of the Mendota research, based on its deviation from the theory and method of psychedelic therapy. This appears to have been distributed only among Savage's colleagues. From the review, it is clear that Savage saw Ludwig, Levine, and Stark's work as a great threat to the significance of their own results and to the future of LSD psychotherapy research.

Savage described Ludwig, Levine, and Stark's research as a "disservice to science and the alcoholic." Instead of employing the scientific method as an "impartial arbiter," Savage saw the clinical trial as representing "bias in, bias out." "What makes the work unscientific is that they make not the slightest effort to replicate the works that they are attacking except by employing the same name, psychedelic. . . . The point is not whether or not the psychedelic hypothesis is correct, but that they made no effort to test it."[85] Savage emphasized that Ludwig, Levine, and Stark had shown a firm understanding of the theory and method of psychedelic therapy in their review of previous research. They had described its goal of producing a transcendental experience through intensive patient preparation and the use of visual and auditory stimuli, which could promote positive changes in the patient in a similar manner to a conversion experience. Yet their form of psychedelic therapy employed minimal preparation; a brief, conventional, insight-oriented psychotherapy session; little regard to "set and setting"; and an antimystical focus. Hypnodelic therapy used hypnosis to improve control over the LSD session, but this did not fundamentally alter the treatment. In essence, both of the Mendota treatments involved a single session of psycholytic therapy. However, that form of therapy usually involved numerous LSD sessions over an extended time, and, as Savage stated, "I know of no one who has ever claimed that a single psycholytic session was curative of anything, least of all alcoholism." It is questionable whether Ludwig, Levine, and Stark could have themselves expected their treatment to be successful: Savage quoted their statement that, with alcoholism, "all forms of insight orientated therapies . . . have been employed with equivocal or inconclusive results being obtained at best." In their monograph, the Wisconsin researchers even acknowledged—although only in passing—that their form of psychedelic therapy was not the mystically oriented treatment that the name usually referred to. They explained that their use of the term was "primarily for convenience."[86] This led Savage to accuse the researchers of designing an intentionally deceptive clinical trial: "It is apparent that they rejected the psychedelic model on moral grounds while pretending to test it."[87]

Savage argued that, in addition to being misleading and ineffective, the Mendota researchers' therapeutic method was intentionally antitherapeutic. He believed that after their early positive research, as "LSD fell out of favor and positive results [became] politically unwise," they "loaded the dice in favour of the null hypothesis." Where Ludwig and Levine had originally found success performing the therapy themselves after having a personal training session with LSD, they now used inexperienced therapists who were denied a personal experience with the drug. Furthermore, Savage argued that elements of the researchers' therapeutic method seemed deliberately unpleasant. He highlighted that the Mendota researchers' practice of placing patients alone in an observation room for the majority of the drug's period of action was "considered contraindicated and antitherapeutic by most other workers in psychedelic research." At the American Psychological Association's third Research in Psychotherapy conference in 1966, Ludwig had described this posttherapy observation room as the "cooker," which had led Savage to comment that the treatment "was not an experience that I suspect he would care to have had himself."[88] Ludwig, Levine, and Stark had reported that two-thirds of their patients had "pleasant reactions" and that 47 percent claimed that the experience had been beneficial.[89] The researchers also commented on a peculiar finding in their analysis of readmission rates for the study participants: while proportionately fewer LSD patients than milieu treatment patients were readmitted to Mendota State Hospital during the follow-up period, when other local institutions were included the total number of readmissions were equivalent for the two groups. They concluded that "patients may have avoided Mendota State Hospital to preclude the possibility of additional therapy with LSD."[90]

Ultimately, Savage argued that the antitherapeutic nature of the Mendota researchers' treatment was evident in their results:

> What is striking about the study is not the low incidence of mystical experience since the very nature of the design programmed them out, but the appallingly low remission rate in all categories. By 6 months, between 70 and 80% of their patients in all categories were drinking, and by a year, between 80 and 90%. One would have expected from the Hawthorne effect alone that the result would have been a little better than that. One can only conclude with [Charles] Truax that therapy is for better or worse and that at Mendota State Hospital it is by and large for worse.[91]

In another unpublished review of Ludwig, Levine, and Stark's study, the Spring Grove researchers contrasted the eighteen-month results in the two trials: 22.2 percent of the Spring Grove high-dose LSD patients had maintained complete sobriety, compared to only 6.8 percent for the Mendota patients. They also emphasized that "morale at Spring Grove was (and is) enthusiastic and each patient looked forward to his treatment; in addition, most patients have stated a willingness for a repeat session if indicated."[92]

In an attempt to preempt critiques of their therapeutic method, Ludwig, Levine, and Stark argued that although only 8.4 percent of their patients had a mystical experience, their data showed that there was no significant correlation between the "peak" response and therapeutic outcome. They also defended their minimal patient preparation on the basis that "virtually all patients seemed sufficiently prepared so as to experience the panoramic, spectacular effects of this drug without marked adverse reactions," and on the positiveness of patients' accounts of their experiences.[93] Savage pointed out the false logic in this assertion, comparing it to "justifying surgery on the basis that the patients did not bleed to death."[94]

While the Spring Grove researchers were critical of the Mendota trial, the reverse was also true. Despite the Spring Grove researchers' attempt to design their alcoholism trial in a way that balanced clinical needs with scientific rigor, the Mendota researchers questioned the level of control achieved: Ludwig and his team criticized their lack of a nondrug control group, as well as a possible nontherapy drug control group.[95] During the course of the Spring Grove trial, Levine had frequently visited the researchers in his role overseeing LSD research for the NIMH, and in retrospect Savage wondered "why he permitted some of the now obvious defects to remain uncorrected, unless he wished to give us plenty of rope."[96] In their final report, the Spring Grove researchers recognized that a nondrug control would have been useful. However, including a nontherapy drug control was a more complex issue. As public policy scholar and contemporary psychedelic research advocate Rick Doblin has argued, if Kurland and colleagues believed that their patient preparation and extensive psychotherapy was necessary to ensure safety and efficacy when administering LSD, giving the drug without these measures would have been unethical.[97]

Ludwig, Levine, and Stark were also dismissive of the Spring Grove results, stating that at the six-month evaluation—for which the researchers reported significant, positive results—high-dose patients had not shown significantly superior improvement rates when uneven prognostic factors in the treatment groups were factored in. This opinion, apparently based on both reported results and informal communication, seems particularly unfair, if not misleading.[98] In their final 1971 report, Kurland and colleagues acknowledged that randomization had failed to control some important variables, but they also stressed that the groups were matched on "IQ, age, occupational status, and most importantly, on the pre-treatment rating of abstinence."[99] They also emphasized that the great success of the low-dose group suggested that this group's patients had not been predisposed to treatment failure. Therefore, although they took the idea into account, the Spring Grove researchers did not conclude that the uneven variables such as marital status accounted for the significant difference in drinking behavior at six months. Nor did they have the data needed to thoroughly assess this proposition.

The Wisconsin researchers were not the only critics of the Spring Grove Study. At Hahnemann Medical College's 1968 "Psychedelic Drugs" symposium, Carl Salzman, program head of the NIMH Psychopharmacology Research Branch's Early Clinical Drug Evaluation Unit, presented a critical overview of controlled research with psychedelics. His comments on the Spring Grove trial, based on preliminary results, focused on flaws in the design of its control condition. Salzman recognized that the low-dose LSD treatment may have been an unintentionally effective treatment and that without a second non-LSD control treatment the efficacy of neither high- nor low-dose treatments could be properly assessed. However, he also downplayed the positive elements of the results: "These results are further corroboration of earlier efforts: all patients in an LSD treatment program initially improved when compared on pre-post [treatment] measurements, and no differences were ultimately observed between treatment and control groups."[100] Salzman then criticized the design of the Spring Grove researchers' analysis of the relationship between profoundness of drug reaction and treatment results, regardless of dosage. He described the use of therapist ratings to assess the intensity of patients' experiences as a "serious methodological problem," arguing that this introduced the potential for biased ratings and that objective observers should have been used instead. Savage strongly objected to this critique, arguing that this was a simple assessment where there was minimal risk of bias creeping in. Salzman was not convinced.[101]

Discussing a number of other LSD therapy trials, Salzman's analysis continued to focus on research design. While he gave limited descriptions of the treatment methods tested in the studies and conceded that psychedelic drugs were "unique" and "particularly sensitive to non-drug factors," he did not speculate as to how such factors may have influenced outcomes in individual studies. He described Ludwig and Levine's trials as "well designed" and as representing "further progression along the controlled psychedelic treatment scale."[102] In fact, seemingly supporting their treatment method, he praised their incorporation of patient preparation, the suggestions for positive expectations of outcome given to patients, and the central place of the patient-therapist interaction in the study. Salzman concluded that studies so far had demonstrated that psychedelic therapies were often effective, although not demonstrably more effective than other treatment forms. The form of psychedelic treatment appeared to Salzman to have no impact on results. Salzman claimed that his critique represented his views as a psychiatrist and researcher, rather than as an NIMH official. However, with his critique so closely aligned with Levine's, it is clear that, at the NIMH, clinical studies purporting to assess the original claims for psychedelic therapy's effectiveness were read with little concern for the role of treatment technique in those claims, but rather with a fixed focus on the level of control achieved through their designs.

Despite the significant flaws in Ludwig, Levine, and Stark's treatment method, the wider psychiatric community also judged the trial on the scientific rigor of its design. In 1970 the American Psychiatric Association granted the study the prestigious Hofheimer Award for "developing a technique for administering a complex but precisely defined schedule for LSD treatment of chronic alcoholic patients, a method for studying it under controlled conditions, and for evaluating the clinical outcome in both qualitative and quantitative terms."[103] For psychiatrists who were not sensitive to the unique theories of psychedelic therapy, the Mendota researchers' method would have indeed seemed watertight, and the inadequacies in treatment technique would have gone unnoticed. In addition, in a discipline that was striving to solidify its scientific basis, a critique based on a lack of mystical focus would have seemed absurd. Although the Spring Grove research was also performed on a large scale and attempted to provide a sophisticated controlled analysis of efficacy, it could more easily be ignored as it provided only inconclusive results that on the surface suggested a lack of long-term effectiveness. The problems with the trial's design that led to this situation could easily be overlooked.

Conclusion

In the mid-1960s, seven research groups set out to systematically evaluate claims of the effectiveness of psychedelic therapy in the treatment of alcoholism. For the Spring Grove researchers, the difficulty of incorporating their complex treatment into a randomized controlled trial study design left them with largely inconclusive results. For Ludwig and colleagues, whether or not elements of their trial were intentionally antitherapeutic, it seems that their biases against the theory of psychedelic therapy left them unwilling adopt its method. They instead favored a method that clung to traditional forms of psychotherapy and unsurprisingly produced negative results. Why the studies led by Hollister, Ditman, Bowen, Tomsovic, and Van Dusen took the directions they did is less clear. Bowen cited a lack of staff time for the absence of psychotherapy in his study. This may have been a factor in the other studies. Psychedelic therapy was a labor-intensive treatment, and it may have been that the other researchers simply did not have the resources to implement its full procedure. The use of nurses or research assistants as session guides in several of the studies supports this interpretation. Even if this was the case, given that the researchers largely did not acknowledge how their treatments deviated from the established techniques of psychedelic therapy—even Bowen gave the lack of psychotherapy only passing mention—it also seems likely that they simply failed to grasp the centrality of psychotherapy and close session guidance to the treatment. Their treatments focused on brief instructive preparation, followed by administration of the drug in a standardized setting. This format more closely resembled a standard drug treatment than a form of psychotherapy, and its standardized nature made objective testing easier. Psychedelic chemotherapy fit dominant perceptions of both how drug treatments functioned and how drug efficacy should be tested.

Ultimately, the controlled trials obscured rather than clarified the efficacy of psychedelic therapy. Each research group promoted the randomized controlled trial methodology as the only reliable tool for obtaining objective data on the efficacy of treatment, because of its ability to eliminate bias from research. Yet the methodology could not account for bias in the design of the treatment, only in the evaluation of its effects. In the six non–Spring Grove studies, the randomized controlled trials did in fact provide an objective appraisal of the researchers' treatments. The problem was that the researchers had expressed their bias when designing their treatments, so their bias was built into the clinical trials, and the negative results were essentially foregone conclusions. For the Spring Grove researchers the problem was almost the opposite: rather than hiding their bias, the methodology hid their treatment's potential efficacy because of their problematic control condition. Therefore, in each study the controlled trial methodology gave the appearance of objectivity while hiding the design flaws that ultimately shaped the results. However, faith in the methodology was so high among scientists that its employment gave the results authority, and the therapeutic methods employed were not scrutinized. With studies appearing to show a consensus that psychedelic therapy was ineffective, research would dwindle before dying out entirely.

CHAPTER SIX

The Quiet Death of Research

Psychedelic Therapy in the 1970s

In the United States, limitations in systematically assessing the role of LSD-type drugs in psychotherapy arise principally from shortages of research funds and specifically trained personnel at most local levels due to the lack of State and Federal support of programs and the general disinterest displayed by the pharmaceutical industry.

O. Lee McCabe and Thomas Hanlon, 1977,
Maryland Psychiatric Research Center

From the early 1970s, the field of LSD psychotherapy research began to rapidly decline, along with the drug's image as a potential medical marvel. In 1970, the Controlled Substances Act listed LSD and other psychedelics on the schedule for drugs with a high potential for abuse and "no currently accepted medical use," resulting in increased regulation over research.[1] In 1972, Jerome Levine, in his position as chief of the Psychopharmacology Research Branch of the National Institute of Mental Health, commented that studies had shown that LSD therapy was "no better than other therapies." His predecessor, Jonathan Cole, who had helped to initiate many of the studies, also described the treatment as "mostly a bomb." The two did, however, concede that in the right hands and with the right patients, it could be useful.[2] The NIMH ceased funding LSD research in 1974, and the following year an NIMH research task force reported that studies had "contributed little to our understanding of the bizarre and potent effects of this drug" and had "not clearly defined a therapeutic use."[3] With no federal funding and increased regulation, psychedelic research faced a bleak future.

Nevertheless, as this chapter explores, the increased regulations did not ban research, and it did not come to a complete halt in the early 1970s. In fact, psychedelic research continued at the Maryland Psychiatric Research Center until 1976, and it finally came to a close there because of a change in the management of the center, rather than problems with regulation, funding, or controversy over LSD. Yet the fate of LSD psychotherapy was set long before it ended by the inability of researchers to convincingly demonstrate its effectiveness through controlled clinical trials.

While this analysis accounts for the demise of LSD psychotherapy research in the mid-1970s, it was not the only factor that held LSD back from becoming an approved tool of psychiatric therapy. Turning a drug into an approved medicine requires both research and development. While complementary, and usually closely intertwined, research and development are ultimately distinct undertakings. Research is the domain of scientists; development is normally the responsibility of pharmaceutical firms. Much research was conducted with LSD in the United States between 1949 and 1976; however, the drug underwent very little development. Sandoz Pharmaceuticals withdrew its sponsorship of LSD research in 1966, and even earlier the company appeared to do little to direct research toward the goal of submitting a New Drug Application to the FDA. The case of LSD research therefore raises questions over the significance and prospects of clinical drug research without the backing of a pharmaceutical company: if the results from the clinical trials of LSD therapy of the 1960s had clearly demonstrated its efficacy and safety in treating alcoholism, would that have resulted in the drug becoming an approved tool of psychiatry?

LSD under the Controlled Substances Act

In 1970, LSD research became subject to new regulations under the Controlled Substances Act. While this act was designed to tackle drug abuse, it had the potential to discourage or even disable psychedelic research, since gaining approval to conduct research became more complex. Part of the Comprehensive Drug Abuse Prevention and Control Act of 1970, the Controlled Substances Act reformed the complex set of federal laws that controlled drugs of abuse. Previous laws—notably the 1914 Harrison Narcotic Act, the 1937 Marihuana Tax Act, and the 1965 Drug Abuse Control Amendments—had each controlled different categories of drugs, in different ways, and through different agencies: the Treasury Department's Federal Bureau of Narcotics controlled opiates, cocaine, and marijuana through taxation, while the Department of Health, Education, and Welfare's Bureau of Drug Abuse Control controlled depressants, stimulants, and hallucinogens through regulating interstate commerce. This complex regulatory system caused significant jurisdictional difficulties for enforcers when, for example, drug traffickers were caught with both heroin and barbiturates.

In 1968 this problem was partly solved through the merger of the Federal Bureau of Narcotics and the Bureau of Drug Abuse Control into the Bureau of Narcotics and Dangerous Drugs, under the Department of Justice. However, while the new agency had jurisdiction over all drugs of abuse, enforcement was still complicated by the different regulatory frameworks and penalty structures for different drugs. The Controlled Substances Act remedied this situation by bringing all drugs of abuse under one regulatory framework, administered and enforced by the Department of Justice.[4]

The Controlled Substances Act created five schedules for drugs, each denoting a different level of regulation. Inclusion in a schedule was based on a determination of the drug's potential for abuse, the severity of physical or psychological dependence it could produce, and whether it had a legitimate medical use. The legislation listed the drugs to initially be included in each schedule, and future additions and changes in scheduling were the responsibility of the attorney general. LSD, along with other psychedelics such as mescaline and psilocybin, was listed in Schedule I. This was the most prohibitive schedule, under which heroin and marijuana were also listed. The criteria for inclusion in Schedule I are the following:

(A) The drug or other substance has a high potential for abuse.
(B) The drug or other substance has no currently accepted medical use in treatment in the United States.
(C) There is a lack of accepted safety for use of the drug or other substance under medical supervision.[5]

It may appear that the Department of Justice was now responsible for making determinations as to the medical use and safety of drugs—a task normally under the jurisdiction of the FDA. In the case of LSD, the last criterion seems to contradict scientific experience with LSD, as the safety record for all forms of LSD psychotherapy had been exemplary when performed under medical supervision.[6] However, officials in the Bureau of Narcotics and Dangerous Drugs considered that—for the purposes of scheduling—determining whether a drug was safe or had a medical use did not require lengthy deliberation or scientific investigation but simply checking the drug's official status with health authorities.[7] Further, in scheduling decisions, the attorney general was required to solicit the advice of the secretary of health, education, and welfare on medical and scientific criteria, and such advice would be binding. In the United States, the FDA's approval of an NDA officially established a drug as having both an approved medical use and accepted safety under medical supervision. Therefore, in effect, the criteria for Schedule I simply meant that a drug had a high potential for abuse and did not have an approved NDA. In fact, as Schedule I was the only schedule for drugs without an accepted medical use, any drug with enough of an abuse potential to warrant scheduling (in the eyes of the Department of Justice) but without an approved NDA would be placed in that schedule. LSD clearly met these criteria.

The regulation of Schedule I drugs equated to almost total prohibition of their manufacture, distribution, administration, and possession. However, as with previous laws, there was an exemption for legitimate scientific research: medical practitioners could use a Schedule I drug in research after obtaining registration from the attorney general. This registration requirement was in addition to the standard FDA approval process to conduct research with an investigational drug. While this provision can appear to have put the ultimate control of research in the hands of the Department of Justice, the attorney general's powers to deny registration were in fact very limited. On receiving an application for registration, the attorney general was required to refer it to the secretary of health, education, and welfare, who judged the adequacy of the researcher's qualifications and the merits of the research proposal. The secretary was also required to consult with the attorney general on the adequacy of measures to prevent diversion of drug supplies to illegitimate channels. If the secretary then recommended registration, the attorney general was permitted to deny it only if applicants had falsified information in the application, had been convicted of a felony related to a controlled substance, or had had their license to practice medicine revoked.[8]

Despite the attorney general's limited powers to deny registration for legitimate research with Schedule I drugs, the intrusion of the Department of Justice into medical research was highly controversial. At congressional hearings considering the proposed legislation, several prominent figures in psychopharmacology research, including Jonathan Cole, Nathan Kline, and Daniel Freedman, as well a representative of the American Psychiatric Association, spoke out against the provisions. They argued that registration would seriously impede research by slowing the approval process, discouraging researchers from investigating Schedule I drugs. They also feared that the Department of Justice might take a harder line in regulating research than intended in the legislation.[9]

Whether the registration requirements of the Controlled Substances Act did indeed impede research in the case of LSD is not easy to determine. As explored below, LSD research at the MPRC did not come to a close until 1976, and then for reasons unrelated to LSD per se. Although the legislation did not immediately terminate LSD research, from the start of the 1970s research was clearly in decline, and it had faded away to almost nothing before its eventual demise. Difficulties in gaining and maintaining approval for research could have influenced this. A 1972 survey of researchers interested in psychedelics found that 81 percent of respondents rated governmental red tape as a "large" obstacle.[10] FDA officials responded to claims of prohibitive regulations by arguing that, in fact, disillusionment with psychedelics had resulted in few researchers actually submitting applications to work with the drugs. They also argued that widespread research with marijuana suggested that registration requirements did not prevent access to Schedule I drugs.[11] More closely examining responses to the survey can reveal possible factors behind these differing perspectives on the role of regulation.

Walter Houston Clark, a psychologist of religion with long-held interests in psychedelics and mysticism, led the survey, which was conducted through a questionnaire published in the journal *Behavior Today* and the newsletter of the Association for Humanistic Psychology. The one hundred respondents thus represented a self-selected group, motivated to voluntarily respond to questions on psychedelic research and mail in their answers. Indeed, 32 percent of respondents were currently involved in psychedelic research, 49 percent had been at some previous time, and 82 percent had personally used a psychedelic. Only one no longer wished to work with the drugs. In addition to governmental red tape impeding research, the respondents rated highly other similar factors such as "other red tape," difficulties in securing clearance, disapproval of administrators and superiors, and lack of funding.[12] But the survey could not reveal how many of these were real rather than perceived hurdles: in part supporting the FDA's claim to receive few applications, many respondents had not actually attempted to initiate psychedelic research, as they had simply assumed they would be unsuccessful.

Aside from this limitation, the survey reveals a great disparity in perspective between the respondents and medical authorities on the qualifications deemed necessary for conducting psychedelic research. Clearly considering psychedelic research to be a unique field of drug research, the survey respondents most frequently mentioned the need for personal experience with the drugs; personal attributes such as empathy, mental balance, and ethical responsibility; and specific training in the field. Only twelve responded that medical or other traditional academic qualifications were a necessary factor, and only two listed approval from regulatory authorities. Clark commented that these differing perspectives on qualifications seemed to reflect generational factors, as well as the impact of personal experience with the drugs: he contrasted a graduate student in social relations' response of "purity of motive" with Jonathan Cole's "IND to FDA only."[13]

The FDA perspective on required qualifications was far more black and white: drug research should be led by medically qualified researchers who were experienced in drug research and had appropriate facilities. Given the questionnaire's distribution, the respondents likely skewed toward being psychologists rather than psychiatrists, and they eschewed the idea that medical credentials were an important qualification for psychedelic researchers. These factors bring into question the proportion of respondents that the FDA would have considered qualified to conduct drug research at all, regardless of whether the drug was as controversial and closely regulated as LSD. Further, although survey respondents most frequently listed psychotherapy as their area of psychedelic research interest, other suggestions such as studies in religion, self-growth in therapists and other healthy individuals, creativity, problem solving, "facilitation of the paranormal," business management, and "apparent X-ray-like effects under the drugs" (mentioned only once) went far beyond the bounds of conventional medical drug research.[14] For the FDA, IND research was meant to establish the safety and efficacy of a drug in the treatment of a specific medical condition.[15] Rather than facilitating broad interdisciplinary investigation, INDs regulated research for the ultimate purpose of developing a new drug into a commercial medical product. For many interested in the research potential of psychedelics, their proposals—and potentially their qualifications—simply did not fit with the formalized framework of drug research under the Drug Amendments of 1962.

Ultimately, although the increased regulation may have had some impact, the decline in LSD research in the 1970s can be more convincingly explained through the outcome of the clinical trials of the late 1960s, as discussed in the previous chapter. With research on the surface appearing to show that LSD therapy was ineffective, institutional and financial support disappeared, and research subsequently dwindled to a close.

Later Research at the Maryland Psychiatric Research Center

As the controlled trials of LSD therapy initiated in the 1960s came to a close in the early 1970s, clinical LSD research in the United States declined. For most of the researchers, the results of their trials had shown that their form of LSD therapy was ineffective so they withdrew from the field. In 1975, the

FDA listed five medical institutions as still authorized to conduct research programs involving LSD administration to human subjects. Besides approved programs at the MPRC, research with LSD and alcoholism was still authorized at the Veterans Administration Hospital in Topeka, Kansas, where Kenneth Godfrey and William Bowen had conducted research, and at the Vista Hill Psychiatric Foundation in California, through which UCLA researcher Keith Ditman had conducted his trial. Additionally, research with psychotic patients was approved at the Medical College of Birmingham, Alabama, as was research involving psychotherapy with chronic LSD users at the Langley Porter Neuropsychiatric Institute in California.[16]

Although LSD research was still permitted at these institutions, it is not clear whether it was actually taking place. In 1975, Levine commented that Godfrey still occasionally administered LSD "even though his own previous studies don't support it."[17] Indeed, Godfrey's interest in LSD had not waned over the early 1970s, despite William Bowen's analysis of his results as being no better than other treatments. In Clark's 1972 survey, he complained of his lack of funding to hire good therapists for research, and in 1975 he told the *New York Times* that he was considering withdrawing from the field altogether because of government pressure and red tape.[18] The other approved research programs were most likely inactive.[19] The MPRC was certainly the only institution from which published reports of systematic studies were still emanating.

At the MPRC, psychedelic research continued despite new internal obstacles, as well as the new registration requirements of the Controlled Substances Act. In the early 1970s, as results were being published for the four original Spring Grove trials of psychedelic therapy, almost the entire senior psychedelic research team departed the MPRC. In July 1971, Walter Pahnke tragically drowned while scuba diving in Maine at the age of forty. Pahnke's close colleague William Richards described him as intellectually brilliant but also impulsive and accident prone. Pahnke had entered the rocky ocean alone, too impatient to wait for his wife to join him, despite it being his first time diving. His body was never recovered.[20] Pahnke was at the time director of clinical sciences research at the MPRC, the division that oversaw psychedelic research. Since his arrival in 1967, Pahnke had been central driving force in the research team; Savage later described the significance of his loss as "incalculable."[21]

Sanford Unger, whose name last appeared on an MPRC publication in 1972, left for medical reasons. Charles Savage departed the MPRC around

1973, taking up the positions of chief of psychiatry and director of drug abuse programs at the Baltimore Veterans Administration Hospital. He was also by then associate professor of psychiatry at the University of Maryland.[22] Why Savage left the MPRC, and in doing so ended his long career with psychedelics, is not clear. Likely, after twenty-four years of research culminated in disappointing results and with the writing on the wall about LSD's future, Savage simply decided it was time to move on. Later in life Savage worked as a psychiatrist for the US Virgin Islands Department of Health, before retiring to become a medical missionary in Guatemala and publishing poetry in Spanish after completing a master's degree in the language. He died in 2007, at the age of eighty-nine.[23] Stanislav Grof also left the MPRC in 1973, motivated by difficulties in obtaining support for new research, disagreements with management, and a lack of employment opportunities for his wife in Baltimore. With extensive unanalyzed data from his years of research and book offers from various publishers, Grof relocated to the Esalen Institute in California to write several monographs on his work.[24]

The loss of these researchers presented a threat to the future of psychedelic research at the MPRC. Not only had they been critical to the initiation, design, and conduct of the Spring Grove and MPRC clinical trials, but they also held many positions of authority in the MPRC. However, Kurland remained superintendent of the center, and he continued to focus much of its research on psychedelics. Additionally, by the early 1970s many of the originally more junior members of the MPRC psychedelic research team, such as Richards, were highly experienced in psychedelic research and were able to sustain the program. Richards, who held masters degrees in psychology and divinity, had joined the Spring Grove research team as a therapist in 1967. In prior years he had also studied under renowned psycholytic therapist Hanscarl Leuner at Georg-August University in Germany and worked as a research assistant to prominent humanistic psychologist Abraham Maslow.[25] At the MPRC Richards had been heavily involved in the research treating terminally ill cancer patients. He led this research after the senior researchers departed and through it earned his PhD in 1975.[26] Other committed researchers included Richard Yensen, John Rhead, and Francesco DiLeo.

The later years of psychedelic research at the MPRC were characterized by experimentation with new forms of psychedelic therapy. The focus of research changed from LSD to the shorter-acting psychedelic dipropyltryptamine. This move was not prompted by either disappointment in the results of their previous LSD studies or overwhelming controversy over the drug,

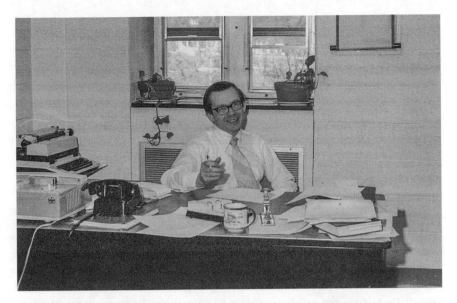

William Richards in his office in the Maryland Psychiatric Research Center, circa 1972. Photo by Richard Yensen.

but was instead a long-planned evolution of the research program. As early as 1966, Kurland had stated that if he found positive results for psychedelic therapy with LSD, then he would look for a shorter-acting psychedelic drug that would render treatment more practical as a routine therapy.[27] The researchers began experimenting with DPT in the early 1970s and found it to have subjective effects similar to those of LSD but with a four- to six-hour period of action (half that of LSD) and a quicker transition back to normal consciousness. If psychedelic therapy with DPT could be as effective as with LSD, then the drug's shorter period of action would make treatment much easier for both therapists and patients, making it a more attractive treatment. While it was not the primary reason to switch, the researchers did also consider the lack of stigma around the drug, which was barely known outside of medicine, as an added benefit.[28]

The MPRC researchers used DPT in a number of studies, some of which were closely related to their previous LSD trials and some of which explored other forms of therapy. In 1973 the researchers published results from an uncontrolled pilot study of psychedelic therapy with DPT in the treatment of fifty-one alcoholic patients. The form of treatment employed was the same as in the LSD study, except that patients received up to 6 drug sessions, with an average of 1.86. Positive results were found, closely mirroring the rate of success for high-dose LSD therapy.[29] Another uncontrolled pilot study, published in 1979, also confirmed that DPT could have a similar therapeutic effect to LSD: thirty cancer patients received a single DPT session in a psychedelic therapy framework, with a comparison of pre- and posttreatment tests showing significant improvements in their psychological states.[30]

In addition to this psychedelic research with DPT, the MPRC researchers explored using the drug in psycholytic therapy. Psycholytic therapy had not previously been employed at Spring Grove State Hospital or the MPRC, and it had not been popular in the United States since the start of the 1960s. Nevertheless, it had remained popular in Europe throughout that decade, and Grof was highly experienced with the treatment from his previous research in Czechoslovakia. Before he left the MPRC, Grof influenced the research team to take a greater interest in using psychedelics to aid conventional forms of psychotherapy.[31] In 1973, the team published results of a partially controlled study of DPT-assisted psychotherapy with eighteen alcoholic patients. After one or two drug-free psychotherapy sessions, the patients underwent six to eight further sessions where they received either a low dose of DPT or an inert placebo, on a randomized double-blind basis. The low dose attenuated both the intensity and the duration of the drug's effects; the sessions lasted just 1.5–2 hours. Based on postsession ratings made by both therapists and patients, the researchers found that DPT significantly enhanced recall of memories, emotional expressiveness, self-exploration, and psychodynamic resolution in psychotherapy sessions.[32]

The researchers also conducted a small pilot study of methylenedioxy-amphetamine (MDA)–assisted psychotherapy with ten outpatients suffering from neuroses. Chemically related to amphetamine, MDA produced milder effects than psychedelics such as LSD or DPT did.[33] It produced therapeutically useful effects such as increased insight, empathy, and openness but with fewer perceptual changes, visions, and peak experiences. The tested treatment saw patients undergo two to four MDA sessions, as part of a two- to six-month course of psychotherapy. The conduct of the drug sessions incorporated elements of both psychedelic and psycholytic therapy. The researchers reported in 1976 that the treatment significantly benefited their patients.[34] Another study saw patients who were undergoing private psychotherapy referred to the MPRC for the full psychedelic therapy procedure (with LSD or DPT), to study whether it could significantly progress their ongoing therapy. Based on clinical impressions, psychoanalytically oriented psychiatrist Margret Berendes reported that the treatment greatly benefited her patients.[35]

The last major controlled study using psychedelics at the MPRC tested the efficacy of DPT therapy in the treatment of alcoholism. Reported in 1977, the researchers attempted to learn from their past research by using both a modified treatment technique and a clearer control condition than low-dose psychedelic therapy. Nevertheless, problems again emerged in the conduct of the trial that led to insignificant results. The trial's design saw 174 patients randomly assigned to one of three treatment groups: routine hospital treatment, or routine hospital treatment plus either DPT therapy or individual psychotherapy. This design had the advantage of providing a clear baseline control group in the form of the routine hospital treatment group and a control for the psychotherapy element of DPT therapy in the individual psychotherapy group. With such distinct comparative treatments, blind administration could not be achieved. However, as in the previous trials, the researchers ensured objective ratings of outcome by having social workers who were blind to patients' treatment groups perform follow-up assessments with standardized psychological tests. Patients in the DPT group received up to six drug sessions at the therapist's discretion. After several preparatory drug-free psychotherapy interviews, patients underwent at least one session of psycholytic therapy with a low dose of DPT. Besides being therapeutic, the researchers considered these sessions as further preparation for later high-dose sessions. Psycholytic sessions were interspersed with further drug-free interviews. When the therapist deemed them ready, patients then received at least one high-dose psychedelic therapy session.[36]

At the six-month follow-up point, the researchers found no significant differences in the results among the three treatment groups. At twelve months, results for occupational adjustment and sobriety significantly favored individual psychotherapy. Although this trial's design had seemed watertight, the researchers ultimately concluded that its open nature likely influenced the insignificant results. Before entering the study, patients were fully informed of the three treatment groups and the fact that they would be randomly allocated to one. This resulted in high and varied dropout rates among the treatment groups, as patients who signed up hoping for one treatment were assigned to another. After the dropouts, each treatment group's population was no longer a representative sample of the original total pool of patients but rather a self-selected group of those most motivated for that treatment. The higher the dropout rate in a group, the more refined the population and therefore the greater the bias toward treatment success. Unsurprisingly, the routine hospital treatment group had the highest dropout rate. The psychotherapy group had a dropout rate similar to that of the DPT group at the conclusion of treatment, but significantly more patients could not be located for follow-up assessment. As it was likely that those who could not be located were leading an unstable life and had not fared well after treatment, those who could be located represented a further refinement of the patient sample: the "cream of the crop." The comparative assessment of results among the groups was thus skewed in favor of the control conditions, as their sample sizes were smaller and more highly refined toward treatment success.[37]

Despite this analysis, in their report the MPRC researchers also more broadly reflected on the largely unrealistic expectations held for psychedelic therapy over the past two decades. Gone was their assumption that a single psychedelic peak experience would reliably lead to lasting changes in behavior, personality, and life adjustment. As they wrote, "The difficulty with this assumption was that it proved to be true on a frequent enough basis to be very seductive and to lure many researchers into naive and almost magical expectations about the efficacy and general application of such a treatment approach, but it proved to be false frequently enough to wash out differential treatment effects in controlled studies."[38] Although the researchers had attempted to move past this approach, by employing multiple sessions of both psycholytic and psychedelic therapy, they still found the treatment had limitations. They reported—as other researchers had also observed—that dramatic positive changes in outlook and self-image resulting from peak experiences could be difficult to maintain and integrate into everyday life when faced with the patient's deeply ingrained attitudes and often insufficient support structures. In fact, the undoing of treatment effects could begin as early as the patients' return to the alcoholic ward immediately after treatment, as other patients undermined their new and unusual insights and perspectives. The researchers now believed that posttreatment support networks, perhaps in the style of Alcoholics Anonymous, could help patients to maintain and integrate their new outlooks.

A 1977 summary of the field of psychedelic research by longtime Spring Grove/MPRC researchers O. Lee McCabe and Thomas Hanlon concluded in even more measured tones. After similarly stressing the need to move beyond the one-shot approach, the researchers played down the ultimate public health implications of psychedelic therapy. Because the treatment procedure was labor intensive and required extensive training to adequately perform, psychedelic therapy was impractical for treating patients on a mass scale. Finally, they stressed that psychedelics could be of value to psychiatry "only insofar as therapists possess the necessary skills to use them."[39] LSD therapy could never have an intrinsic level of treatment efficacy, as its effectiveness was ultimately a reflection of the therapist using it. LSD was a tool—a useful tool in the right hands, but not a miracle cure.

The End of Psychedelic Research

Psychedelic research at the MPRC finally came to a close in 1976 for reasons essentially unrelated to LSD. Over the 1960s, LSD research had flourished in Maryland partly because Kurland had been able to facilitate it through his roles as director of research for both Spring Grove State Hospital and the state Department of Mental Hygiene, as well as superintendent of the MPRC. However, in 1973 a controversy began over the apparently poor management of the MPRC under Kurland and the state commissioner of mental hygiene. Over the next three years prolonged disputes over the MPRC raged in public, judicial, and legislative arenas, eventually resulting in the transfer of its management to the University of Maryland. In this transfer, the MPRC was reorganized, Kurland and many other staff members were replaced, the research focus of the center was changed, and psychedelic research was terminated. Despite this eventuality, the psychedelic research at the MPRC was not a focus of the uproar, which was closely covered in the *Baltimore Sun*. The final demise of psychedelic research was not due to restrictive regulations or controversy over LSD's nonmedical use. Instead, after the disappointments of the controlled clinical trials of LSD psychotherapy, research had survived at a diminished scale purely because of the continued enthusiasm of researchers such as Kurland. With the lack of wider interest and support, the future of LSD research was tied to the careers of its champions.

Kurland first became the subject of controversy in January 1973, as part of a state audit of Friends Medical Science Research Center. Kurland, with the support of the state, had founded the nonprofit organization (commonly referred to simply as Friends) in 1955 for the purpose of obtaining and administering federal and private funding for psychiatric research in Maryland. By the early 1970s, Friends handled all federal research grants for Maryland's state hospitals, as well as private and state grants; employed 150 professional staff; and ran a neurological laboratory, group homes, and clinics. Kurland retained the position of director of research in the organization and was a member of its board of directors and central research authority. State legislative auditor Pierce J. Lambdin criticized many aspects of Friends' management of state funds, including failure to account for how they were spent, running at a significant cash deficit, and making large payouts to state employees. His report singled out payments totaling almost $14,000 to Kurland, who was also receiving a salary from the state as superintendent of the MPRC. Lambdin's report criticized the relationship between Friends and state employees for being so confused that it was impossible to tell whether state employees such as Kurland were performing work for Friends on the state's time. The executive director of Friends defended the organization's financial practices and stated that Kurland had been made director of research at the insistence of the state Health Department; however, Kurland was forced to resign his positions at Friends.[40]

Four months later, the *Baltimore Sun* again reported on criticism against Kurland; this time it was over the management of the MPRC. The state commissioner of mental health Bertram Pepper was investigating the research center after having received a letter from former MPRC medicinal chemist Reuben Sawdaye accusing Kurland and the director of the MPRC's biochemistry department Richard Von Korff of "mismanagement of state funds and mistreatment of employees." Specifically, Sawdaye made complaints regarding management's purchase of expensive, unnecessary equipment; the poor management and lack of productivity in the biochemistry department; Kurland's censorship of all staff communication with the outside world; the close relationship between the MPRC and Friends; and the treatment of staff under Von Korff, stating, "Never during my scientific career have I seen such lack of co-operation between departments and individuals, and so much suspicion and distrust." Kurland had recently fired Sawdaye from the MPRC, which Sawdaye believed had been done to make way for a Friends scientist. He subsequently filed a complaint with the state Department of Personnel, complaining that the firing was "arbitrary, capricious, unlawful and personally motivated."[41] Soon after Sawdaye, MPRC educational psychologist John Lenox also wrote to the commissioner of mental health accusing Kurland of wasting taxpayer money. Lenox had also recently been dismissed from the center by Kurland. Lenox criticized Kurland's dismantling of a recently completed $80,000 physiology laboratory because he had "lost interest" in it, as well as his "devoting most of his energies to promoting 'a dream of a $10 million cancer project in which psychedelics are given to cancer patients.'"[42] Significantly, this was the only time that psychedelic research at the MPRC was mentioned in the newspaper's extensive coverage of the center's management controversy.

As a result of these disputes, in June 1973 an MPRC management committee fired Von Korff. The state health department also conducted an investigation into the center that resulted in Sawdaye and Lenox's reinstatement and a limited reorganization of management. However, these developments did not settle the matter, and in March 1974 MPRC researchers began again voicing complaints. In May, Kurland again fired Sawdaye and Lenox, along with biochemist Mishrilal Jain and psychologist Lawrence Gaines, shortly after they had called for the replacement of both Kurland and the MPRC's associate director T. Glyne Williams, both publicly and in writing to the state secretary of health and mental hygiene Neil Solomon. In terminating their employment, Kurland cited poor performance and "taking public actions which were not in the best interest of the center." Throughout the controversy, Kurland declined to publicly defend his management of the MPRC. While the researchers complained that their dismissals were simply a "reprisal" for their criticism, Solomon backed Kurland's decision. Robert Campbell, the health department's coordinator of psychological services and research, also defended the management of the center. In response to their firings, the four MPRC scientists filled a federal lawsuit for reinstatement and damages, with Kurland, Solomon, and Campbell named as defendants. The lawsuit would not be settled until August 1975, when an arbiter ordered that Jain, Sawdaye, and Lenox be reinstated to their positions at the MPRC.[43]

In the intervening period, the state House Appropriations Subcommittee on Health and Education responded to the controversy by ordering an audit of the MPRC. In March 1975, auditor Lambdin, who had performed the 1973 audit of Friends, reported that the center's management was "inadequate," and had resulted in low staff morale. He criticized the close relationship between the center and Friends and argued that the Health Department's attempts to remedy the problems at the center had been ineffective. Lambdin recommended that control of the MPRC be transferred from the state commissioner of mental hygiene to the University of Maryland School of Medicine, and that "a clear separation" be made between the center and Friends.[44]

Despite protests from Campbell and Solomon, in May 1976 the state legislature went through with the recommendations, passing legislation that transferred control of the MPRC to the University of Maryland as of 1 January 1977. They also ordered the new management to focus the center's research on schizophrenia—a recommendation that had come from the American Psychiatric Association.[45] The association had recently completed a review of the state's mental health programs at the request of Governor Marvin Mandel. The review reported that the MPRC was isolated from the state's other mental health facilities and "appears to be an ivory tower, where work is done in eso-

teric areas such as the use of LSD in psychotherapy." This work did not seem
to be "particularly relevant" to the mental health needs of the state.[46] By the
late 1970s, therefore, the nation's leading psychiatric organization considered
LSD research not as a controversial area of bunk science but rather as a purely
intellectual curiosity with limited public health implications.

In the MPRC's transition over to the University of Maryland, Kurland was
replaced, and the new management dismissed many of the staff, on the basis
that "the expertise of the men was not appropriate for the new goals of the
center."[47] A committee of the university's School of Medicine terminated the
center's psychedelic research program and disbanded the clinical sciences department. Richards was the last member of the psychedelic research team to
leave the MPRC. He left later in 1977, after being invited to stay on part time
for one year so that he could retain his health insurance benefits, as his wife
had recently been diagnosed with cancer. Even at the end, Richards maintained FDA approval to conduct psychedelic research at the center, but the
lack of funding and institutional support prevented it.[48]

The University of Maryland School of Medicine's termination of the
MPRC psychedelic research program may have been influenced by a controversy over clandestine army and CIA LSD research that erupted in the
press in 1975. Reports accused the School of Medicine of participating in
army LSD research in the 1950s, where the drug had been given to subjects
without their knowledge.[49] Therefore, the medical school may have wished
to distance itself from the drug. However, coverage in the *Baltimore Sun* had
been careful to distinguish between the unethical forms of research conducted by the army and CIA, and legitimate medical research. Editorials and
reports contrasted the murky motives and lack of informed consent in the
CIA and army research with the admirable motives, careful attention to informed consent, and extensive patient preparation and support in the MPRC
research: as one editorial author commented, "That federal institutions have
sponsored LSD experiments is not a scandal, but the circumstances of some
experiments might be."[50] Indeed, the paper continued to publish articles on
the MPRC research that not only presented it in a positive or neutral light
but that lamented its demise: according to one editorial, treatment results
so far suggested that "research not only should not be halted but should be
expanded."[51] Whether or not this controversy played a role in the School of
Medicine's decision to terminate psychedelic research at the MPRC, LSD research was ultimately unlikely to survive the change in the center's management, as a result of the general declining prospects of psychedelic research,

the absence of a strong champion in Kurland, and the mandate to overhaul the center and focus on schizophrenia.

Psychedelic Research and Development

As this book has established, the difficulties in convincingly demonstrating LSD psychotherapy's efficacy through randomized controlled trials, as required under the Drug Amendments of 1962, was the primary issue that frustrated research and led to its demise. Without proof of efficacy, LSD could not be become an approved tool of psychiatry. However, proof of efficacy would still not have automatically resulted in LSD becoming a marketable pharmaceutical—a sponsor was still needed to collate all the necessary data on the drug's safety and efficacy for a specific indication and submit it to the FDA in the form of a New Drug Application. Besides research, LSD needed development. A developer's role was not only turning the results of scientists' research into an NDA, but also directing and coordinating research toward that goal. The case of LSD research highlights the distinctions between the usually intertwined processes of drug research and development.

Since LSD research began in the United States in 1949, it had progressed with little developmental oversight. Prior to 1962, Sandoz had distributed the drug widely and free of charge to interested researchers, with recommendations that it be explored as a tool to facilitate psychotherapy and to study psychoses. Other than this, it appears that the company's only effort to stimulate research was providing some funding for conferences.[52] Sandoz did not submit an NDA for LSD, despite needing only to supply proof of safety when used as directed on the label. After the passage of the Drug Amendments of 1962, Sandoz took a somewhat more active approach in overseeing LSD research, by formally acting as the drug's sponsor and voluntarily restricting research to hospital-based studies funded or approved by federal or state agencies. While the field of LSD research became more organized in the mid-1960s, with numerous researchers conducting controlled trials of LSD therapy with alcoholics, this does not appear to be primarily a result of Sandoz's influence. Instead, independent researchers initiated the studies on the basis of the great scientific and medical significance of the results reported from earlier uncontrolled research. That the new research took the form of larger-scale controlled trials appears symptomatic of the formalization of pharmaceutical research under the 1962 amendments, rather than a result of Sandoz's sponsorship. Sandoz withdrew its sponsorship of LSD research before these studies concluded because of the negative publicity surrounding the drug. It is thus difficult to determine what intentions the company had for LSD, if any.

In the absence of evidence, it can be reasoned that commercial as well as scientific factors would have influenced Sandoz to take a backseat in LSD's development. While there was much scientific and clinical interest in LSD as a potential tool in psychiatry, its effects were clearly unconventional. There were precedents for drug-assisted psychotherapy; however, the barbiturates and amphetamines used in those treatments had been established in the market on the basis of their other conventional uses. There was therefore no precedent for developing a drug through FDA approval on the basis of its variable subjective effects. Even if Sandoz had successfully developed LSD into an approved pharmaceutical, it was unlikely to be a hugely profitable product for the company. Psychedelic therapy usually involved only one administration of LSD. Psycholytic therapy involved a greater number of drug sessions, but the number was still relatively small, typically less than fifty. The commercial potential of LSD paled in comparison to tranquilizers, antidepressants, and anxiolytics that were commonly taken every day for extended periods. After Sandoz's patent for LSD expired in 1963, there was even less financial incentive for developing the drug, as generic manufacturers could reap the profits of Sandoz's investment.[53]

Ultimately, LSD's potential in psychiatry was of greater medical and scientific significance than commercial. Faced with an unconventional drug with a difficult development path and limited potential profitability, the prudent approach was to release it to the scientific community and see whether a marketable use for it emerged. If so, then a more limited investment could turn the independent researchers' work into an NDA. Officials at Sandoz must not have believed that this point had been reached, at least not before the controversy over LSD's nonmedical use made the drug's commercial potential even less worth pursuing. While the public controversy over the drug did not end clinical LSD research in the United States, by influencing Sandoz to withdraw from the field, it did make the drug's development into an approved pharmaceutical much less likely.

The importance of a pharmaceutical firm's role in developing an experimental drug into an approved medicine went beyond sponsoring research and collating the results into an NDA, to determining how efficacy should be conceptualized for that specific drug. The Drug Amendments of 1962 required that an NDA contain "substantial evidence that the drug will have the effect it purports or is represented to have under the conditions of use prescribed, recommended, or suggested *in the proposed labeling.*"[54] How the drug was to be labeled defined the kind of treatment effect that needed to be demonstrated through controlled trials. As historian Peter Temin has explained, this had profound implications for drug development: "Experts, by insisting on changes in the drug's label, can change the effectiveness of that drug. . . . If a drug has any desirable effect at all, the process of getting FDA approval will be centered on the label."[55]

Of the post-1962 controlled trials of LSD therapy with alcoholics, all except Keith Ditman's evaluated the long-term effects of treatment on drinking behavior, and often aspects of psychopathology and social adjustment—their research questions all equated to "does LSD therapy cure alcoholism?"[56] This may have been the most medically significant question, but it was necessary to establish such an ambitious effect only if that was the claim to be made on the labeling. This is illustrated in the case of Antabuse (disulfiram), another drug used to treat alcoholism. Ludwig, Levine, and Stark had tested the efficacy of Antabuse as well as LSD in their clinical trial. They found that it was also an ineffective treatment for alcoholism. The drug was, however, unquestionably effective at causing alcohol consumption to produce severely unpleasant physical effects in patients. This effect was useful in helping alcoholics to abstain from drinking, but only insofar as they were motivated to stay on the drug. Ayerst Laboratories therefore labeled Antabuse as "an aid in the management of selected chronic alcoholic patients," rather than as a cure for alcoholism. Indeed, the labeling explicitly stated the drug's limitations in treatment: "Used alone, without proper motivation and without supportive therapy, it is not a cure for alcoholism, and it is unlikely that it will have more than a brief effect on the drinking pattern of the chronic alcoholic." Reviewing the drug's efficacy in 1969, the FDA concluded that Antabuse was "an effective adjunct in the management of selected chronic alcoholic patients."[57] By promoting it as simply an "aid in management," the drug was approved despite its very limited efficacy as an actual treatment. Physicians were then left to decide for themselves how useful it ultimately was.

Such a tactic might have been possible with LSD. Rather than focus on the disappointing long-term results of treatment, a developer could have analyzed clinical trial results for what effects treatment reliably did have on patients. The Spring Grove researchers found significant results in favor of high-dose psychedelic therapy at the six-month follow-up point, and even Leo Hollister found his chemotherapeutic form of LSD therapy effective at the two-month follow-up point. Additionally, patients in many of the studies reported that their drug experience was beneficial and had motivated them to stop drinking but then returned to drinking when faced with life's difficulties after discharge. As with Antabuse, a developer's claim of effect for LSD could have focused on it being a tool of treatment, rather than a treatment in itself: an aid in motivating patients to stop drinking, rather than a treatment that causes them to stop drinking. For LSD, this would still have been a more difficult path to approval than it had been for Antabuse, as that drug's potential usefulness was based on an objective physiological response—it was a magic bullet drug. Using LSD as a tool to promote patient motivation still required crafting a subjective drug experience to inspire a change in the patient's personality. This would be a highly unorthodox use for a drug in medicine, and proving that it could reliably be achieved through controlled trials would still be very difficult. Nevertheless, it could potentially have been less difficult than proving that LSD therapy cured alcoholism.

Without a developer, LSD research moved sideways instead of forward. Each research team employed a different treatment method and clinical trial design, so results were not directly comparable. Furthermore, each research team set out to test a hypothesis that was needlessly ambitious, at least for the sake of FDA approval. Even had the researchers established the efficacy of some form of LSD therapy for some indication, that still would not have resulted in FDA approval unless someone used the results to support an NDA. Establishing LSD as an approved therapeutic tool clearly required the skills of a developer as well as those of researchers. But did this developer have to be a pharmaceutical company? As discussed in chapter 4, the Spring Grove researchers did at least briefly consider submitting an NDA for LSD when Sandoz withdrew its sponsorship of research. Charles Savage mentioned the significant costs involved as a major obstacle to this idea. As commercial distributors, pharmaceutical companies were in the best position to act as a drug's developer, as they were both motivated and equipped to make the necessary investment in the interests of turning it into profit. However, in the case of a drug with limited profit potential but great medical significance, there was nothing theoretically stopping a nonprofit government or private organization from acting as a developer and sponsoring an NDA.

In practice, though, the case of lithium's development as a mood stabilizer for manic-depressive patients suggests that the cooperation of a pharmaceutical company was necessary to develop a drug through to FDA approval. Lithium had been in limited use in medicine in the United States since the mid-nineteenth century, but the FDA banned it in 1949 because of dangers that appeared when it was used as a salt substitute in diets for cardiac patients. Unfortunately, this happened just as its usefulness in treating mania was discovered in Australia. Over the next two decades, evidence of its efficacy mounted, despite vigorous debate over how to evaluate it as a prophylactic for recurrent bouts of mania and depression. Rowell Laboratories, a small pharmaceutical firm in Minnesota, had been manufacturing supplies for American investigators. However, as the drug was unpatentable, there was little incentive for firms to push it through the NDA process. The drug was finally licensed in 1970, after several prominent psychopharmacologists, including Jonathan Cole, Nathan Kline, and Frank Ayd, publicly promoted the drug and pressured the FDA to approve it. Kline even attempted to convince the American College of Neuropsychopharmacology to sponsor the drug. Responding to the pressure, the FDA finally persuaded major pharmaceutical firms Smith, Kline, and French and Pfizer, to submit NDAs, which they did along with Rowell.[58]

Lithium therefore came to market through the combined effort of independent researchers, FDA officials, and pharmaceutical companies. For LSD, had the results of the controlled trials of the 1960s clearly demonstrated the efficacy of treatment, such a development path could have been possible. Sandoz or another pharmaceutical firm may have been convinced to sponsor the drug if it had the support of the government and the scientific community. However, FDA and NIMH officials were unconvinced of its efficacy, psychiatry was increasingly focused on magic bullet drug treatments, and the public controversy over the drug's nonmedical use continued. Considering LSD's unfavorable status in both medicine and the public, and the lack of a clear financial incentive, there was little chance that a firm could be convinced to aid in the drug's development. By the time psychedelic research came to a halt at the MPRC in 1976, there had long been little prospect of LSD becoming an approved tool of psychiatry in the United States.

Conclusion

In the 1970s, LSD psychotherapy research died a slow and quiet death. Having fallen from its previous status as a potential medical marvel, research continued out of the public eye in Maryland. There, unimpeded by further restrictions placed on LSD, researchers continued to advance their treatment techniques yet still struggled to find a way to demonstrate their effectiveness through controlled clinical trials. While Clark's survey shows that there was certainly still interest in psychedelics in niche circles, mainstream psychiatry had moved on and funding had dried up, leaving Kurland the lone champion capable of facilitating an FDA-approved psychedelic research program. Kurland's powerful administrative positions in the state's organizations for psychiatric research underlay the successes and continuation of his program. Yet his managerial style with some staff members led to a revolt that ultimately brought his thirteen-year psychedelic research program down. Nevertheless, despite being stripped of his roles and facilities, Kurland's quest to prove the therapeutic potential of psychedelics was still not finished.

Epilogue

Resurrection

On the basis of this preliminary investigation, L.S.D. 25 may offer a means for more readily gaining access to the chronically withdrawn patients. It may also serve as a new tool for shortening psychotherapy. We hope further investigation justifies our present impression.

Anthony Busch and Warren Johnson, 1950

Despite the promise that LSD's unique and dramatic effects have held out, experiments seeking to use the powerful psychological forces of the LSD experience for man's benefit have been engulfed in uncertainty. . . .

. . . [I]t can be hoped that more research will lead eventually to effective therapies that will heal—more quickly and comfortably—the psychic wounds that leave so many people handicapped and alienated.

Albert Kurland, 1979

Comparing the reports of LSD researchers from the time the drug first arrived in the United States to those from the end of the period of its widespread investigation, it can appear that little progress was made in more than twenty-five years of study: the conclusion remained that LSD had therapeutic potential but that more research was needed to confirm this. The continuing uncertainty over LSD's therapeutic efficacy was not due to a lack of research: as early as 1960, a survey of forty-four LSD researchers found that they had administered the drug on more than 25,000 occasions to almost 5,000 patients and volunteer subjects.[1] Albert Kurland's team alone treated more than 700 patients over a thirteen-year period.[2] LSD psychotherapy was the subject of hundreds of research reports and numerous major conferences.[3] With seven controlled studies evaluating the use of LSD in the treatment of alcoholism published between 1967 and 1971, the question of its efficacy should have been resolved by the early 1970s.

Regulatory developments in the 1960s and early 1970s certainly impacted

LSD research, but not in the manner typically depicted. The Drug Amendments of 1962 radically changed the nature of pharmaceutical research and development in the United States—for all drugs, not just LSD—resulting in LSD research becoming a smaller-scale but more sophisticated venture. However, neither this legislation nor the increasing prohibition of LSD that followed banned research. Officials of the FDA and NIMH may have held a skeptical attitude toward the unconventional methods and astounding results that many LSD psychotherapists promoted; yet they actively supported research until the point where it seemed that the data produced had debunked the treatment. Ultimately, as Kurland explained in 1979, the uncertainty over LSD's utility in psychiatry "arises from scientific disagreement, journalistic excess, and the limitations imposed by current research methods in carrying out controlled studies."[4] The increasingly rigid mode of pharmaceutical research and development in the 1960s may not have prohibited research, but it did install a research framework that was inhospitable to such a unique treatment form as psychedelic therapy. Without the financial and strategic backing of a pharmaceutical company, LSD research faded away in the 1970s after researchers struggled to convincingly demonstrate treatment efficacy through the methods required.

The transfer of the Maryland Psychiatric Research Center to the University of Maryland in 1976 ended the sole surviving psychedelic research program in the United States. Yet it did not end Kurland's efforts to explore the therapeutic effects of the drugs. In 1979, Kurland teamed up with ex-MPRC researchers Richard Yensen and Francesco DiLeo to revive LSD research, and their initial application to the FDA to amend Kurland's long-standing IND to include a new study met with approval. They subsequently began working on a small study with cancer patients in collaboration with North Charles General Hospital and the University of Maryland, where from 1980 Kurland held the position of research professor of psychiatry. Over the following years they treated approximately ten patients.[5]

In 1982 their run of success with the FDA hit its first major hurdle. In August Kurland again submitted an application to amend his IND, this time for a project that aimed to improve the researchers' understanding of the psychedelic experience and its role in treatment outcome, as well as their ability to predict which patients were most likely to respond to treatment. They hoped that this research would develop knowledge and assessment procedures that would assist in future controlled studies of treatment efficacy. In October, the FDA's Paul Leber replied that he was not satisfied that it was safe to administer LSD to psychiatric patients and that in fact "current staff of the agency question the use of psychotomimetic agents in any population."[6] After Kurland replied with a full outline of his considerable experience with the drug, Leber backtracked somewhat but still maintained that the IND amendment could not be approved on several grounds.

First, he and his staff were still not satisfied with the safety of LSD psychotherapy and requested that Kurland present his safety data before the Psychopharmacologic Drugs Advisory Committee. Second, he highlighted that the IND regulations required that drug sponsors not "unduly prolong distribution of drugs for investigational use" and argued that Kurland's long history of research with the drug could constitute "prolonged use." Therefore, a close examination of Kurland's proposal was justified. Lastly, and most significantly, Leber questioned whether a study of LSD psychotherapy could be justified at all, because of the methodological difficulties in evaluating its efficacy: "A sine qua non of any meaningful research on psychotherapy is the existence of valid and reliable outcome measures to assess the effects of psychotherapy. Thus, even if I were convinced that LSD posed no immediate hazard to most patients who are exposed it, I would still be unable to conclude, on the basis of what I know about research in psychotherapy, that a valid and meaningful experiment to assess LSD as an adjunct to psychotherapy could be conducted."[7] Later in the letter, Leber elaborated that his skepticism over the possibility of a "bona fide experiment" to assess LSD psychotherapy related to it being "unlikely that an effective blind control for an active CNS [central nervous system] substance is possible." At the ensuing meeting of the Psychopharmacologic Drugs Advisory Committee, Kurland and his colleagues satisfied the committee that their research plan was acceptably safe and that the prolonged nature of their research program was justified. However, the committee still rejected the proposal on the basis that the assessment procedures in the study were too subjective and therefore could not demonstrate efficacy. This was despite the fact that the study was not designed to evaluate efficacy, and that it was indeed aimed at improving the precision of future efficacy studies.[8]

With Leber's comments and the committee's decision, the framework for pharmaceutical research and development set out under the Drug Amendments of 1962 reached a new level of rigidity, but one that highlights the tensions that had frustrated research over the previous decades. The difficulties of demonstrating the efficacy of LSD psychotherapy through controlled trials had led to inconclusive or negative results and the subsequent demise of research. Now, the FDA, acknowledging the difficulties, instead of suggesting alternative forms or standards of evidence for efficacy, simply dismissed LSD psychotherapy as a legitimate research direction, as its effectiveness could not be established. Further, the scope of legitimate drug research narrowed, to include only studies that could directly demonstrate effectiveness in medical use. While this book has focused on attempts at this form of research, to many researchers the potential of psychedelics went far beyond treating mental illness—from broad explorations of human psychology and religion to increasing creativity and promoting wellbeing in healthy individuals. Indeed, later in life Charles Savage lamented that "careful psychological investigations were shoved aside by simplistic outcome research," resulting in LSD research contributing "little to a general psychology or metapsychology."[9]

Congress passed the Drug Amendments of 1962 to ensure that clinical drug research progressed in a safe and scientifically sound manner toward the goal of developing medicines that were both safe and effective. Although this book has explored the complexity of the concept of drug efficacy and many of the theoretical and practical limitations of randomized controlled trials, in intent, the 1962 amendments were clearly in the best interests of American society. Ineffective treatments had the potential not only to waste the time and money of patients and health care providers but also to cause harm by replacing other more effective treatments. The randomized controlled trial was an ideal methodology for evaluating most conventional drug treatments. Yet, while the long and rigorous process of efficacy evaluation can protect patients from ineffective treatments, it can also harm them by excessively delaying their access to new effective treatments. Regulating efficacy in the best interest of patients involves balancing complex risk-versus-benefit equations.

This book has shown that the negative reports of efficacy for psychedelic therapy in alcoholism were based on flawed research. However, it is ultimately still unclear whether the end result was the public being denied an effective treatment or spared an ineffective one. Prior to 1962, careful uncontrolled empirical research, performed by responsible scientists, led to the discovery of many effective drug treatments. Ultimately, how useful a drug was became clear over time through its widespread routine clinical use. As historian Edward Shorter has emphasized, requiring proof of efficacy through comparison to an inert placebo does not ensure that drugs approved for sale are useful, as they may be effective but less so than other drugs already on the market.[10] Therefore, the market will often remain the ultimate site of efficacy evaluation.

However, the power of pharmaceutical marketing can counteract any survival-of-the-fittest nature of the marketplace, and regardless the sheer quantity of modern pharmaceutical options would seem to render commercial competition an inefficient, if at all effective, arbiter. Therefore, regulatory oversight of drug efficacy does seem necessary. Yet, the case of LSD psychotherapy draws into relief the disadvantages of requiring evidence of efficacy to take too rigid a form. It highlights the need to consider alternative forms of evidence and to sensitively weigh the need for definitive research against the potential significance of treatments, when standard research techniques are problematic. Alcoholism was, and remains, a severely debilitating illness, to both the individual and society, associated with considerable mortality and with limited treatment options. With such an illness, it would seem necessary to ask whether the risk to patients in leaving them untreated outweighs the risk that the apparent benefits from treatment may be due to nonspecific factors.

In fact, in 1962, the Senate Committee on the Judiciary reflected this perspective in its report on the amendment bill, expressing that the intent was not to restrict the availability of new medicines until a scientific consensus had formed but rather simply to protect the public from products marketed on unfounded claims of effect:

> When a drug has been adequately tested by qualified experts and has been found to have the effect claimed for it, this claim should be permitted even though there may be preponderant evidence to the contrary based upon equally reliable studies. There may also be a situation in which a new drug has been studied in a limited number of hospitals and clinics and its effectiveness established only to the satisfaction of a few investigators qualified to use it. There may be many physicians who would deny the effectiveness simply on the basis of a disbelief growing out of their past experience with other drugs or with the diseases involved. Again, the studies may show that the drug will help a substantial percentage of the patients in a given disease condition but will not be effective in other cases. What the committee intends is to permit the claim for this new drug to be made to the medical profession with a proper explanation of the basis on which it rests.
>
> In such a delicate area of medicine, the committee wants to make sure that safe new drugs become available for use by the medical profession so long as they are supported as to effectiveness by a responsible body of opinion.[11]

The scenario outlined by the committee here in many ways describes the state of LSD psychotherapy research in the early 1970s: a minority of qualified and responsible investigators supported the efficacy of psychedelic therapy, based on a limited number of both controlled and uncontrolled studies that showed it to be significantly effective in a substantial subset of patients, but the results of which were contested by other, equally qualified researchers and their studies. Although the FDA never banned or significantly restricted research (at least until the 1980s), and in fact saved it from extinction in 1966, it set the bar for evidence of efficacy higher than had been intended—too high for LSD psychotherapists to reach given the unique challenges that research with the drug entailed.

Yet in one way this analysis is unfair—as no one ever submitted a New Drug Application for LSD, the FDA never had the opportunity to make an official determination on the adequacy of the evidence for its efficacy in treatment. Undoubtedly, much of the responsibility for the failure of LSD psychotherapy rests with Sandoz, which had the resources and expertise to potentially develop the drug through the NDA process, either before or after 1962. Nevertheless, the FDA's expectations for research standards after 1962 were clear, and, in the absence of a strong developmental sponsor in Sandoz, researchers struggled to meet them while maintaining the psychotherapy-focused treatment methods on which the original reports of effectiveness were based.

The Drug Amendments of 1962 did not simply rein in the worst of pharmaceutical research and development but fundamentally reshaped its landscape, in line with the goals, theories, and methods of biomedicine and the highest research standards that had been promoted by experts. This had a particularly significant impact on psychiatry, perhaps the greatest outlier discipline of mainstream medicine. With the lack of clear evidence for the origins of mental illness, psychiatry encompassed a wide variety of divergent and even contradictory etiological theories and treatment approaches. Psychological theories and treatments enjoyed high status in psychiatry for a time in the postwar period, yet psychological approaches always sat awkwardly within psychiatry's broader medical context. Nevertheless, psychiatrists were driven to experiment with all tools at their disposal in the hopes of providing some relief to their patients.

LSD psychotherapy's emergence in the 1950s reflected this eclectic and pragmatic nature of psychiatry, where psychiatrists frequently blended psychological, physical, and pharmacological treatment methods. The Drug Amendments of 1962 changed this scenario, as they required psychiatry's drug treatments to conform to efficacy standards that the unregulated psychotherapies were not. The conceptual and practical difficulties in evaluating LSD psychotherapy through randomized double-blind controlled trials reveals the problematic complexity of the notion of objectivity in clinical research, as underlying the technique was an assumption that a drug's thera-peutic use was based solely on its biological activity. This reflected the magic bullet antibiotics that were pharmacology's greatest success story and that randomized controlled trials had been developed and popularized alongside. The breakthrough psychiatric drugs of the 1950s—the tranquilizers, anti-depressants, and anxiolytics—conformed to the magic bullet form of drug therapy, and their efficacy was easily established through double-blind trials. By contrast, LSD psychotherapy faded from psychiatry as researchers strug-gled to demonstrate the efficacy of their neither purely pharmacological nor psychological treatments. Increasingly, psychopharmacology became solely oriented toward magic bullet treatments, while psychiatrists focusing on psy-chological forms of treatment abandoned their use of drugs as facilitators. Even without the passage of the Drug Amendments of 1962, the success of the magic bullet psychoactive drugs would have led to a tightening of the relationship between psychopharmacology and biological concepts of drug efficacy in mainstream psychiatry. Nevertheless, without the regulation, re-searchers interested in drug-assisted psychotherapy would have faced less-insurmountable obstacles in establishing their niche in psychiatry.

The case of LSD psychotherapy under the Drug Amendments of 1962 highlights the complex interplay among clinical science, regulation, and ther-apeutics in postwar American medicine. Clinical scientists' rising concern for objectivity in research and their experience with the wildly successful magic bullet drugs led them to develop and promote the randomized controlled trial as the ideal form of efficacy testing. Legislators and regulators, concerned that drugs available to the public be effective, incorporated the methodology into the required development path for drugs. In doing so, however, they did not simply ensure that efficacy testing would be objective but shaped future drug research to conform to the magic bullet concept of drug efficacy. For psychi-atry, this drove a wedge between pharmacology and psychology in research and treatment: psychoactive drugs were regulated in a way that presumed they acted objectively on the brain, while psychotherapy remained unregu-lated as it acted subjectively on the mind. The hitherto purely theoretical rift between biological and psychological treatments in psychiatry thus became formalized. Drug-assisted psychotherapy subsequently faded from psychia-try.[12] Clinical science influenced regulation, which in turn influenced clinical science and therapeutics in profound and unintentional ways.

Moreover, by wedding the concept of treatment efficacy to the randomized controlled trial and standardized outcome measures, the amendments more generally helped to steer psychiatry away from focusing on subjective "meaning" in patients' experiences of their illnesses and, in the process and outcome of treatment, toward simply the identification and alleviation of symptoms. With the dominance of psychodynamic forms of psychiatry in the immediate postwar period, the ideal of psychiatric treatment—if frequently not the reality, particularly in understaffed state hospitals—was to focus on patients as individuals with pathologies stemming from unique psychological conflicts, which had roots stretching back into childhood. Psychiatrists uncovered patients' conflicts, helped them to understand their "meaning," and guided them to find new, more constructive interpretations for the life events and feelings that underlay them. Symptoms of pathology were not the target of treatment; their alleviation was a by-product of resolving the conflicts that had produced them. Treatment efficacy was not limited to the alleviation of symptoms but encompassed resolving conflicts, increasing insight, and fostering personal growth. However, as symptoms were the only outcome criteria that could reliably be measured in controlled trials, the focus on randomized controlled trials in medicine after the 1962 amendments reduced the scope of psychiatry's treatments to reducing overt signs of psychopathology, rather than promoting psychological health and growth.

While this was initially true only of psychiatry's drug treatments, by the 1990s even psychotherapy research became primarily focused on randomized controlled trials. To conform to this research standard, studies have primarily involved evaluations of short-term, standardized forms of psychotherapy—primarily cognitive and behavioral forms—in reducing the symptoms of mental disease, based on the increasingly discrete and symptom-focused disease categories defined by the American Psychiatric Association's *Diagnostic and Statistical Manual of Mental Disorders* since its third, 1980 edition (*DSM-III*). Even psychotherapy—at least in its "evidence-based" forms —ultimately came to mimic the model of conventional drug treatment. Psychiatry's increasingly tight focus on the diagnosis and treatment of specific mental diseases—based on the evaluation of symptoms—in the late twentieth century reflected a general return to dominance of biologically oriented psychiatry. Indeed, the practice and evaluation of psychotherapy became largely the domain of clinical psychologists, rather than psychiatrists. This biological turn was influenced by many factors, including the success of drug treatments and the influence of the pharmaceutical industry, the desire for psychiatry to realign with the other "scientific," evidence-based medical disciplines—including through using the same research methods—and the preference of the insurance industry for funding drug treatments.[13] But the amendments helped to cement the notion of what constituted the methodological standards for evidence in clinical evaluation, and this limited the kinds of treatment forms that could be scientifically evaluated.

Despite being blocked by the FDA in 1982, Kurland and Yensen did not give up trying to revive their psychedelic research. In 1991, the FDA finally approved a new research protocol, under their dormant IND, for a double-blind controlled study assessing the relationship between peak experiences and outcome in LSD therapy with substance abusers. To carry out the research, Kurland, Yensen, and psychiatrist Donna Dryer (Yensen's wife) established the Orenda Institute, a nonprofit organization incorporated in 1993. Yensen was director, Dryer medical director, and the institute was based in the couple's large Baltimore home. The trio proceeded to order supplies of LSD from the National Institute on Drug Abuse (NIDA), which had taken over from the NIMH as the custodian of research supplies of LSD, and in 1995 the Drug Enforcement Administration (DEA) approved the Orenda Institute as a site for research with the Schedule I drug. NIDA, however, dragged out its approval, ordering further reviews of the research protocol, and cast doubt on whether it would supply the drug.[14] Eventually the researchers bypassed NIDA and received permission from the DEA to import 100 milligrams of LSD from the University of Bern, Switzerland in 1996.[15]

However, in 1997, as the researchers were recruiting patients and preparing to commence their study, the FDA again had a change of heart, and their research ground to a halt. In July, the researchers had submitted a further amendment to their IND, to allow for research with cancer patients under a new protocol. In October, the FDA's Cynthia McCormick responded by placing the IND on "clinical hold." This hold was for all research under the IND, which included the previously approved study with substance abusers. She was in fact unaware of the 1991 approval, claiming that the IND had already been on clinical hold since 1986. McCormick included in her response a long list of the deficiencies in both the design of the cancer study, and the safety and chemical information provided. These included a lack of controls in the study and extensive further information required on medical monitoring, potential drug interactions, the method of preparation for the LSD, the nature of its packaging, and even whether molecules of LSD could become trapped

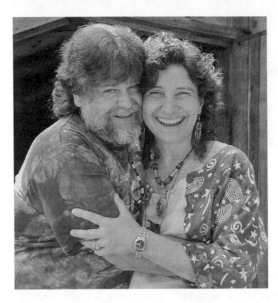

Richard Yensen and Donna Dryer. Courtesy of Richard Yensen, photo by Rita Cantu.

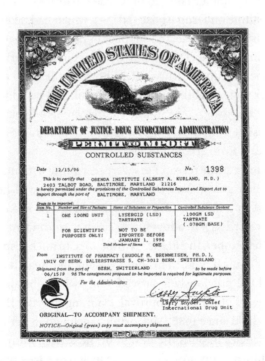

FOR SCIENTIFIC PURPOSES ONLY! This 1996 permit from the US Drug Enforcement Administration allowed the Orenda Institute to import 100 milligrams of LSD from Switzerland for use in their FDA-approved clinical research. Courtesy of Richard Yensen.

in the walls of its packaging, affecting the miniscule doses.[16] McCormick's concern over the study may have been influenced by an article on Yensen and the planned research published in *Esquire* in September. Written in a frequently mocking tone, it featured a sensationalistic imaginary scenario, where a patient "sent straight to hell" on LSD breaks out of the unsecured treatment room, takes a carving knife from the kitchen and "tries to cut the soul out of his own body—or out of Yensen's two-year-old daughter"—or escapes into the neighborhood.[17]

In 2001, the Orenda researchers submitted an amended protocol that attempted to address the FDA's concerns, but McCormick still judged it as lacking and continued the clinical hold. Despite claiming in a teleconference with the researchers that she would "like to help" them "proceed out of this dilemma" and that she believed they had within their experience and resources "the ability to get off clinical hold," McCormick continued to insist that they furnish extensive safety and chemical data that was exceedingly difficult for the independent, privately funded researchers to produce and that was arguably unnecessary in light of their extensive experience of safely administering the drug. This data included details from animal studies and safety data from their previous decades of research of a kind that they had not been required to collect at the time.[18] In many ways, their situation reflected that of Harold Abramson in the 1960s, as he had struggled to submit the safety and chemical data required for his independent IND, when the safety of the drug was never truly in question. A follow-up letter from McCormick further detailed deficiencies in the study design that included patient inclusion criteria being too broad, a lack of adequate justification for drug doses, and the use of clinical judgment rather than objective criteria in determining the number of drug sessions patients received.[19]

Ultimately, Yensen and Dryer believed that the level of safety and chemical data that the FDA requested was simply a method of deliberately obstructing their research and that they would never be able to satisfy the FDA's requirements. They reluctantly let go of the project, moved to British Columbia, and became Canadian citizens. Before doing so, they handed their hundreds of vials of LSD to the DEA, having held onto them for years without using a single one.[20] Kurland retired in 2002 and died at the age of ninety-four in 2008. At the time of his death he was working on a book, entitled "LSD: An Investigational Odyssey."[21]

Yet this was still not the end. Although the Orenda researchers' efforts to revive psychedelic research in the 1990s had been thwarted, others had been more successful. Why these researchers were able to satisfy the FDA where the Orenda researchers were not is unclear. In 1990, psychiatrist Rick Strassman from the University of New Mexico received FDA and DEA approval to conduct research exploring the effects of the short-acting psychedelic di-methyltryptamine (DMT) in healthy volunteers. The study ran until 1995, with sixty volunteers receiving approximately four hundred doses.[22] More significantly, two further nonprofit organizations were founded in the 1980s and 1990s that successfully reignited clinical research with increasing pace from the first decade of the 2000s. The Multidisciplinary Association for Psychedelic Studies (MAPS) was founded by Rick Doblin in 1986 to facilitate the development of methylenedioxymethamphetamine (MDMA) through FDA approval as an adjunct to psychotherapy. A number of therapists had been using the drug in treatment since the mid-1970s—outside of the IND process—but the DEA halted this practice in 1986, when it placed the drug in Schedule I because of its growing recreational use. Like MDA, the drug produced milder effects than classical psychedelics such as LSD and was un-likely to produce peak experiences, but had many beneficial effects including increased openness, empathy, and ability to confront traumatic emotions and past experiences.[23]

After negotiations with the FDA and preliminary work stretched out over the late 1980s and 1990s, the first MAPS-sponsored clinical study with MDMA in the United States received FDA approval in 2001 and commenced in 2004. Led by psychiatrist Michael Mithoefer, the pilot randomized, double-blind controlled trial assessed the drug's use in treating twenty patients with chronic, treatment-resistant posttraumatic stress disorder (PTSD). The trial utilized an inert placebo in the control condition. Nineteen of the twenty patients could accurately guess whether MDMA had been administered, as could the therapists in all cases. Nevertheless, Mithoefer reported extremely promising results.[24] This was the first of a series of MAPS-sponsored Phase 2 clinical studies with PTSD patients, some of which took place internationally. Through one such Canadian study, commenced in 2013, Yensen finally got the chance to participate again in clinical research with psychedelics, while Dryer participated for the first time. The couple acted as therapists in the small study, which took place in Vancouver. Psychiatrist Ingrid Pacey led the study, but Yensen took over as acting principal investigator for much of its duration. The study included six patients and concluded in 2016; results are yet to be published.[25] In November 2016, the FDA approved MAPS to move on to Phase 3 clinical trials that would establish the treatment's safety and efficacy in larger patient populations, providing the data necessary for NDA approval.[26]

Research sponsored by a second nonprofit organization, the Heffter Research Institute, more directly picked up where the LSD research of the 1970s left off. Purdue University pharmacologist David Nichols founded Heffter in 1993 with a group of his colleagues. Nichols—who manufactured the DMT and MDMA for Strassman and MAPS—had completed his PhD on the structure-activity relationships of psychedelics in 1973, as clinical research with the drugs was dwindling to a close. Nevertheless, he continued his laboratory research with psychedelics, and his interest in the potential of clinical research grew as he met other like-minded researchers in the 1980s, spurring him to work to reestablish the field. Early on, the researchers decided to use psilocybin rather than LSD in their studies, because of the stigma surrounding LSD and psilocybin's shorter period of action. Heffter-sponsored clinical research began in 2001, with a small study using psilocybin to treat obsessive-compulsive disorder, led by Francisco Moreno at the University of Arizona, which reported positive results. Subsequently, Heffter focused its efforts on clinical research using psilocybin to treat anxiety and depression in patients suffering from cancer—research that extended directly from the Spring Grove / MPRC studies.[27]

In fact, this link to the past went beyond the research indication, as William Richards—Kurland and Yensen's old MPRC colleague—coestablished the most significant Heffter-sponsored clinical research program, at Johns Hopkins University. Planning for the program began in 1999, when Richards met Johns Hopkins psychopharmacologist Roland Griffiths. Griffiths had spent several decades of his career engaged in conventional drug research; however, his personal practice of meditation had sparked an interest in mystical and spiritual experiences. On meeting Richards, the two decided to collaborate.[28]

The researchers first conducted two preliminary studies, examining the effects of psilocybin in healthy volunteers who had religious or spiritual backgrounds, the first of which was published in 2006. With these studies, the FDA appears to have relaxed its policy to only approve INDs for research that directly assessed efficacy in treatment, even if proposed nonefficacy studies were in fact intended as background for future efficacy studies (as was the case with Kurland's rejected 1982 proposal). The studies in effect replicated and extended Walter Pahnke's 1963 PhD research on the ability of psilocybin to produce mystical-type experiences, and the studies even employed rating scales based on those devised by Pahnke and Richards in the 1960s and 1970s to assess such experiences. The Johns Hopkins drug sessions were conducted in the same manner as they had been at the MPRC, with a living room–type setting, eyeshades, and headphones playing a special program of classical music. Richards conducted the sessions with a female colleague.[29]

Both studies were double-blind and placebo controlled. The first study included thirty-six volunteers and used the stimulant methylphenidate as an active placebo. The session guides correctly guessed which drug was administered 77 percent of the time. But they incorrectly guessed the study design, believing that varying doses of psilocybin, and drugs other than those employed, were administered. The researchers therefore argued that the blind was adequately maintained. The second trial used an inert placebo and a variety of psilocybin doses given in varying order, with eighteen volunteers. This design better maintained the blind. The studies both confirmed that, under their conditions, psilocybin reliably produced mystical-type experiences—in up to 72 percent of volunteers—which subjects rated as among the most meaningful experiences of their lives and to which they attributed sustained positive benefits.[30]

The Heffter-sponsored Johns Hopkins study of the efficacy of psilocybin in treating distress associated with a life-threatening cancer diagnosis was published in 2016. The trial featured fifty-one patients, who were randomly assigned to receive either a high or low (placebo) dose of psilocybin, on a double blind, crossover basis. This meant that all patients received both high and low doses, but in random order, approximately five weeks apart. Both patients and therapists were unaware of the study design, other than that it involved two unspecified doses of psilocybin, with one being moderate to high. The researchers reported that significant confusion among many of the therapists as to the study design and doses suggested that the blinding procedures "provided some protection" against bias. Prior to their first psilocybin session, patients underwent an average of eight hours of preparation with their therapists and had further postsession and follow-up meetings. The study featured a comparative assessment of the effects of the two doses, by comparing results five weeks after patients received their first, randomly determined dose (just before they received their second, alternative dose). It also gave a noncomparative assessment of the effects of the high dose measured six months after its administration. Results found that the high dose produced a large and statistically significant advantage over the low dose on ratings of both depression and anxiety at the five-week assessment, and that the high-dose effects were sustained at the six-month follow-up point.[31]

In addition to this study, the Johns Hopkins researchers also explored using psilocybin to treat tobacco addiction, and Heffter-sponsored researchers at the University of New Mexico conducted a pilot study of psilocybin in the treatment of alcoholism, bringing psychedelic therapy back to its origins. Both have reported positive results.[32] Further, parallel to the Johns Hopkins cancer study, a closely affiliated group of Heffter-sponsored researchers led by Stephen Ross at New York University conducted a very similar cross-over trial with twenty-nine cancer patients. The study utilized niacin instead of low-dose psilocybin in the control treatment, which the therapists could distinguish from psilocybin in all but one of the patients. The researchers reported similar positive results.[33]

Yet, despite the rigor and consistent positive results from these two cancer studies, the old objections remain. In a 2017 *New York Times* opinion piece entitled "LSD to Cure Depression? Not So Fast," Richard A. Friedman, professor of clinical psychiatry and director of the psychopharmacology clinic at Weill Cornell Medical College, warned against being "seduced by preliminary research." He highlighted Ross's study for its "serious design flaws." These included the use of niacin as a placebo, as it was unlikely to maintain blind administration, and the cross-over design, as patients who received niacin second may have still been experiencing the effects of their earlier psilocybin session, impacting the assessment of niacin's effects. While these may be valid critiques, Friedman concluded his piece with the same tone-deaf solution that had been brought out for close to sixty years: "Psychedelics might turn out to have real promise, but that needs to be proven through large, rigorous, placebo-controlled trials. We're not there yet." As might be expected, he did not suggest how such studies could be accomplished, given the difficulties in placebo comparison he had just highlighted. Ultimately, he dismissed the likelihood that psychedelics would become useful treatment tools, stating, "What they tell us about our brain is probably more valuable than what they can do for us."[34]

From this point, it is unclear whether the current era of psychedelic research will succeed where the previous failed. So far, it looks promising. The number and frequency of new studies is increasing, and all have reported positive results. One major area of benefit for the current era is the existence of organizations such as Heffter and MAPS to take over the role of pharmaceutical companies. While funding pharmaceutical research and development through public donations is certainly a challenge, given the fate of the independent research of the 1960s and 1970s, the importance of having organizations that can strategically initiate and coordinate multiple studies toward the goal of submitting an NDA can hardly be overstated.

However there are also areas where it is not clear that the lessons of the past have been learned: the role of psychotherapy in treatment and the difficulties of research design. The fate of research in the 1960s and 1970s clearly demonstrates the importance of maintaining and highlighting psychedelic therapy as a form of drug-assisted psychotherapy rather than as a simple drug treatment. Researchers in the recent psilocybin studies have certainly maintained the form of drug session guidance developed in the 1950s in Canada and perfected at the MPRC, and all involve preparation sessions involving some form of therapy as well as specific preparation for the drug session. Griffiths's patients spent approximately eight hours in preparation and Ross's six. This is roughly equivalent to the duration of preparation in the Spring Grove / MPRC cancer trials, where patients received less psychotherapy than in the other studies. However, the Heffter-sponsored alcoholism and tobacco studies involved similar periods of preparation, so there seems to be a trend toward more limited psychotherapy in contemporary psychedelic research. Nevertheless, the treatments remain much closer to the classic psychedelic therapy technique than to the chemotherapeutic approach of some 1960s researchers such as Leo Hollister. As long as there is a targeted psychotherapeutic framework, it may not be too significant to count the exact number of hours patients spend in preparation. More significant is how the role of psychotherapy is sidelined in the reports. Griffiths's report briefly describes the nature of the preparation, but it does not use the term "psychotherapy" and does not highlight its centrality to the overall treatment procedure and efficacy. Ross's study more explicitly stresses that the treatment is psilocybin administered "in conjunction with targeted psychotherapy," but details of the psychotherapeutic procedures are relegated to an online-only supplementary appendix and could easily be overlooked by many readers.[35]

This lack of focus on the psychotherapeutic elements of treatment is reflected in the many positive media reports on the cancer studies. These reports also present the treatment as an almost magic one-shot cure, as early researchers in the 1950s and 1960s had, but that MPRC researchers such as O. Lee McCabe by the mid-1970s saw as naïve and damaging to the field. A 2016 *Time* article, entitled "Just One Dose of this Psychedelic Drug Can Ease Anxiety," reported the dramatic results of the cancer trials while giving no mention of psychotherapy or session preparation. In fact, it reported that the study authors had suggested that psilocybin worked by activating "parts

of the brain that are impacted by serotonin"—known to play a role in anxiety and depression—implying a biological basis for the treatment. A similar
article in the *Atlantic*, entitled "The Life Changing Magic of Mushrooms,"
also speculated on the potential biological basis of treatment, although it
did acknowledge in passing that Ross's study involved psychotherapy.[36] Perspectives such as these could again steer the treatment away from its psychotherapeutic roots, which past studies suggest is the key to psychedelic
therapy's efficacy. Further, a focus on obtaining remarkable results from a
single session could again set up unrealistic treatment expectations, upon
which later studies could flounder.

In regard to research design, the cyclical nature of psychedelic research
is even more apparent. In relating to the past era, modern reports largely
defer to the standard narrative of its demise, seeing it as cut short by controversy and prohibitive regulation before it reached scientific maturity. From
this perspective, the lessons of the past are fairly simple: avoid controversy
by maintaining a cautious, tempered approach; ensure that all research con-
forms to rigorous scientific standards; and hope that recreational use of the
drugs does not again spike, leading to a less favorable sociopolitical context.
Indeed, in a 1998 article on the lessons from past research, Heffter board
member and UCLA psychiatrist Charles Grob stressed that, "in the future,
the putative value of hallucinogens in psychiatry can no longer rest on claims
deriving from anecdotal case studies, as inspiring as they may be, but rather
must evolve out of the findings of well-structured, controlled, scientific investigation."[37] Missing from his discussion is recognition that this statement
almost exactly mirrors many made by researchers in the early 1960s. Further
missing is recognition that those researchers did in fact attempt such rigorous
research, but the problematic practical and theoretical relationships between
psychedelic therapy and the randomized controlled trial prevented a clear
picture of treatment efficacy from emerging.[38] Grob conducted his own pilot
study treating cancer patients with psilocybin, published in 2011, and like
Ross used niacin as a placebo. Unsurprisingly, investigators and subjects alike
could differentiate between the two drugs.[39]

Therefore, in most of the recent studies it appears that the difficulty of
designing a placebo treatment that successfully maintains double-blind administration has been largely sidestepped rather than resolved—the studies
simply employ blinds that frequently do not work. Perhaps this is no longer a major problem—including a double-blind placebo control in a study
is more important than whether that control achieves its intended aim. This

would mean that research design has become a simple checklist of required techniques such as randomization and placebo control, rather than these techniques being merely tools to achieve a scientific ideal. This is a long way from the vision of the research experts and FDA officials who in the late 1950s and early 1960s promoted randomized controlled trials as the favored clinical trial format. Furthermore, aside from the practical difficulty of finding an adequate placebo condition, the theoretical complexity of attempting to control for a psychological placebo effect in the context of a psychological treatment and the possibility that an effective placebo condition would mimic the experimental treatment too closely to demonstrate differential treatment effects are not acknowledged in modern research reports.

Ultimately, it will be up to the FDA to determine whether the issue of sufficient blinding in future Phase 3 trials is problematic enough to undermine any evidence of efficacy. While it may not have become a major issue so far, there is no guarantee that avoiding the problem will remain an effective strategy. Indeed, while Grob argued that "to maintain an iconoclastic insistence that the very nature of these substances transcends standard research designs would be to prolong their marginalization," equally, ignoring the problematic relationship between psychedelics and controlled trials could again lead to cycles of inconclusive research and calls for more research.[40]

Introduction

Epigraph: [Charles Savage], untitled manuscript, n.d., folder 10, box 7, Charles Savage Papers, MSP 70, Archives and Special Collections, Purdue University Libraries, West Lafayette, Indiana (hereafter Savage Papers).

1. The patient's name has been changed for confidentiality.

2. "Post-Session Notes," n.d., folder 18, box 9, Savage Papers. See also Stanislav Grof and Joan Halifax, *The Human Encounter with Death* (New York: E. P. Dutton, 1977), p. 21.

3. "Post-Session Notes."

4. "My LSD Experience," 19 August 1965, folder 18, box 9, Savage Papers.

5. Sidney Wolf, "Reminisces [*sic*] of Dr. Sidney Wolf with Dr. Kurland," 22 July 1975, folder "LSD Cancer Papers Kurland," Orenda Institute, Cortes Island, British Columbia, Canada.

6. Ibid.

7. "My LSD Experience."

8. Albert A. Kurland, "LSD-Assisted Psychotherapy in Terminal Cancer," application for research grant to Department of Health, Education and, Welfare, MH CA 12916-01, received 1 February 1966, folder 4, box 9, Savage Papers, p. 8.

9. Wolf, "Reminisces."

10. Abram Hoffer, "A Program for the Treatment of Alcoholism: LSD, Malvaria and Nicotinic Acid," in Harold A. Abramson (ed.), *The Use of LSD in Psychotherapy and Alcoholism* (Indianapolis: Bobbs-Merrill, 1967), p. 351.

11. For the growth of psychopharmacology in the 1950s, see David Healy, *The Antidepressant Era* (Cambridge, MA: Harvard University Press, 1997); David Healy, *The Creation of Psychopharmacology* (Cambridge, MA: Harvard University Press, 2002); Jonathan Michel Metzl, *Prozac on the Couch: Prescribing Gender in the Era of Wonder Drugs* (Durham, NC: Duke University Press, 2003); Edward Shorter, *Before Prozac: The Troubled History of Mood Disorders in Psychiatry* (New York: Oxford University Press, 2009); Andrea Tone, *The Age of Anxiety: A History of America's Turbulent Affair with Tranquilizers* (New York: Basic Books, 2009); and David Herzberg, *Happy Pills in America: From Miltown to Prozac* (Baltimore: Johns Hopkins University Press, 2009). Nicolas Rasmussen has argued that the modern era of psychopharmacology began earlier, with amphetamine in the 1930s. See Nicolas Rasmussen, "Making the First Anti-Depressant: Amphetamine in American Medicine, 1929–1950," *Journal of the History of Medicine and Allied Sciences* 64, no. 3 (2006), pp. 288–323; and Nicolas Rasmussen, *On Speed: The Many Lives of Amphetamine* (New York: New York University Press, 2008).

12. For a discussion of the complex politics of the 1960s psychedelic movement, see Chris Elcock, "The Fifth Freedom: The Politics of Psychedelic Patriotism," *Journal for the Study of Radicalism* 9, no. 2 (2015), pp. 17–40.

13. A complete list of works that predominantly reflect this perspective is far too long to list here. The first major retrospective account of LSD research—a scientific review—clearly established the prohibitionist analysis of LSD psychotherapy's downfall. See Lester Grinspoon and James B. Bakalar, *Psychedelic Drugs Reconsidered* (1979; new ed., New York: Lindesmith Center, 1997). Two prominent journalistic general histories of LSD further built on this narrative and have remained the most influential histories of the drug. See Martin A. Lee and Bruce Shlain, *Acid Dreams: The Complete Social History of LSD; The CIA, the Sixties, and Beyond* (New York: Grove Press, 1985); and Jay Stevens, *Storming Heaven: LSD and the American Dream* (London: Heinemann, 1987). Subsequent works have focused more specifically on aspects of LSD's medical history yet have stayed within a prohibitionist analysis. See Robert F. Ulrich and Bernard M. Patten, "The Rise, Decline, and Fall of LSD," *Perspectives in Biology and Medicine* 34,

no. 4 (1991), pp. 561–578; Steven J. Novak, "LSD before Leary: Sidney Cohen's Critique of 1950s Psychedelic Research," *Isis* 88, no. 1 (1997), pp. 87–110; Richard Elliot Doblin, "Regulation of the Medical Use of Psychedelics and Marijuana" (PhD diss., Harvard University, 2000); Erika Dyck, *Psychedelic Psychiatry: LSD from Clinic to Campus* (Baltimore: Johns Hopkins University Press, 2008); Lana Cook, "Empathetic Reform and the Psychedelic Aesthetic: Women's Accounts of LSD Therapy," *Configurations* 22, no. 1 (2014), pp. 79–111; Sarah Shortall, "Psychedelic Drugs and the Problem of Experience," *Past and Present* 222, suppl. 9 (2014), pp. 187–206; and Kim Hewitt, "Rehabilitating LSD History in Postwar America: Dilworth Wayne Woolley and the Serotonin Hypothesis of Mental Illness," *History of Science* 54, no. 3 (2016), pp. 307–330.

14. Historian of journalism Stephen Siff has found that news media coverage of LSD rapidly declined after 1968, having reaching its peak in the preceding years. See Stephen Siff, *Acid Hype: American News Media and the Psychedelic Experience* (Urbana: University of Illinois Press, 2015), pp. 185, 13.

15. Lee and Shlain, *Acid Dreams*. The CIA and military LSD research was first exposed in John Marks, *The Search for the "Manchurian Candidate": The CIA and Mind Control* (New York: Times Books, 1979).

16. This narrative, through these four actors, is most clearly and completely laid out in Stevens, *Storming Heaven*; and Lee and Shlain, *Acid Dreams*. The following summary of the narrative is based on these works.

17. Dyck, *Psychedelic Psychiatry*, p. 2.

18. Aldous Huxley, *Brave New World* (London: Chatto & Windus, 1932); Aldous Huxley, *The Doors of Perception* (New York: Harper, 1954); Aldous Huxley, *Heaven and Hell* (New York: Harper, 1956); Aldous Huxley, *Island: A Novel* (New York: Harper, 1962). For more on Huxley's association with Osmond and his role in influencing interest in psychedelics outside of strictly clinical applications, see Novak, "LSD Before Leary," pp. 87–110.

19. For more on Leary and Alpert, see Don Lattin, *The Harvard Psychedelic Club: How Timothy Leary, Ram Dass, Huston Smith, and Andrew Weil Killed the Fifties and Ushered in a New Age for America* (New York: HarperOne, 2011); and Siff, *Acid Hype*.

20. This quote is widely reproduced in discussions of Leary; however, this author was unable to find its original source or date. See Lattin, *Harvard Psychedelic Club*, pp. 61, 133; and Laura Mansnerus, "Timothy Leary, Pied Piper of Psychedelic 60's, Dies at 75," *New York Times*, 1 June 1996, https://nyti.ms/2jFSnjS. Jay Stephens attributes the quote to a federal judge, but he also leaves it unreferenced. See Stephens, *Storming Heaven*, p. 121. Whether or not the quote is genuine and accurate, it does accurately convey the hysteria surrounding Leary in the late 1960s.

21. Ken Kesey, *One Flew Over the Cuckoo's Nest* (New York: Viking Press, 1962).

22. Tom Wolfe, *The Electric Kool-Aid Acid Test* (New York: Farrar, Straus, and Giroux, 1968).

23. For histories of pharmaceutical research and regulation in the mid-twentieth century, see Peter Temin, *Taking Your Medicine: Drug Regulation in the United States* (Cambridge, MA: Harvard University Press, 1980); Harry. M. Marks, *The Progress of Experiment: Science and Therapeutic Reform in the United States, 1900–1990* (Cambridge: Cambridge University Press, 1997); John P. Swann, "Sure Cure: Public Policy on Drug Efficacy before 1962," in Gregory J. Higby and Elaine C. Stroud (eds.), *The Inside Story of Medicines: A Symposium* (Madison, WI: American Institute of the History of Pharmacy, 1997), pp. 223–261; Philip J. Hilts, *Protecting America's Health: The FDA, Business, and One Hundred Years of Regulation* (New York: Alfred A. Knopf, 2003); Arthur Daemmrich, *Pharmacopolitics: Drug Regulation in the United States and Germany* (Chapel Hill: University of North Carolina Press, 2004); Jeremy A. Greene, *Prescribing by Numbers: Drugs and the Definition of Disease* (Baltimore: Johns Hopkins University Press, 2007); Daniel Carpenter, *Reputation and Power: Organizational Image and Pharmaceuti-*

cal Regulation at the FDA (Princeton: Princeton University Press, 2010); Dominique A. Tobbell, *Pills, Power, and Policy: The Struggle for Drug Reform in Cold War America and Its Conse-quences* (Berkeley: University of California Press, 2012); and Scott H. Podolsky, *The Antibiotic Era: Reform, Resistance, and the Pursuit of a Rational Therapeutics* (Baltimore: Johns Hopkins University Press, 2015).

24. Drug Amendments of 1962, 87 P.L. 781, 76 Stat. 780, 10 October 1962. The law amended the Federal Food, Drug, and Cosmetic Act of 1938.

25. See Dyck, *Psychedelic Psychiatry*, pp. 47–51, 73–78, 120. For further works that more briefly acknowledge the difficulties in clinically evaluating LSD therapies, see Lee and Shlain, *Acid Dreams*, p. 90; and Kimberly Allyn Hewitt, "Psychedelics and Psychosis: LSD and Chang-ing Ideas of Mental Illness, 1943–1966" (PhD diss., University of Texas, 2002), p. 214. Nicholas Langlitz has recognized that the decline and demise of LSD research was a result of number of complex factors—including changing regulatory frameworks for pharmaceutical research, lack of funding, and professional discouragement—rather than simple prohibition. However, his work has not explored these factors in any depth. Nicolas Langlitz, *Neuropsychedelia: The Revival of Hallucinogen Research since the Decade of the Brain* (Berkeley: University of Califor-nia Press, 2013).

26. While drug efficacy had been a provision of the original bill, Kefauver's primary con-cern had always been high drug prices due to industry price fixing. In its final form, however, the bill was rewritten to focus on drug safety and effectiveness, and provisions such as patent law reform were left out. For recent works that focus particular attention on the Drug Amend-ments of 1962, see Carpenter, *Reputation and Power*; Daemmrich, *Pharmacopolitics*; Tobbell, *Pills, Power, and Policy*; Temin, *Taking Your Medicine*; Hilts, *Protecting America's Health*; and Jeremy A. Greene and Scott H. Podolsky, "Reform, Regulation, and Pharmaceuticals—the Kefauver-Harris Amendments at 50," *New England Journal of Medicine* 367, no. 16 (2012), pp. 1481–1483. For an account of the amendments' history written soon after its passage, see Rich-ard Harris, *The Real Voice* (New York: Macmillan, 1964). For a critical account of the amend-ments from a pharmacologist who testified before Kefauver's congressional hearings as an influential supporter, see Louis Lasagna, "Congress, the FDA, and New Drug Development: Before and after 1962," *Perspectives in Biology and Medicine* 32, no. 3 (1989), pp. 322–343; and William M. Wardell and Louis Lasagna, *Regulation and Drug Development* (Washington, DC: American Enterprise Institute for Public Policy Research, 1975). For more on the thalidomide tragedy, see also Leslie J. Reagan, *Dangerous Pregnancies: Mothers, Disabilities, and Abortion in Modern America* (Berkeley: University of California Press, 2010), pp. 57–63.

27. Drug Amendments of 1962, Title 1, Part A, Sec. 102 (c).

28. For histories of the randomized controlled trial, see Abraham M. Lilienfeld, "Ceteris Paribus: The Evolution of the Clinical Trial," *Bulletin of the History of Medicine* 56, no. 1 (1982), pp. 1–18; Marks, *Progress of Experiment*; Arthur K. Shapiro and Elaine Shapiro, *The Powerful Placebo: From Ancient Priest to Modern Physician* (Baltimore: Johns Hopkins University Press, 1997); Ted J. Kaptchuk, "Intentional Ignorance: A History of Blind Assessment and Placebo Controls in Medicine," *Bulletin of the History of Medicine* 72, no. 3 (1998), pp. 389–433; Harry M. Marks, "Trust and Mistrust in the Marketplace: Statistics and Clinical Research, 1945–1960," *History of Science* 38, no. 3 (2000), pp. 343–355; Scott H. Podolsky, "Antibiotics and the Social History of the Controlled Clinical Trial, 1950–1970," *Journal of the History of Medicine and Allied Sciences* 65, no. 3 (2010), pp. 327–367; Podolsky, *Antibiotic Era*; Laura E. Bothwell et al., "Assessing the Gold Standard—Lessons from the History of RCTs," *New England Journal of Medicine* 374, no. 22 (2016), pp. 2175–2181.

29. For overviews of some of aspects of this historiography, see Andrew Scull, "Somatic Treatments and the Historiography of Psychiatry," *History of Psychiatry* 5, no. 17 (1994), pp. 1–12; Don R. Lipsitt, "Psyche and Soma: Struggles to Close the Gap," in Roy W. Menninger and

John C. Nemiah (eds.), *American Psychiatry after World War II (1944–1994)* (Washington, DC: American Psychiatry Press, 2000), pp. 152–186. For works that to a greater or lesser extent chart the divide and competing interests of these two factions of psychiatry, see Nathan G. Hale Jr., *The Rise and Crisis of Psychoanalysis in the United States: Freud and the Americans, 1917–1985* (Oxford: Oxford University Press, 1995); Edward Shorter, *A History of Psychiatry: From the Era of the Asylum to the Age of Prozac* (New York: John Wiley & Sons, 1997); Gerald N. Grob, "Psychiatry's Holy Grail: The Search for the Mechanisms of Mental Diseases," *Bulletin of the History of Medicine* 72, no. 2 (1998), pp. 189–219; Jack D. Pressman, *Last Resort: Psychosurgery and the Limits of Medicine* (Cambridge: Cambridge University Press, 1998); Joel T. Braslow, "Therapeutics and the History of Psychiatry," *Bulletin of the History of Medicine* 74, no. 4 (2000), pp. 794–802; Healy, *Creation of Psychopharmacology*; Mark S. Micale, "The Psychiatric Body," in Roger Cooter and John Pickstone (eds.), *Companion to Medicine in the Twentieth Century* (London: Routledge, 2003), pp. 323–346; Joel Paris, *The Fall of an Icon: Psychoanalysis and Academic Psychiatry* (Toronto: University of Toronto Press, 2005); Leon Eisenberg and Laurence B. Guttmacher, "Were We All Asleep at the Switch? A Personal Reminiscence of Psychiatry from 1940 to 2010," *Acta Psychiatrica Scandinavica* 122, no. 2 (2010), pp. 89–102; Hannah S. Decker, *The Making of DSM-III: A Diagnostic Manual's Conquest of American Psychiatry* (New York: Oxford University Press, 2013); and Andrew Scull, *Madness in Civilization: A Cultural History of Insanity from the Bible to Freud, from the Madhouse to Modern Medicine* (Princeton: Princeton University Press, 2015).

30. See Rasmussen, *On Speed*; Tone, *Age of Anxiety*; Jonathan Sadowski, "Beyond the Metaphor of the Pendulum: Electroconvulsive Therapy, Psychoanalysis, and the Styles of American Psychiatry," *Journal of the History of Medicine and Allied Sciences* 61, no. 1 (2006), pp. 1–25; Mical Raz, "Between the Ego and the Icepick: Psychosurgery, Psychoanalysis, and Psychiatric Discourse," *Bulletin of the History of Medicine* 82, no. 2 (2008), pp. 387–420.

Chapter 1 · Free Experiment

Epigraph: Louis S. Cholden (ed.), *Lysergic Acid Diethylamide and Mescaline in Experimental Psychiatry* (New York: Grune & Stratton, 1956), pp. 68–69.

1. See Albert Hofmann, *LSD: My Problem Child; Reflections on Sacred Drugs, Mysticism and Science*, trans. Jonathan Ott (Santa Cruz: Multidisciplinary Association for Psychedelic Studies, 2009), pp. 35–52. See also Erika Dyck, *Psychedelic Psychiatry: LSD from Clinic to Campus* (Baltimore: Johns Hopkins University Press, 2008), p. 13; Lester Grinspoon and James B. Bakalar, *Psychedelic Drugs Reconsidered* (New York: Lindesmith Center, 1997), p. 60; Stanislav Grof, *LSD Psychotherapy* (Pomona: Hunter House, 1980), pp. 17–20; Martin A. Lee and Bruce Shlain, *Acid Dreams: The Complete Social History of LSD; The CIA, the Sixties, and Beyond* (New York: Grove Press, 1985), p. xvii–xix; Jay Stevens, *Storming Heaven: LSD and the American Dream* (London: Heinemann, 1987), pp. 3–12 .

2. Hofmann, *LSD*, p. 47.

3. Ibid., pp. 32–52.

4. Annelie Hintzen and Torsten Passie, *The Pharmacology of LSD: A Critical Review* (Oxford: Oxford University Press, Beckley Foundation Press, 2010), p. 4. For Stoll's report see W. A. Stoll, "Lysergsäure-Diäthylamid, Ein Phantastikum Aus Der Mutterkorngruppe," *Schweizer Archiv für Neurologie und Psychiatrie* 60 (1947), pp. 279–323.

5. Hofmann, *LSD*, pp. 73, 85.

6. Frances O. Kelsey, "Symposium on Investigational Drugs—the Government," presentation to the American College of Apothecaries and American Society of Hospital Pharmacists, Miami Beach, Florida, 15 May 1963, in FDA (comp.), *Speeches and Papers, 1963*, Part 1 (Rockville, MD: Food and Drug Administration, 1979), FDA Biosciences Library, Silver Spring, Maryland.

7. Nicolas Rasmussen has explored the relationships between researchers and pharmaceu-

tical companies in America in the early to mid-twentieth century. He has dubbed this form the "free-lancer" relationship; one of three common relationships he delineates in the period. Nicolas Rasmussen, "The Drug Industry and Clinical Research in Interwar America: Three Types of Physician Collaborator," *Bulletin of the History of Medicine* 70, no. 1 (2005), pp. 61–66, 76.

8. Ethical standards and guidelines for human research—such as the Nuremburg Code of 1947—did of course exist; however, these were neither legislated nor enforced through regulatory oversight. For the role of the FDA and the Drug Amendments of 1962 in formalizing the need for patient consent in clinical research, see Daniel Carpenter, *Reputation and Power: Organizational Image and Pharmaceutical Regulation at the FDA* (Princeton: Princeton University Press, 2010), pp. 546–549. For research ethics in the first half of the twentieth century, see Susan E. Lederer, *Subjected to Science: Human Experimentation in America before the Second World War* (Baltimore: Johns Hopkins University Press, 1995).

9. S. Weir Mitchell, "Remarks on the Effects of Anhelonium Lewinii (the Mescal Button)," *British Medical Journal* 2, no. 1875 (1896), pp. 1625–1629. For subsequent similar but expanded studies, see Heinrich Klüver, *Mescal: The "Divine" Plant and its Psychological Effects* (London: Kegan Paul, Trench, Trubner, 1928); and E. Lowell Kelly, "Individual Differences in the Effects of Mescal," *Journal of General Psychology* 8 (January 1933), pp. 462–471.

10. Erich Lindemann and William Malamud, "Experimental Analysis of the Psychopathological Effects of Intoxicating Drugs," *American Journal of Psychiatry* 90, no. 4 (1934), pp. 853–881.

11. Jack D. Pressman, *Last Resort: Psychosurgery and the Limits of Medicine* (Cambridge: Cambridge University Press, 1998), pp. 147–154.

12. For discussions of drug therapy in psychiatry prior to the psychopharmacological revolution, see Edward Shorter, *Before Prozac: The Troubled History of Mood Disorders in Psychiatry* (New York: Oxford University Press, 2009), pp. 19–21; Andrea Tone, *The Age of Anxiety: A History of America's Turbulent Affair with Tranquilizers* (New York: Basic Books, 2009), pp. 22–23. For the use of amphetamines specifically, see Nicolas Rasmussen, "Making the First Anti-Depressant: Amphetamine in American Medicine, 1929–1950," *Journal of the History of Medicine and Allied Sciences* 64, no. 3 (2006), pp. 288–323.

13. Ken Kesey's novel *One Flew over the Cuckoo's Nest* is probably the most famous and influential depiction of ECT and psychosurgery as brutal, oppressive, and therapeutically useless treatments. See Ken Kesey, *One Flew over the Cuckoo's Nest* (New York: Viking Press, 1962). For a historical account critical of somatic therapies, see Joel Braslow, *Mental Ills and Bodily Cures: Psychiatric Treatment in the First Half of the Twentieth Century* (Berkeley: University of California Press, 1997). For works that challenge these depictions, reevaluating the treatments in their historical context, see Pressman, *Last Resort*; Edward Shorter and David Healy, *Shock Therapy: A History of Electroconvulsive Treatment in Mental Illness* (Toronto: University of Toronto Press, 2007).

14. Nathan G. Hale Jr., *The Rise and Crisis of Psychoanalysis in the United States: Freud and the Americans, 1917–1985* (New York: Oxford University Press, 1995), pp. 115–134; Edward Shorter, *A History of Psychiatry: From the Era of the Asylum to the Age of Prozac* (New York: John Wiley & Sons, 1997), pp. 166–170.

15. Hale, *Psychoanalysis in the United States*, p. 188.

16. Gerald N. Grob, *From Asylum to Community: Mental Health Policy in Modern America* (Princeton: Princeton University Press, 1991), pp. 10–17.

17. Jonathan Michel Metzl, *Prozac on the Couch: Prescribing Gender in the Era of Wonder Drugs* (Durham, NC: Duke University Press, 2003), p. 201n3; Grob, *Asylum to Community*, p. 32; Shorter, *History of Psychiatry*, pp. 162–163.

18. Committee on Nomenclature and Statistics of the American Psychiatric Association, *Diagnostic and Statistical Manual: Mental Disorders* (Washington, DC: American Psychiatric Association, 1952), pp. 9, 31. For more on the origin of *DSM-I*, see Gerald N. Grob, "Origins of

DSM-I: A Study in Appearance and Reality," *American Journal of Psychiatry* 148, no. 4 (1991), pp. 421–431; Robert Cancro, "Functional Psychoses and the Conceptualization of Mental Illness," in Roy W. Menninger and John C. Nemiah (eds.), *American Psychiatry after World War II (1944–1994)* (Washington DC: American Psychiatry Press, 2000), pp. 413–429.

19. Gerald N. Grob, "From Hospital to Community: Mental Health Policy in Modern America," *Psychiatric Quarterly* 62, no. 3 (1991), pp. 192–193.

20. Ralph R. Greenson, "The Classic Psychoanalytic Approach," in Silvano Arieti (ed.), *American Handbook of Psychiatry*, vol. 2 (New York: Basic Books, 1959), p. 1405.

21. Mical Raz, "Between the Ego and the Icepick: Psychosurgery, Psychoanalysis, and Psychiatric Discourse," *Bulletin of the History of Medicine* 82, no. 2 (2008), pp. 387–420. For a similar argument for the case of ECT, see Jonathan Sadowski, "Beyond the Metaphor of the Pendulum: Electroconvulsive Therapy, Psychoanalysis, and the Styles of American Psychiatry," *Journal of the History of Medicine and Allied Sciences* 61, no. 1 (2006), pp. 1–25.

22. W. J. Bleckwenn, "Production of Sleep and Rest in Psychotic Cases: A Preliminary Report," *Archives of Neurology & Psychiatry* 24, no. 2 (1930), p. 368; W. J. Bleckwenn, "Sodium Amytal in Certain Nervous and Mental Conditions," *Wisconsin Medical Journal* 29 (December 1930), p. 695; Erich Lindemann, "Psychological Changes in Normal and Abnormal Individuals under the Influence of Sodium Amytal," *American Journal of Psychiatry* 88, no. 6 (1932), p. 1086.

23. For a discussion of war neuroses, see Hale, *Psychoanalysis in the United States*, p. 192. Techniques similar to narcosynthesis were at the same time being developed by British psychiatrists, especially William Sargant and Eliot Slater. See Elizabeth Roberts-Pederson, "The Hard School: Physical Treatments for War Neurosis in Britain during the Second World War," *Social History of Medicine* 29, no. 3 (2016), pp. 611–632.

24. Roy R. Grinker and John P. Spiegel, "Brief Psychotherapy in War Neuroses," *Psychosomatic Medicine* 6, no. 2 (1944), p. 127.

25. Ibid., p. 128

26. For positive case studies, see Roy R. Grinker and John P. Spiegel, *Men under Stress* (Philadelphia: Blakiston, 1945), pp. 396–405.

27. *The Snake Pit*, dir. Anatole Litvak (1948; Beverly Hills: Twentieth Century Fox, 2004), DVD. The movie was an adaption of Mary Jane Ward's novel of the same name (1946), although narcosynthesis does not feature in the book. See Mary Jane Ward, *The Snake Pit* (New York: Random House, 1946). The book and film's depictions of the crowded and often poor conditions in state psychiatric hospitals influenced public perceptions of hospital psychiatry.

28. Leonard Tilkin, "The Present Status of Narcosynthesis Using Sodium Pentothal and Sodium Amytal," *Diseases of the Nervous System* 10, no. 7 (1949), p. 217.

29. Nicolas Rasmussen, *On Speed: The Many Lives of Amphetamine* (New York: New York University Press, 2008), fig. 24, p. 122. The use of amphetamines as facilitators for psychotherapy is explored in greater detail in Nathan William Moon, "The Amphetamine Years: A Study of the Medical Applications and Extramedical Consumption of Psychostimulant Drugs in the Postwar United States, 1945–1980" (PhD diss., Georgia Institute of Technology, 2009), pp. 95–153.

30. Tone, *Age of Anxiety*, pp. 44–45, 74–75.

31. Rinkel first reported his research briefly in Edwin Gildea (moderator), "Endocrinologic Orientation to Psychiatric Disorders: Discussion," *Journal of Clinical and Experimental Psychopathology* 12, no. 1 (1951), p. 42. For more detailed reports, see Six Staff Members of Boston Psychopathic Hospital, "Experimental Psychoses," *Scientific American* 192, no. 6 (1955), pp. 34–39; Max Rinkel, "Pharmacodynamics of LSD and Mescaline," *Journal of Nervous and Mental Disease* 125, no. 3 (1957), pp. 424–427.

32. Anthony K. Busch and Warren C. Johnson, "L.S.D. 25 as an Aid in Psychotherapy," *Diseases of the Nervous System* 11, no. 8 (1950), p. 241.

33. Ibid., p. 243.

34. Ibid., p. 243.

35. Charles Savage, "Biographical Data," folder 4, box 9, Charles Savage Papers, MSP 70, Archives and Special Collections, Purdue University Libraries, West Lafayette, Indiana (hereafter Savage Papers).

36. [Charles Savage], untitled manuscript, n.d., folder 10, box 7, Savage Papers.

37. Klüver, *Mescal*, pp. 107, 109.

38. Charles Savage, "Hypnagogic Hallucinations" (MS diss., University of Chicago, 1943).

39. [Savage], untitled manuscript.

40. Savage, "Biographical Data"; Charles Savage, untitled speech, n.d., folder 13, box 8, Savage Papers.

41. Harold A. Abramson (ed.), *The Use of LSD in Psychotherapy: Transactions of a Conference on D-Lysergic Acid Diethylamide (LSD-25)* (New York: Josiah Macy, Jr. Foundation, 1960), p. 9.

42. Charles Savage, "Lysergic Acid Diethylamide (LSD-25): A Clinical-Psychological Study," *American Journal of Psychiatry* 108, no. 12 (1952), pp. 897, 896.

43. Ibid., p. 900.

44. Charles Savage, "Variations in Ego Feeling Induced by D-Lysergic Acid Diethylamide (LSD-25)," *Psychoanalytic Review* 42, no. 1 (1955), pp. 1–16.

45. Louis S. Cholden, Albert Kurland, and Charles Savage, "Clinical Reactions and Tolerance to LSD in Chronic Schizophrenia," *Journal of Nervous and Mental Disease* 122, no. 3 (1955), pp. 211–221. Although the researchers experimented with administering LSD in a double-blind fashion, they did not actually use that term, which was not yet in widespread use.

46. Ibid., pp. 213, 217.

47. Constantine J. Falliers, "In Memoriam: Harold A. Abramson, M.D. 1899–1980," *Journal of Asthma* 18, no. 1 (1981), pp. 83–84; Arthur H. Aufses Jr. and Barbara Niss, *This House of Noble Deeds: The Mount Sinai Hospital, 1852–2002* (New York: New York University Press, 2002), p. 54.

48. Abramson, *LSD in Psychotherapy*, p. 8.

49. See H. A. Abramson et al., "Lysergic Acid Diethylamide (LSD-25): I. Physiological and Perceptual Responses," *Journal of Psychology* 39 (1955), pp. 3–60; H. A. Abramson et al., "Lysergic Acid Diethylamide (LSD-25): V. Effect on Spatial Relations Abilities," *Journal of Psychology* 39 (1955), pp. 435–442; H. A. Abramson, M. E. Jarvik, and M. W. Hirsch, "Lysergic Acid Diethylamide (LSD-25): VII. Effect upon Two Measures of Motor Performance," *Journal of Psychology* 39 (1955), pp. 455–464; M. E. Jarvik et al., "Lysergic Acid Diethylamide (LSD-25): VIII. Effect on Arithmetic Test Performance," *Journal of Psychology* 39 (1955), pp. 465–474.

50. John Marks, *The Search for the "Manchurian Candidate": The CIA and Mind Control* (New York: Times Books, 1979), pp. 59–64.

51. See M. E. Jarvik, H. A. Abramson, and M. W. Hirsch, "Lysergic Acid Diethylamide (LSD-25): VI. Effect upon Recall and Recognition of Various Stimuli," *Journal of Psychology* 39 (1955), pp. 443–454; A. Levine et al., "Lysergic Acid Diethylamide (LSD-25): XIV. Effect on Personality as Observed in Psychological Tests," *Journal of Psychology* 40 (1955), pp. 351–66; M. E. Jarvik, H. A. Abramson, and M. W. Hirsch," Lysergic Acid Diethylamide (LSD-25): IV. Effect on Attention and Concentration," *Journal of Psychology* 39 (1955), pp. 373–384. Marks briefly cites a funding proposal from Abramson to the CIA in which he suggests giving LSD to healthy individuals without their knowledge for "psychotherapeutic purposes." The precise plan, its purpose, and whether it was put into place is not clear. See Marks, *Search*, p. 83. Abramson was also brought in as a psychiatric consultant by the CIA to assess and treat Frank Olsen, a scientist from the Army Chemical Corps' Special Operations Division who worked with biological weapons and who was collaborating with the CIA. According to Marks, based

largely on CIA records released in 1975, Olsen had become mentally unstable after receiving a covert dose of LSD from the CIA and ultimately committed suicide by jumping out of his hotel window while in New York under the care of the CIA to see Abramson. According to Marks, Abramson participated in initially covering up the circumstances surrounding Olsen's mental breakdown and death. See ibid., pp. 73–86. After uncovering further evidence, Olsen's son, Eric Olsen, believes that even this narrative was a cover-up, and that his father was killed by the CIA because his colleagues there believed he was a security risk after he objected to the apparent use of biological weapons in the Korean war. See *Wormwood*, directed by Errol Morris, miniseries (Los Gatos, CA: Netflix Studios, 2017), https://www.netflix.com/title/80059446. Ultimately, the precise level of Abramson's involvement in the events preceding Olsen's death and any subsequent cover-up is unclear.

52. Harold A. Abramson (ed.), *The Use of LSD in Psychotherapy and Alcoholism* (Indianapolis: Bobbs-Merrill, 1967), pp. 474–475; Harold A. Abramson, "Some Observations on Normal Volunteers and Patients," in Cholden, *Lysergic Acid Diethylamide and Mescaline*, pp. 52–53.

53. Harold A. Abramson, "Lysergic Acid Diethylamide (LSD-25): III. As an Adjunct to Psychotherapy with Elimination of Fear of Homosexuality," *Journal of Psychology* 39 (1955), pp. 127–155; Abramson, *LSD in Psychotherapy*, pp. 25, 34; Harold A. Abramson, "Lysergic Acid Diethylamide (LSD-25): XIX. As an Adjunct to Brief Psychotherapy, with Special Reference to Ego Enhancement," *Journal of Psychology* 41 (1956), pp. 199–230.

54. Abramson, "(LSD-25): III," pp. 127–155.

55. Cholden, *Lysergic Acid Diethylamide and Mescaline*, p. x.

56. For reference to Sandison's coining of the term "psycholytic therapy," see Hanscarl Leuner, "Present State of Psycholytic Therapy and Its Possibilities," in Abramson, *LSD in Psychotherapy and Alcoholism*, p. 101.

57. R. A. Sandiaon, "The Clinical Uses of Lysergic Acid Diethylamide," in Cholden, *Lysergic Acid Diethylamide and Mescaline*, pp. 31–32.

58. Ibid., p. 28. For more on Sandison's research, see R. A. Sandison, A. M. Spencer, and J. D. A. Whitelaw, "The Therapeutic Value of Lysergic Acid Diethylamide in Mental Illness," *Journal of Mental Science* 100, no. 479 (1954), pp. 491–507; and R. A. Sandison, "Psychological Aspects of the LSD Treatment of the Neuroses," *Journal of Mental Science* 100, no. 419 (1954), pp. 508–515.

59. Charles Savage, "The LSD Psychosis as a Transaction between the Psychiatrist and Patient," in Cholden, *Lysergic Acid Diethylamide and Mescaline*, p. 41.

60. For Leary's use of the term, see Timothy Leary, Ralph Metzner, and Richard Alpert, *The Psychedelic Experience: A Manual Based on the Tibetan Book of the Dead* (1964; repr., New York: Citadel Press, 1992), p. 11. For a history of the term that reflects the common belief that it was coined in the 1960s by Leary, see Ido Hartogsohn, "Constructing Drug Effects: A History of Set and Setting," *Drug Science, Policy and Law* 3, published electronically, 1 January 2017, doi:10.1177/2050324516683325.

61. Aldous Huxley, "Mescaline and the 'Other World,'" in Cholden, *Lysergic Acid Diethylamide and Mescaline*, p. 46.

62. Ibid., p. 49.

63. Cholden, *Lysergic Acid Diethylamide and Mescaline*, pp. 67, 77–78.

64. Erika Dyck has most extensively explored the history of LSD research in Saskatchewan. See Dyck, *Psychedelic Psychiatry*; Erika Dyck, "'Hitting Highs at Rock Bottom': LSD Treatment for Alcoholism, 1950–1970," *Social History of Medicine* 19, no. 2 (2006), pp. 313–329; Erika Dyck, "Land of the Living Sky with Diamonds: A Place for Radical Psychiatry?," *Journal of Canadian Studies* 41, no. 3 (2007), pp. 42–66; and Erika Dyck, "Spaced-out in Saskatchewan: Modernism, Anti-psychiatry, and Deinstitutionalization, 1950–1968," *Bulletin of the History of Medicine* 84, no. 4 (2010), pp. 640–666.

65. Dyck, *Psychedelic Psychiatry*, pp. 15–19; David Healy, *The Creation of Psychopharmacology* (Cambridge, MA: Harvard University Press, 2002), pp. 182–185.

66. Dyck, *Psychedelic Psychiatry*, pp. 26–31, 39–40.

67. Abram Hoffer, "A Program for the Treatment of Alcoholism: LSD, Malvaria and Nicotinic Acid," in Abramson, *LSD in Psychotherapy and Alcoholism*, pp. 343–344.

68. Ibid., pp. 343–344; Humphry Osmond, "Alcoholism: A Personal View of Psychedelic Treatment," in Richard E. Hicks and Paul Jay Fink (eds.), *Psychedelic Drugs* (New York: Grune & Stratton, 1969), pp. 217–218.

69. Hoffer, "Treatment of Alcoholism," p. 344.

70. Colin M. Smith, "A New Adjunct to the Treatment of Alcoholism: The Hallucinogenic Drugs," *Quarterly Journal of Studies on Alcohol* 19 (1958), pp. 406–417.

71. Ibid., p. 415.

72. Ibid., p. 414.

73. Abram Hoffer, "Treatment of Alcoholism with Psychedelic Drugs," in Bernard Aaronson and Humphry Osmond (eds.), *Psychedelics: The Uses and Implications of Hallucinogenic Drugs* (Garden City, NY: Anchor Books, 1970), p. 360; Abram Hoffer and Humphry Osmond, *New Hope for Alcoholics* (New York: University Books, 1968), p. 57.

74. A. Hoffer and H. Osmond, with a contribution by T. Weckowicz, *The Hallucinogens* (New York: Academic Press, 1967), p. 155. In 1956 Hoffer, Osmond, and colleagues Duncan Blewett and Teddy Weckowicz participated in a local peyote ceremony held by the Red Pheasant Band. They were invited to participate in order to help build support for continued legal access to peyote for religious use among Native Americans in the face of political challenges. See Dyck, *Psychedelic Psychiatry*, pp. 81–89; and Fannie Kahan, with contributions from Abram Hoffer et al., *A Culture's Catalyst: Historical Encounters with Peyote and the Native American Church in Canada*, ed. and with an introduction by Erika Dyck (Winnipeg: University of Manitoba Press, 2016).

75. For references to James, see Smith, "Treatment of Alcoholism," p. 407; Colin M. Smith, "Some Reflections on the Possible Therapeutic Effects of the Hallucinogens," *Quarterly Journal of Studies on Alcohol* 20 (1959), pp. 294–296. For James's discussion, see William James, *The Varieties of Religious Experience: A Study in Human Nature* (1902; reprint, New York: Modern Library, n.d.), pp. 198–200, 262–263. For reference to Bill W., see Hoffer, "Treatment of Alcoholism," p. 344.

76. Stevens, *Storming Heaven*, pp. 43–46; Aldous Huxley, *The Doors of Perception* (New York: Harper, 1954). For Huxley's interest in mysticism, see Aldous Huxley, *The Perennial Philosophy* (New York: Perennial Library, 1970).

77. Humphry Osmond, "A Review of the Clinical Effects of Psychotomimetic Agents," *Annals of the New York Academy of Sciences* 66 (March 1957), p. 418.

78. Ibid., pp. 420, 429, 430.

79. Ibid., p. 429.

80. See Lee and Shlain, *Acid Dreams*, pp. 44–53; Stevens, *Storming Heaven*, pp. 53–60.

81. Hubbard's PhD was from Taylor University of Bio-Psycho-Dynamic Sciences. The American Medical Association recognized this institution as a diploma mill. See Oliver Field to Lynn Gunn, 10 September 1959, folder 9, box 482, collection 471, Historical Health Fraud and Alternative Medicine Collection, American Medical Association, Chicago, Illinois.

82. Hoffer and Osmond, *New Hope for Alcoholics*, pp. 58–60. For Hubbard's full therapeutic method, see J. Ross MacLean et al., "The Use of LSD-25 in the Treatment of Alcoholism and Other Psychiatric Problems," *Quarterly Journal of Studies on Alcohol* 22 (1961), pp. 34–45.

83. N. Chwelos et al., "Use of d-Lysergic Acid Diethylamide in the Treatment of Alcoholism," *Quarterly Journal of Studies on Alcohol* 20 (1959), pp. 577–590.

84. Ibid., pp. 584, 588.

85. Stevens, *Storming Heaven*, pp. 58–69. For Watts's description and interpretation of his LSD experience, see Alan W. Watts, *The Joyous Cosmology: Adventures in the Chemistry of Consciousness* (New York: Pantheon Books, 1962).

86. Dyck, *Psychedelic Psychiatry*, pp. 96–98.

87. Betty Grover Eisner and Sidney Cohen, "Psychotherapy with Lysergic Acid Diethylamide," *Journal of Nervous and Mental Disease* 127 (1958), p. 538.

88. Betty Grover Eisner, "Remembrances of LSD Therapy Past" (unpublished manuscript, 2002), p. 5, http://www.maps.org/images/pdf/books/remembrances.pdf; Sidney Cohen, *The Beyond Within: The LSD Story*, 2nd ed. (New York: Atheneum, 1967), pp. 106–108, 286. Cohen's experience is also described in Steven J. Novak, "LSD before Leary: Sidney Cohen's Critique of 1950s Psychedelic Research," *Isis* 88, no. 1 (1997), p. 92.

89. Eisner, "Remembrances of LSD Therapy Past," pp. 26–28; Novak, "LSD before Leary," p. 97.

90. James Terrill, "The Nature of the LSD Experience," *Journal of Nervous and Mental Disease* 135 (1962), p. 428.

91. Donald D. Jackson, "LSD and the New Beginning," *Journal of Nervous and Mental Disease* 135 (1962), p. 438.

92. Charles Savage, "LSD, Alcoholism and Transcendence," *Journal of Nervous and Mental Disease* 135 (1962), p. 430n10.

93. Ibid., p. 430. The original quote from James was, "The only radical remedy I know for dipsomania is religiomania," and James credited it to "some medical man." James, *Varieties of Religious Experience*, p. 263n1.

94. Savage, "LSD, Alcoholism and Transcendence," p. 431.

95. James, quoted in ibid., p. 432.

96. Ibid., pp. 432–433.

97. [Charles Savage], untitled manuscript, n.d., folder 10, box 7, Savage Papers. The incident is also briefly alluded to in Terrill, "Nature of the LSD Experience," p. 427n4.

Chapter 2 · Regulating Research

Epigraph: *Organization and Coordination of Federal Drug Research and Regulatory Programs: LSD*, Hearings before the Subcommittee on Executive Reorganization of the Committee on Government Operations, United States Senate, 89th Congress, 2nd Session, May 24, 25, 26, 1966 (Washington, DC: US Government Printing Office, 1966), p. 2.

1. Ibid., p. 59.

2. Myron J. Stolaroff, *Thanatos to Eros: Thirty-Five Years of Psychedelic Exploration* (Berlin: VWB—Verlag für Wissenschaft und Bildung, 1994), p. 29; Harold A. Abramson, "Will the Legal Supply of LSD to the Private Medical Practitioner be Stopped Indefinitely?," *Mademoiselle* (January 1967), folder "National Institute of Mental Health," box 10, Peter G. Stafford Papers, Rare Book and Manuscript Library, Columbia University Libraries, New York. Emphasis original.

3. Daniel Carpenter, *Reputation and Power: Organizational Image and Pharmaceutical Regulation at the FDA* (Princeton: Princeton University Press, 2010), pp. 173–175.

4. Arthur A. Daemmrich, *Pharmacopolitics: Drug Regulation in the United States and Germany* (Chapel Hill: University of North Carolina Press, 2004), p. 66.

5. Earl L. Meyers, "The Food and Drug Administration's View of Investigational Drugs," presentation to the Annual Pharmacy Congress, St. John's University, Jamaica, New York, 18 April 1963, folder 505.51 April–May, box 3572, General Subject Files 1938–1974, Division of General Services, RG 88—Records of the Food and Drug Administration, National Archives at College Park, Maryland (hereafter RG 88), p. 1. The case of thalidomide, and its influence on the passage of the Drug Amendments of 1962, is discussed in detail in Carpenter, *Reputation and Power*, pp. 213–260; and Philip J. Hilts, *Protecting America's Health: The FDA, Business, and One Hundred Years of Regulation* (New York: Alfred A. Knopf, 2003), pp. 144–165.

6. Drug Amendments of 1962, 87 P.L. 781; 76 Stat. 780, 10 October 1962, Title 1, Part A, Sec. 103 (b).

7. Meyers, "Investigational Drugs," p. 3.

8. Bureau of Enforcement to Directors of Bureaus and Divisions, and Directors of Districts, 7 May 1963, folder 505.51 April—May, box 3572, RG 88.

9. George P. Larrick, "Procedural and Interpretative Regulations; Investigational Use," *Federal Register* 28, no. 5 (8 January 1963), pp. 179–182. The three-phase structure of drug investigation was an FDA invention that would thereafter fundamentally shape the nature of drug research. See Carpenter, *Reputation and Power*, pp. 275–280, 292–297.

10. Meyers, "Investigational Drugs," p. 8.

11. For the discovery and synthesis of psilocybin, see Albert Hofmann, *LSD: My Problem Child; Reflections on Sacred Drugs, Mysticism and Science*, trans. Jonathan Ott (Santa Cruz: Multidisciplinary Association for Psychedelic Studies, 2009), pp. 117–129.

12. J. F. Reilly to Kelsey re. IND #311—Psilocybin Tablets, 15 August 1963, folder 505.51 August, box 3570, RG 88; William D'Aguanno to Kelsey re IND #305—LSD-25 Substance, 19 September 1963, folder 505.51 Sept., box 3570, RG 88. The LSD dose of 200–300 mcg/kg is so huge as to suggest an error—by 1967, 1500 mcg was the largest single dose that had been reported, and 200–300 mcg was a standard single high dose. Similarly, the dose of 1 to 5 mcg seems infinitesimal even for children—25 mcg was considered the threshold dose for adults, and standard doses were frequently given to children. Therefore, 1–5 mcg/kg may have been the correct dose range. However, these doses are listed in several versions of the FDA report and could merely represent the dose range considered nontoxic. For dose ranges, see A. Hoffer and H. Osmond, with a contribution by T. Weckowicz, *The Hallucinogens* (New York: Academic Press, 1967), pp. 103–104, 178.

13. *Drug Safety* (Part 5, Appendixes, and Index), Hearings before a Subcommittee on Government Operations, House of Representatives, 89th Congress, 2nd Session, March 9, 10; May 25, 26; June 7, 8, and 9, 1966 (Washington, DC: US Government Printing Office, 1966), p. 2134.

14. Reilly to Kelsey re. IND #311, 15 August 1963; D'Aguanno to Kelsey re IND #305, 19 September 1963.

15. *Drug Safety*, pp. 2134–2135. The psilocybin IND was also approved, presumably after similar deliberation.

16. The investigators are listed in George P. Larrick to L. R. Fountain, 17 September 1963, box 3587, RG 88. For their research, see Keith S. Ditman and John R. B. Whittlesey, "Comparison of the LSD-25 Experience and Delirium Tremens," *A.M.A. Archives of General Psychiatry* 1 (1959), pp. 47–57; Keith S. Ditman, Max Hayman, and John R. B. Whittlesey, "Nature and Frequency of Claims Following LSD," *Journal of Nervous and Mental Disease* 134, no. 4 (1962), pp. 346–52; Dietrich W. Heyder, "LSD-25 in Conversion Reaction," *American Journal of Psychiatry* 120, no. 4 (1963), pp. 396–397; Eric C. Kask, "The Analgesic Action of Lysergic Acid Diethylamide Compared with Dihydromorphinone and Meperidine," *Bulletin on Drug Action and Narcotics* 27 (1963), pp. 3517–3529; L. Bender, L. Goldschmidt, and D. V. S. Siva, "Treatment of Autistic Schizophrenic Children with LSD-25 and UML-491," *Recent Advances in Biological Psychiatry* 4 (1962), pp. 170–177; A. Kurland et al., "LSD in the Treatment of Alcoholics," *Pharmakopsychiatrie-Neuro-Psychoparmakologie* 4, no. 2 (1971), pp. 83–94; Wilson Van Dusen et al., "Treatment of Alcoholism with Lysergide," *Quarterly Journal of Studies on Alcohol* 28, no. 2 (1967), pp. 295–303.

17. *Organization and Coordination: LSD*, p. 62.

18. Harold A. Abramson (ed.), *The Use of LSD in Psychotherapy and Alcoholism* (Indianapolis: Bobbs-Merrill, 1967), p. xiii.

19. Craig Burrell to Frances Kelsey, 5 March 1964, folder 521.6-525.091, box 3758, RG 88.

20. Harold A. Abramson to FDA, 9 May 1963, box 3750, RG 88.

21. C. E. Beisel to Harold A. Abramson, 13 June 1963, box 3750, RG 88; C. E. Beisel to Harold A. Abramson, 22 August 1963, box 3750, RG 88.

22. Memorandum of Interview between Harold A. Abramson, Merle L. Gibson, and Francis O. Kelsey, 8 November 1963, folder 521.6-525.091, box 3758, RG 88.

23. Harold A. Abramson and Llewellyn T. Evans, "Lysergic Acid Diethylamide (LSD 25): II. Psychobiological Effects on the Siamese Fighting Fish," *Science* 120, no. 3128 (1954), pp. 990–991.

24. Interview between Abramson, Gibson, and Kelsey, 8 November 1963.

25. Harold A. Abramson to Rudolph Bircher, 11 November 1963, folder 521.6-525.091, box 3758, RG 88. For sections 1–6 of the IND form, see Larrick, "Regulations; Investigational Use," p. 179.

26. Leonard B. Achor to Harold A. Abramson, 18 November 1963, folder 521.6-525.091, box 3758, RG 88. Emphasis original.

27. Harold A. Abramson to Leonard B. Achor, 21 November 1963, folder 521.6-525.091, box 3758, RG 88.

28. Leonard B. Achor to Harold A. Abramson, 12 December 1963, folder 521.6-525.091, box 3758, RG 88.

29. Harold A. Abramson to Frances O. Kelsey, 2 January 1964, folder 521.6-525.091, box 3758, RG 88.

30. Frances O. Kelsey to C. J. Karadimos, 23 March 1964, folder 521.6-525.091, box 3758, RG 88; Burrell to Kelsey, 5 March 1964.

31. Frances O. Kelsey to Charles J. Karadimos, 24 January 1964, box 3750, RG 88; Kelsey to Karadimos, 23 March 1964.

32. C. J. Karadimos to Director, New York District Division of Field Operations, 15 April 1964, folder 521.6-525.091, box 3758, RG 88.

33. Irwin Schorr to Director, New York District, 29 June 1964, folder 521.6-525.091, box 3758, RG 88.

34. Ibid.

35. Ibid.

36. Ibid.

37. Geo. P. Larrick to Harold A. Abramson, 11 May 1965, box 3750, RG 88.

38. Geo. P. Larrick to Harold A. Abramson, 23 July 1965, box 3750, RG 88.

39. Robert T. Dee to Director, New York District, 10 August 1965, folder 521.6-525.091, box 3758, RG 88.

40. Ibid.; A. Harris Kenyon to A. E. Rayfield, 10 September 1965, folder 521.6-525.091, box 3758, RG 88.

41. Merle L. Gibson to Harold A. Abramson, 18 June 1969, folder 505.51 June, box 4247, RG 88.

42. *Drug Safety*, p. 2202.

43. Stolaroff, *Thanatos to Eros*, pp. 18–24.

44. Ibid., p. 25.

45. Ibid., p. 26.

46. *Drug Safety*, p. 2212. For the date Savage joined the foundation, see Abram Hoffer to Al Hubbard, 23 November 1961, II. A. 106, S-A1101, Abram Hoffer Fonds F 410, Provincial Archives of Saskatchewan, Saskatoon, Canada (hereafter Hoffer Fonds).

47. Stolaroff, *Thanatos to Eros*, p. 26.

48. As discussed in chapter 1, Hubbard claimed to have a PhD in Bio-Psycho-Dynamic Sciences, but the granting institution was considered a diploma mill.

49. "Research Program of the International Foundation for Advanced Study," undated, folder 1, box 8, Charles Savage Papers, MSP 70, Archives and Special Collections, Purdue University Libraries, Indiana (hereafter Savage Papers), p. 3; Charles Savage, "LSD-25: Value

Changes in the Psychedelic Experience," application for research grant to the U.S. Department of Health, Education, and Welfare, MH 07221-01, received 2 July 1962, folder 1, box 8, Savage Papers, p. 11.

50. "Research Program," p. 5. For Hoffer and Osmond's placement on the Foundation's advisory board, see Myron J. Stolaroff to Abram Hoffer, 26 February 1963, II. A. 107, S-A1101, Hoffer Fonds.

51. Savage, "LSD-25," p. 6.

52. "Research Program," p. 4.

53. J. N. Sherwood, M. J. Stolaroff, and W. W. Harman, "The Psychedelic Experience—a New Concept in Psychotherapy," *Journal of Neuropsychiatry* 4 (1962), p. 74. Lead author John Sherwood was the foundation's medical supervisor, while Savage was medical director.

54. Ibid., p. 72.

55. Ibid., p. 74.

56. Savage, "LSD-25," p. 6.

57. Ibid., pp. 7–8.

58. Ibid., p. 9.

59. Ibid., p. 9.

60. Charles Savage, "A Controlled Study of LSD-25 and Alcoholism," draft application for research grant to the US Department of Health, Education and Welfare, 27 December 1962, folder 3, box 8, Savage Papers.

61. Charles Savage and Willis Harman, "A Controlled Investigation of the Psychedelic (LSD-25) Approach to Alcoholism," undated draft proposal, folder 1, box 8, Savage Papers.

62. Charles Savage et al., "The Effects of Psychedelic (LSD) Therapy on Values, Personality, and Behavior," *International Journal of Neuropsychiatry* 2 (May–June 1966), pp. 241–254. For other reports of the same research, see Robert E. Mogar and Charles Savage, "Personality Change Associated with Psychedelic (LSD) Therapy: A Preliminary Report," *Psychotherapy* 1 (1964), pp. 154–162; Charles Savage et al., "LSD: Therapeutic Effects of the Psychedelic Experience," *Psychological Reports* 14 (1964), pp. 111–120. The Public Health Service was the direct parent organization of the FDA and National Institutes of Health, under the Department of Health, Education, and Welfare.

63. *Drug Safety*, p. 2206.

64. William D'Aguanno to Kelsey re. IND #486–-d-lysergic acid diethylamide, psilocybin, 7 October 1963, folder 505.51 October, box 3570, RG 88.

65. *Drug Safety*, pp. 2202–2203.

66. Myron J. Stolaroff to Abram Hoffer, 26 August 1964, II. A. 107, S-A1101, Hoffer Fonds; Albert A. Kurland to Charles Savage, 28 September 1964, folder 2, box 2, Savage Papers.

67. Stolaroff to Hoffer, 26 August 1964; Don D. Jackson, memorandum to members of the division of psychiatry, Palo Alto-Stanford Hospital Center, 1 July 1964, enclosed with ibid.; Charles Savage, "Biographical Data," folder 4, box 9, Savage Papers. For Jackson's career in family therapy, see Wendel A. Ray, Ryan J. Stivers, and Courtney Brasher, "Through the Eyes of Don D. Jackson M.D.," *Journal of Systemic Therapies* 30, no. 1 (2011), pp. 38–58.

68. *Drug Safety*, p. 2203.

69. Ibid., p. 2204.

70. Food and Drug Administration, Summary of Proceedings, Thirteenth Meeting, Advisory Committee on Investigational Drugs, 3 December 1964, Washington, DC, folder 1, box 13, Frances Oldham Kelsey Papers, Manuscript Division, Library of Congress, Washington, DC (hereafter Kelsey Papers), p. 5.

71. *Drug Safety*, p. 2137; Minutes of telephone call between Abram Hoffer and Myron Stolaroff, 2 November 1964, II. A. 107, S-A1101, Hoffer Fonds.

72. John L. Harvey to Myron J. Stolaroff, 6 January 1965, box 3750, RG 88.

73. *Drug Safety*, p. 2202. For a discussion of psychoanalytic asthma research see Nathan G. Hale Jr., *The Rise and Crisis of Psychoanalysis in the United States: Freud and the Americans, 1917–1985* (New York: Oxford University Press, 1995), pp. 257–263.

74. Stolaroff, *Thanatos to Eros*, p. 26; Savage et al., "Effects of Psychedelic (LSD) Therapy."

75. See J. Ross MacLean et al., "The Use of LSD-25 in the Treatment of Alcoholism and Other Psychiatric Problems," *Quarterly Journal of Studies on Alcohol* 22 (1961), pp. 34–45; and Abram Hoffer, "A Program for the Treatment of Alcoholism: LSD, Malvaria and Nicotinic Acid," in Abramson, *LSD in Psychotherapy and Alcoholism*, pp. 343–406.

76. Drug Abuse Control Amendments of 1965, 89 P.L. 74; 79 Stat. 226, 19 July 1965, Sec. 3.

77. John P. Swann, "Drug Abuse Control under FDA, 1938–1968," *Public Health Reports* 112, no. 1 (1997), pp. 84–86.

78. *Drug Abuse Control Amendments of 1965*, Hearings before the Committee on Interstate and Foreign Commerce, House of Representatives, 89th Congress, 1st Session, January 27, 28; February 2, 9, 10, 1965 (Washington, DC: US Government Printing Office, 1965), p. 1.

79. See *Drug Abuse Control Amendments of 1965*, Hearings; "House Report No. 130, 2 March 1965 [to accompany H.R. 2]," Calendar No. 48, 89th Congress, 1st Session, 1965; "Senate Report No. 337, 21 June 1965 [to accompany H.R. 2]," Calendar No. 326, 89th Congress, 1st Session, 1965. For a discussion of the Drug Abuse Control Amendments as they related to depressant and stimulant drugs, see Nicolas Rasmussen, *On Speed: The Many Lives of Amphetamine* (New York: New York University Press, 2008), pp. 208–212.

80. *Drug Abuse Control Amendments of 1965*, Hearings, p. 23.

81. Drug Abuse Control Amendments of 1965, Sec. 3 (a).

82. For the first notice proposing LSD's control under the amendments, see Winton B. Rankin, "Depressant and Stimulant Drugs: Proposed Listing of Additional Drugs Subject to Control," *Federal Register* 31, no. 11 (18 January 1966), p. 565. For the final notice, see James L. Goddard, "Listing of Additional Drugs Subject to Control: Temporary Exemption from Record Keeping Requirements," *Federal Register* 31, no. 54 (19 March 1966), pp. 4679–4680. Other drugs brought under the control of the amendments included further psychedelics such as mescaline and psilocybin; depressants such as chloral hydrate, diazepam, and meprobamate; and the stimulant methamphetamine. For the reasons behind the delay, see *The Narcotic Rehabilitation Act of 1966*, Hearings before a Special Subcommittee of the Committee on the Judiciary, United States Senate, 89th Congress, 2nd Session, January 25, 26, and 27; May 12, 13, 19, 23, and 25; June 14 and 15; July 19, 1966 (Washington, DC: US Government Printing Office, 1966), pp. 351–352.

83. Legislation passed in 1968 criminalized personal possession of LSD and increased the penalties for other LSD related offences. See 90 P.L. 639, 82 Stat. 1361, 24 October 1968.

84. *Narcotic Rehabilitation Act*, Hearings, pp. 304, 166–168.

85. Ibid., p. 354.

86. Ibid., p. 359, 366.

87. Ibid., pp. 193–194, 208–209.

88. Ibid., p. 239.

89. Ibid., p. 246.

90. Ibid., pp. 326, 322–326.

91. Ibid., pp. 327, 335–339.

92. Ibid., p. 337, 351.

93. Memorandum of conference between representatives of Sandoz Pharmaceuticals, the NIMH, and the FDA, 7 December 1965, folder 521.6-525.091, box 3758, RG 88. A 23 August 1965 letter from Sandoz halting the production and distribution of LSD is reproduced in Hofmann, *LSD*, pp. 85–87. The letter cites this move as due to the drug's growing abuse, resulting from increasing publicity, inadequate legal control, and increased availability after the expiration of

the drug's patent in 1963. It is unclear, however, who this letter was sent to, and what impact it had, as Sandoz did not withdraw its sponsorship of LSD in the United States at this time.

94. Larrick, "Regulations; Investigational Use," p. 180.

95. Conference between Sandoz, the NIMH, and the FDA, 7 December 1965.

96. *Organization and Coordination: LSD*, pp. 80–81.

97. Ibid., pp. 62–62; *Drug Safety*, pp. 2135–2136.

98. *Organization and Coordination: LSD*, p. 94, 57.

99. Ibid., p. 57.

100. Ibid., pp. 55–57, 73, 77.

101. James L. Goddard, "Certain Hallucinogenic Drugs; Conditions for Investigational Use," *Federal Register* 31, no. 135 (14 July 1966), p. 9540.

102. Records of the establishment and activity of this committee are scarce. For an overview of its role, written by its executive secretary, see John A. Scigliano, "Psychotomimetic Agents," *Journal of the American Pharmaceutical Association*, n.s., 8, no. 1 (1968), pp. 28–29. Planning for the committee began at the FDA in May 1964, though it is not clear when it began operating. See Food and Drug Administration, Summary of Proceedings, Tenth Meeting of the Advisory Committee on Investigational Drugs, Washington, DC, 28 May 1964, folder 1, box 13, Kelsey Papers.

103. For a list of the FDA's public advisory committees in 1967, see Carpenter, *Reputation and Power*, p. 314.

104. An initial list of suggested committee members included several prominent LSD psychotherapy researchers, including Humphry Osmond and Albert Kurland; however, for unknown reasons their names had subsequently been crossed out. See Joseph F. Sadusk to Clem O. Miller, 27 July 1964, folder 4, box 13, Kelsey Papers. A 1969 list of committee members included only one member who had published a report on therapeutic research with psychedelics. That researcher, Sidney Merlis, appears to have done only limited psycholytic therapy research in the 1950s. For the list of members, see Members FDA-PHS Psychotomimetic Agents Advisory Committee, 21 January 1969, Savage Papers. For Merlis's research, see Herman C. B. Denber and Sidney Merlis, "A Note on Some Therapeutic Implications of the Mescaline-Induced State," *Psychiatric Quarterly* 28, no. 1 (1954), pp. 635–640. Other members, such as Daniel X. Freedman, Joel Elkes, and Carl Pfeiffer, had used LSD in biological and other nonclinical research, see Daniel X. Freedman, "Psychotomimetic Drugs and Brain Biogenic Amines," *American Journal of Psychiatry* 119 (March 1963), pp. 843–850; P. B. Bradley and J. Elkes, "The Effect of Amphetamine and D-Lysergic Acid Diethylamide (LSD 25) on the Electrical Activity of the Brain of the Conscious," *Journal of Physiology* 120, supplement (1953), pp. 13P–14P; Carl C. Pfeiffer et al., "Time-Series, Frequency Analysis, and Electrogenesis of the EEGs of Normals and Psychotics before and after Drugs," *American Journal of Psychiatry* 121, no. 12 (1965), pp. 1147–1155.

105. Scigliano, "Psychotomimetic Agents," p. 29.

106. Drug Amendments of 1962, Title 1, Part A, Sec. 102 (c).

Chapter 3 · *Proof of Efficacy*

Epigraph: Drug Safety (Part 5, Appendixes, and Index), Hearings before a Subcommittee on Government Operations, House of Representatives, 89th Congress, 2nd Session, March 9, 10; May 25, 26; June 7, 8, and 9, 1966 (Washington, DC: US Government Printing Office, 1966), p. 2135.

1. *The Narcotic Rehabilitation Act of 1966*, Hearings before a Special Subcommittee of the Committee on the Judiciary, United States Senate, 89th Congress, 2nd Session, January 25, 26, and 27; May 12, 13, 19, 23, and 25; June 14 and 15; July 19, 1966 (Washington, DC: US Government Printing Office, 1966), p. 345.

2. Drug Amendments of 1962, 87 P.L. 781, 76 Stat. 780, 10 October 1962, Title 1, Part A, Sec. 102 (c).

3. FDA commissioner Herbert Ley first published a description of the expected research standards for evidence of efficacy in 1969, following debates with drug manufacturers. See Herbert L. Ley Jr., "Antibiotic Drugs: Procedural and Interpretative Regulations," *Federal Register* 34, no. 108 (19 September 1969), pp. 14596–14598. His successor Charles Edwards finalized the standards the following year, see Charles C. Edwards, "Hearing Regulations and Regulations Describing Scientific Content of Adequate and Well-Controlled Clinical Investigations," *Federal Register* 35, no. 90 (8 May 1970), pp. 7250–7253. For the debates and events that led to the publication of these research standards, see Scott H. Podolsky, *The Antibiotic Era: Reform, Resistance, and the Pursuit of a Rational Therapeutics* (Baltimore: Johns Hopkins University Press, 2015), pp. 94–111.

4. Harry Marks has most authoritatively explored the evolution of clinical drug research, but he focuses largely on the role of "therapeutic reformers" in promoting high standards of research methodology, paying little attention to the role of regulation before 1970. Harry M. Marks, *The Progress of Experiment: Science and Therapeutic Reform in the United States, 1900–1990* (Cambridge: Cambridge University Press, 1997). Laura Bothwell and colleagues have also indicated 1970 as the point by which randomized controlled trials were required by the FDA. Laura E. Bothwell et al., "Assessing the Gold Standard—Lessons from the History of RCTs," *New England Journal of Medicine* 374, no. 22 (2016), p. 2175. Daniel Carpenter has performed the most significant study of the Drug Amendments of 1962 and the role of the FDA in the evolution of clinical research. However, he focuses on the FDA's concern for efficacy and preference for controlled trials prior to 1962, rather than the impact of the legislation on research. Daniel Carpenter, *Reputation and Power: Organizational Image and Pharmaceutical Regulation at the FDA* (Princeton: Princeton University Press, 2010). Arthur Daemmrich has most closely examined the FDA's regulation of efficacy after the amendments, revealing careful scrutiny over levels of control in studies of propanolol in the late 1960s and early 1970s. Arthur A. Daemmrich, *Pharmacopolitics: Drug Regulation in the United States and Germany* (Chapel Hill: University of North Carolina Press, 2004), pp. 74–77.

Several authors have explored the issue of efficacy though the FDA's Drug Efficacy Study, commenced in 1966. Contracted out to the National Academy of Sciences, this study was initiated to evaluate the efficacy of the thousands of drugs that had received NDAs between 1938 and 1962, without supplying proof of efficacy. Faced with the impractical prospect of requiring new clinical trials for all of the drugs under review, the review panels opted to assess all available evidence, consider expert opinion, and designate drugs "probably" and "possibly" effective when evidence was not of a high caliber. Although the study is of great significance in the history of drug efficacy regulation, its format meant that it did not necessarily reflect the standards to which developers of new drugs in the same period would have had to conform. See Carpenter, *Reputation and Power*, pp. 345–357; Philip J. Hilts, *Protecting America's Health: The FDA, Business, and One Hundred Years of Regulation* (New York: Alfred A. Knopf, 2003), pp. 171–177; Peter Temin, *Taking Your Medicine: Drug Regulation in the United States* (Cambridge, MA: Harvard University Press, 1980), pp. 128–140; Edward Shorter, *Before Prozac: The Troubled History of Mood Disorders in Psychiatry* (New York: Oxford University Press, 2009), pp. 130–149. Scott Podolsky has most carefully explored the problematic relationship between methods for adjudicating efficacy in the Drug Efficacy Study and developing expectations for "adequate and well-controlled investigations" under the 1962 amendments. See Podolsky, *Antibiotic Era*, pp. 94–111.

5. "Proceedings, FDA Conference on the Kefauver-Harris Drug Amendments and Proposed Regulations, February 15, 1963," folder "FDA—Methodologies Used since New Drug Laws 1961–69," box 6, Harry Filmore Dowling Papers, MS. C 372, Modern Manuscripts Collection, History of Medicine Division, National Library of Medicine, Maryland, p. 25.

6. Ibid., p. 26.

7. Carpenter, *Reputation and Power*, pp. 271–273. For the FDA's strategic use of ambiguity, see Daniel P. Carpenter and Colin Moore, "Robust Action and the Strategic Use of Ambiguity in a Bureaucratic Cohort: FDA Officers and the Evolution of New Drug Regulations, 1950–70," in Stephen Skowronek and Matthew Glassman (eds.), *Formative Acts: American Politics in the Making* (Philadelphia: University of Pennsylvania, 2007), pp. 340–362.

8. Joseph F. Sadusk, "The Definition of the Efficacy of a Drug under the Law," presented to the American College of Physicians, Los Angeles, California, 8 October 1964, in FDA (comp.), *Speeches and Papers, 1964* (Rockville, MD: Food and Drug Administration, 1979), FDA Biosciences Library, Silver Spring, Maryland (hereafter FDA Library).

9. Ibid.

10. For the early use of comparative controls, see Abraham M. Lilienfeld, "Ceteris Paribus: The Evolution of the Clinical Trial," *Bulletin of the History of Medicine* 56, no. 1 (1982), pp. 1–18. For the French studies, see Ted J. Kaptchuk, "Intentional Ignorance: A History of Blind Assessment and Placebo Controls in Medicine," *Bulletin of the History of Medicine* 72, no. 3 (1998), pp. 389–433. For more on the history of clinical trials prior to the twentieth century, see J. Rosser Matthews, *Quantification and the Quest for Medical Certainty* (Princeton: Princeton University Press, 1995); and J. P. Bull, "The Historical Development of Clinical Therapeutic Trials," *Journal of Chronic Diseases* 10, no. 3 (1959), pp. 218–248.

11. For Gold's research, see Arthur K. Shapiro and Elaine Shapiro, *The Powerful Placebo: From Ancient Priest to Modern Physician* (Baltimore: Johns Hopkins University Press, 1997), pp. 140–145; Harry Gold, Nathaniel T. Kwit, and Harold Otto, "The Xanthines (Theobromine and Aminophylline) in the Treatment of Cardiac Pain," *Journal of the American Medical Association* 108, no. 26 (1937), pp. 2173–2179. For Hill's research, see Medical Research Council, "Streptomycin Treatment of Pulmonary Tuberculosis," *British Medical Journal* 2, no. 4582 (1948), pp. 769–782. For more on Hill's clinical trials and their place in the development of the randomized controlled trial, see Shapiro and Shapiro, *Powerful Placebo*, pp. 157–159; Peter Armitage, "Bradford Hill and the Randomized Controlled Trial," *Pharmaceutical Medicine* 6 (1992), pp. 23–37; Matthews, *Quantification*, pp. 127–140; Daemmrich, *Pharmacopolitics*, p. 51; David Healy, *The Antidepressant Era* (Cambridge, MA: Harvard University Press, 1997), p. 89; Mark Parascandola, "Clinical Testing: New Developments and Old Problems," in Gregory J. Higby and Elaine C. Stroud (eds.), *The Inside Story of Medicines: A Symposium* (Madison, WI: American Institute of the History of Pharmacy, 1997), p. 201. The origins of randomization are commonly traced to Roland Fisher's 1920s agricultural research, which advanced understandings of statistical theory and experimental design. However, Hill's use of randomization was not based on such statistical theory but was simply intended to avoid bias in patient allocation between treatment and control groups. See Marks, *Progress of Experiment*, pp. 141–148; and Iain Chalmers, "Statistical Theory Was Not the Reason That Randomization Was Used in the British Medical Research Council's Clinical Trial of Streptomycin for Pulmonary Tuberculosis," in Gérard Jorland, Annick Opinel, and George Weisz (eds.), *Body Counts: Medical Quantification in Historical and Sociological Perspective* (Montréal: McGill-Queen's University Press, 2005), pp. 309–334.

12. A. Bradford Hill, "The Clinical Trial," *British Medical Bulletin* 7, no. 4 (1951), pp. 278–282; A. Bradford Hill, "The Clinical Trial," *New England Journal of Medicine* 247, no. 4 (1952), pp. 113–119.

13. Henry K. Beecher, "The Powerful Placebo," *Journal of the American Medical Association* 159, no. 17 (1955), pp. 1603.

14. Ibid., pp. 1602–1606. For the initial reports of Beecher and colleagues' research into placebo response in postoperative pain, see Henry K. Beecher et al., "The Effectiveness of Oral Analgesics (Morphine, Codeine, Acetylsalicylic Acid) and the Problem of Placebo 'Reactors' and 'Non-Reactors,'" *Journal of Pharmacology and Experimental Therapeutics* 109, no. 4 (1953),

pp. 393–400; and Louis Lasagna et al., "A Study of the Placebo Response," *American Journal of Medicine* 16, no. 6 (1954): 770–779. Beecher later published a landmark book concerning the quantitative study of the subjective effects of drugs (such as sedation) and their effects on subjective symptoms such as pain, hunger, and nausea. The work included a significant discussion on LSD and similar drugs, based on Beecher's own work with LSD as well as that of others. This was primarily a phenomenological and physiological analysis of the drugs' effects, from the general perspective that they caused an artificial psychosis, although Beecher did conclude that the profound mental changes caused by LSD were largely "not striking conversions of normal to psychotic, but rather consistent expansive exaggerations of the pre-drug personality in which structural weaknesses and immature factors are magnified." From this perspective, psychotic reactions were "a release of existing tendencies rather than a creation of new elements." See Henry K. Beecher, *Measurement of Subjective Responses: Quantitative Effects of Drugs* (New York: Oxford University Press, 1959), p. 319. For more on Beecher's work with LSD, see John M. von Felsinger, Louis Lasagna, and Henry K. Beecher, "The Response of Normal Men to Lysergic Acid Derivatives (Di-and Mono-Ethyl Amid): Correlation of Personality and Drug Reactions," *Journal of Clinical and Experimental Psychopathology* 17, no. 4 (1956), pp. 414–428.

15. Scott H. Podolsky, *Pneumonia before Antibiotics: Therapeutic Evolution and Evaluation in Twentieth-Century America* (Baltimore: Johns Hopkins University Press, 2006), pp. 37–42; Scott H. Podolsky, "Antibiotics and the Social History of the Controlled Clinical Trial, 1950–1970," *Journal of the History of Medicine and Allied Sciences* 65, no. 3 (2010), pp. 354–360.

16. Harry M. Marks, "Trust and Mistrust in the Marketplace: Statistics and Clinical Research, 1945–1960," *History of Science* 38, no. 3 (2000), pp. 343–355. Marks's analysis is further advanced in Podolsky, "Antibiotics," pp. 327–367.

17. Over the 1960s some progress was made in developing animal models that could be used to screen new drugs for potential psychoactive effects—such as antidepressant effects—based on factors such as the drugs' effects on behavior and their interaction with other drugs in animals. See Lucie Gerber, "Marketing Loops: The Development of Psychopharmacological Screening at Geigy in the 1960s and 1970s," in Jean-Paul Gaudillière and Ulrike Thoms (eds.), *The Development of Scientific Marketing in the Twentieth Century: Research for Sales in the Pharmaceutical Industry* (London: Pickering and Chatto, 2015), pp. 191–212.

18. Jonathan O. Cole and Ralph W. Gerard (eds.), *Psychopharmacology: Problems in Evaluation* (Washington, DC: National Academy of Sciences—National Research Council, 1959), pp. 1–5.

19. Louis Lasagna and Victor G. Laties, "Problems Involved in the Study of Drug-Modified Behavior in Normal Humans," in Cole and Gerard, *Psychopharmacology*, p. 89. For Lasagna's placebo research with Beecher, see Beecher et al., "Effectiveness of Oral Analgesics," pp. 393–400; Lasagna et al., "Study of the Placebo Response," pp. 770–779. Lasagna also collaborated on Beecher's psychotomimetic LSD research. See von Felsinger, Lasagna, and Beecher, "Response of Normal Men to Lysergic Acid Derivatives," pp. 414–428.

20. Jonathan O. Cole, "The Evaluation of the Effectiveness of Treatment in Psychiatry," in Cole and Gerard, *Psychopharmacology*, pp. 97–102; Cole and Gerard, *Psychopharmacology*, pp. 624, 629–630.

21. Cole and Gerard, *Psychopharmacology*, pp. 605–606.

22. Ibid., p. 607.

23. Cole, "Evaluation of Effectiveness," p. 97; Howard F. Hunt, "Effects of Drugs on Emotional Responses and Abnormal Behavior in Animals," in Cole and Gerard, *Psychopharmacology*, p. 278; Cole and Gerard, *Psychopharmacology*, p. 607.

24. Cole and Gerard, *Psychopharmacology*, pp. 609–610, 618–619.

25. Ibid., p. 327.

26. Ibid., p. 624.

27. Ibid., pp. 327–328.

28. Ibid., p. 626.

29. Ibid., pp. 605, 615.

30. Jonathan Cole, "The Evaluation of Psychotropic Drugs," interview by David Healy, in David Healy (ed.), *The Psychopharmacologists* (London: Altman, 1996), p. 239.

31. Cole and Gerard, *Psychopharmacology*, p. 626.

32. Ibid., p. 627.

33. John Swann and Daniel Carpenter have highlighted this and other early efforts to regulate drug efficacy to argue that the 1962 amendments represented a continuation and codification of efficacy policy, rather than its introduction. See Carpenter, *Reputation and Power*, pp. 149–156, 175–177; John P. Swann, "Sure Cure: Public Policy on Drug Efficacy before 1962," in Higby and Stroud, *Inside Story of Medicines*, pp. 235–250.

34. Earl L. Meyers, "The Food and Drug Administration's View of Investigational Drugs," presented at the Annual Pharmacy Congress, St. Johns University, Jamaica, New York, 18 April 1963, in FDA (comp.), *Speeches and Papers, 1963*, Part 1 (Rockville, MD: Food and Drug Administration, 1979), FDA Library, p. 2.

35. Cole and Gerard, *Psychopharmacology*, p. 589.

36. For chlorpromazine's status in the history of psychiatry and psychopharmacology, see David Healy, *The Creation of Psychopharmacology* (Cambridge, MA: Harvard University Press, 2002).

37. Judith P. Swazey, *Chlorpromazine in Psychiatry: A Study of Therapeutic Innovation* (Cambridge: MIT Press, 1974), pp. 170–190.

38. Vernon Kinross-Wright, "Chlorpromazine—a Major Advance in Psychiatric Treatment," *Postgraduate Medicine* 16 (1954), pp. 297–299; H. E. Lehmann and G. E. Hanrahan, "Chlorpromazine: New Inhibiting Agent for Psychomotor Excitement and Manic States," *A.M.A. Archives of Neurology and Psychiatry* 71, no. 2 (1954), pp. 227–237; N. W. Winkelman Jr., "Chlorpromazine in the Treatment Neuropsychiatric Disorders," *Journal of the American Medical Association* 155, no. 1 (1954), pp. 18–21.

39. Henry Rosner et al., "A Comparative Study of the Effect on Anxiety of Chlorpromazine, Reserpine, Phenobarbital and a Placebo," *Journal of Nervous and Mental Disease* 122, no. 6 (1955), pp. 505–512; H. Freeman, A. L. Arnold, and H. S. Kline, "Effects of Chlorpromazine and Reserpine in Chronic Schizophrenic Patients," *Diseases of the Nervous System* 17, no. 7 (1956), pp. 213–219; Sarah Shtoffer Tenenblatt and Anthony Spagno, "A Controlled Study of Chlorpromazine Therapy in Chronic Psychotic Patients," *Quarterly Review of Psychiatry and Neurology* 17, no. 1 (1956), pp. 81–92; William W. Zeller et al., "Use of Chlorpromazine and Reserpine in the Treatment of Emotional Disorders," *Journal of the American Medical Association* 160, no. 3 (1956), pp. 179–184.

40. Robert A. Hall and Dorothy J. Dunlap, "A Study of Chlorpromazine: Methodology and Results with Chronic Semi-Disturbed Schizophrenics," *Journal of Nervous and Mental Disease* 122, no. 4 (1955), p. 314.

41. Jesse F. Casey et al., "Drug Therapy in Schizophrenia: A Controlled Study of the Relative Effectiveness of Chlorpromazine, Promazine, Phenobarbital, and Placebo," *A.M.A. Archives of General Psychiatry* 2, no. 2 (1960), pp. 210–220.

42. Swazey, *Chlorpromazine in Psychiatry*, p. 160–161.

43. Several of the studies acknowledged the assistance of pharmaceutical companies in supplying the drugs, and Hall and Dunlap also acknowledged financial and other assistance. See Hall and Dunlap, "Study of Chlorpromazine," p. 301; Casey et al., "Drug Therapy in Schizophrenia," p. 210.

44. Shorter, *Before Prozac*, p. 52.

45. Nicholas Weiss, "No One Listened to Imipramine," in Sarah W. Tracy and Caroline

Jean Acker (eds.), *Altering American Consciousness: The History of Alcohol and Drug Use in the United States, 1800–2000* (Amherst: University of Massachusetts Press, 2004), p. 333. Several psychiatric researchers had experimented earlier with the drug, but they had struggled to clearly identify its usefulness. See Healy, *Antidepressant Era*, pp. 62–63; Merton Sandler, "Monoamine Oxidase Inhibitors in Depression: History and Mythology," *Journal of Psychopharmacology* 4, no. 3 (1990), pp. 136–137.

46. Harry P. Loomer, John C. Saunders, and Nathan S. Kline, "A Clinical and Pharmacodynamic Evaluation of Iproniazid as a Psychic Energizer," *Psychiatric Research Reports* 8 (1957), pp. 133–134.

47. Ibid., p. 136.

48. Colin M. Smith, "A New Adjunct to the Treatment of Alcoholism: The Hallucinogenic Drugs," *Quarterly Journal of Studies on Alcohol* 19 (1958), pp. 406–417. For another close comparison, see J. Ross MacLean et al., "The Use of LSD-25 in the Treatment of Alcoholism and Other Psychiatric Problems," *Quarterly Journal of Studies on Alcohol* 22 (1961), pp. 34–45.

49. Nathan S. Kline, "Monoamine Oxidase Inhibitors: An Unfinished Picaresque Tale," in Frank J. Ayd and Barry Blackwell (eds.), *Discoveries in Biological Psychiatry* (Philadelphia: J. B. Lippincott, 1970), pp. 200–202; Nathan S. Kline, "Antidepressant Drugs and Liver Damage," *British Medical Journal* 1, no. 5384 (1964), p. 694.

50. Kline, "Monoamine Oxidase Inhibitors," pp. 200–201; Healy, *Antidepressant Era*, pp. 66–68; Weiss, "No One Listened to Imipramine," pp. 334–335, 338–340.

51. Debate subsequently ensued over whether credit for the discovery should have gone to Kline, Saunders, or Loomer. After several court cases, one-third of Kline's award was given to Saunders. See Healy, *Antidepressant Era*, pp. 68–69. This was the second Lasker Award Kline received. His first was awarded in 1957, for his research with the tranquilizer reserpine. See ibid., p. 64.

52. The FDA laid out requirements such as assignment of subjects to treatment groups "in such a way as to minimize bias," comparative controls that permit "quantitative evaluation," documentation of the level and methods of "blinding" utilized, and the "appropriate statistical methods" used. The FDA stipulated that, in addition to placebo or active treatment control groups, patients left untreated or even historical data on the natural progression of an illness could form an adequate control group. However, no-treatment controls were applicable only in certain cases where "objective measurements of effectiveness are available and placebo effect is negligible," and historical controls only where the course of the disease was highly predictable, such as in diseases with high mortality rates. Like in the earlier statements of FDA officials, in special cases where the required research techniques were not appropriate, the FDA could make an exemption. Yet, as discussed below, it appears that FDA officials would not have considered LSD psychotherapy such a special case. Edwards, "Adequate and Well-Controlled Clinical Investigations," pp. 7251–7252.

53. Harold A. Abramson (ed.), *The Use of LSD in Psychotherapy and Alcoholism* (Indianapolis: Bobbs-Merrill, 1967), pp. ix–x, 233.

54. Ibid., p. 221.

55. Abram Hoffer, "A Program for the Treatment of Alcoholism: LSD, Malvaria and Nicotonic Acid," in Abramson, *LSD in Psychotherapy and Alcoholism*, p. 365.

56. Abramson, *LSD in Psychotherapy and Alcoholism*, p. 495. For more on Hoffer's critique of the double-blind method, see Abram Hoffer and Humphry Osmond, "Double Blind Clinical Trials," *Journal of Neuropsychiatry* 2 (May–June 1961), pp. 221–227; A. Hoffer, "A Theoretical Examination of Double-Blind Design," *Canadian Medical Association Journal* 97, no. 3 (July 15 1967), pp. 123–127; Erika Dyck, *Psychedelic Psychiatry: LSD from Clinic to Campus* (Baltimore: Johns Hopkins University Press, 2008), pp. 47–51, 73–78.

57. John Mann, *Life Saving Drugs: The Elusive Magic Bullet* (Cambridge: Royal Society of

Chemistry, 2004), p. 3; John E. Lesch, *The First Miracle Drugs: How the Sulfa Drugs Transformed Medicine* (New York: Oxford University Press, 2007), pp. 15–19. For a detailed discussion of Ehrlich's chemotherapy concept, see John Parascandola, "The Theoretical Basis of Paul Ehrlich's Chemotherapy," *Journal of the History of Medicine and Allied Sciences* 36, no. 1 (1981), pp. 19–43.

58. For the history of sulfonamides, see Lesch, *First Miracle Drugs.* For penicillin, see Robert Bud, *Penicillin: Triumph and Tragedy* (Oxford: Oxford University Press, 2007).

59. For the history of the concepts of specificity and nonspecificity in medicine, see Michael Shepherd, "The Placebo: From Specificity to the Non-specific and Back," *Psychological Medicine* 23, no. 3 (1993), pp. 569–578.

60. Robert E. Mogar, "Research in Psychedelic Drug Therapy: A Critical Analysis," in John M. Shlien (ed.), *Research in Psychotherapy: Proceedings of the Third Conference* (Washington, DC: American Psychological Association, 1968), p. 504.

61. Ibid., p. 505.

62. Ibid., p. 508.

63. Ibid., pp. 507–509.

64. Lester Luborsky and Hans H. Strupp, "Research Problems in Psychotherapy: A Three-Year Follow-Up," in H. H. Strupp and L. Luborsky (eds.), *Research in Psychotherapy*, vol. 2 (Washington, DC: American Psychological Association, 1962), p. 314.

65. Jerome D. Frank, *Persuasion and Healing: A Comparative Study of Psychotherapy*, rev. ed. (New York: Schocken Books, 1974), p. 332.

66. Jerome D. Frank, "Problems of Controls in Psychotherapy as Exemplified by the Psychotherapy Research Project of the Phipps Psychiatric Clinic," in Eli A. Rubinstein and Morris B. Parloff (eds.), *Research in Psychotherapy* (Washington, DC: American Psychological Association, 1959), pp. 15–16.

67. Lester Luborsky, Barton Singer, and Lise Luborsky, "Comparative Studies of Psychotherapies: Is It True That 'Everyone Has Won and All Must Have Prizes'?," *Archives of General Psychiatry* 32, no. 8 (1975), pp. 995–1008.

68. Morris B. Parloff and Eli A. Rubinstein, "Research Problems in Psychotherapy," in Rubinstein and Parloff, *Research in Psychotherapy*, pp. 277–278.

69. Shapiro and Shapiro, *Powerful Placebo*, pp. 98–107; Michael J. Lambert, "Psychotherapy Research and Its Achievements," in John C. Norcross, Gary R. VandenBos, and Donald K. Freedheim (eds.), *History of Psychotherapy: Continuity and Change* (Washington, DC: American Psychological Association, 2011), p. 304.

70. For a prominent early study that challenged the efficacy of psychotherapy through a comparative study of treatment outcome and that called for more sophisticated controlled studies, see H. J. Eysenck, "The Effects of Psychotherapy: An Evaluation," *Journal of Consulting Psychology* 16, no. 5 (1952), pp. 319–324. For an early work that challenged the notion that the placebo effect was not relevant for psychotherapy research, see Arthur K. Shapiro, "Factors Contributing to the Placebo Effect: Their Implications for Psychotherapy," *American Journal of Psychotherapy* 18 (1964), pp. 73–88. By the mid-1990s, the need to establish the efficacy of the various forms of psychotherapy through randomized controlled trials became a major focus of academic psychology and the American Psychological Association. However, the applicability of the research methods and their impact on limiting the forms of psychotherapy that can be evaluated and subsequently promoted as "evidence-based" remains a contested issue. See Glenn Shean, "Limitations of Randomized Control Designs in Psychotherapy Research," *Advances in Psychiatry* (2014), doi:10.1155/2014/561452; Martin E. P. Seligman, "The Effectiveness of Psychotherapy: The Consumer Reports Study," *American Psychologist* 50, no. 12 (1995), pp. 965–974; Bothwell et al., "Assessing the Gold Standard," pp. 2175–2181. For histories of psychotherapy research into the modern era, see also Hans H. Strupp and Kenneth I. Howard, "A Brief History of Psychotherapy Research," in Donald K. Freedheim (ed.), *History of Psychotherapy: A*

Century of Change (Washington, DC: American Psychological Association, 1992), pp. 309–334; Lambert, "Psychotherapy Research," pp. 299–332.

71. Betty Grover Eisner, "Remembrances of LSD Therapy Past" (unpublished manuscript, 2002), p. 108, http://www.maps.org/images/pdf/books/remembrances.pdf.

72. Harold A. Abramson (ed.), *The Use of LSD in Psychotherapy* (New York: Josiah Macy, Jr. Foundation, 1960), p. 25.

73. Ibid., pp. 26, 225–226.

74. Ibid., pp. 34–35, 48–49, 152–153.

75. Ibid., pp. 94–98.

76. Ibid., p. 132.

77. Ibid., p. 84

78. Ibid., pp. 239–240.

79. *Organization and Coordination of Federal Drug Research and Regulatory Programs: LSD,* Hearings before the Subcommittee on Executive Reorganization of the Committee on Government Operations, United States Senate, 89th Congress, 2nd Session, May 24, 25, 26, 1966 (Washington, DC: US Government Printing Office, 1966), p. 33. Emphasis mine. The quote was originally from the New York County Medical Society; Yolles reproduced it as a representation of the NIMH's view.

Chapter 4 · Against the Tide

Epigraph: [Charles Savage], untitled manuscript, n.d., folder 10, box 7, Charles Savage Papers, MSP 70, Archives and Special Collections, Purdue University Libraries, West Lafayette, Indiana (hereafter Savage Papers).

1. The only previous substantial discussion of the history of LSD research at Spring Grove was co-authored by Spring Grove researcher Richard Yensen. See Richard Yensen and Donna Dryer, "Thirty Years of Psychedelic Research: The Spring Grove Experiment and Its Sequels," *Jahrbuch des Europäischen Collegiums für Bewußtseinsstudien / Yearbook of the European College for the Study of Consciousness* (1993–1994), pp. 73–102. A more limited discussion also appears in Richard Elliot Doblin, "Regulation of the Medical Use of Psychedelics and Marijuana" (PhD diss., Harvard University, 2000), pp. 52–54, 242–245.

2. Albert A. Kurland, interview by Leo E. Hollister, transcript, 15 April 1997, Washington DC, American College of Neuropsychopharmacology Oral History Project, http://www.acnp .org/programs/history.aspx#; Albert A. Kurland, "Curriculum Vitae," n.d., folder 3, box 8, Savage Papers. For the history of Spring Grove State Hospital, see David S. Helsel and Trevor J. Blank, *Spring Grove State Hospital* (Charleston, SC: Arcadia. 2008).

3. Albert A. Kurland, "An Evaluation of Drama Therapy," *Psychiatric Quarterly Supplement* 26, no. 2 (1952), pp. 210–229; Albert A. Kurland, Jacob Morgenstern, and Carolyn Sheets, "A Comparative Study of Wife Murderers Admitted to a State Psychiatric Hospital," *Journal of Social Therapy* 1 (1955), pp. 7–15.

4. Albert A. Kurland, "Chlorpromazine in the Treatment of Schizophrenia: A Study of 75 Cases," *Journal of Nervous and Mental Disease* 121, no. 4 (1955), p. 328.

5. Louis S. Cholden, Albert Kurland, and Charles Savage, "Clinical Reactions and Tolerance to LSD in Chronic Schizophrenia," *Journal of Nervous and Mental Disease* 122, no. 3 (1955), pp. 211–221.

6. Sanford M. Unger, "Curriculum Vitae," n.d., folder 4, box 9, Savage Papers.

7. Sanford Unger, "The Psychedelic Use of LSD: Reflections and Observations," in Richard E. Hicks and Paul Jay Fink (eds.), *Psychedelic Drugs* (New York: Grune & Stratton, 1969), p. 200.

8. Sanford M. Unger, "LSD, Mescaline, Psilocybin, and Personality Change: A Review," *Psychiatry* 26 (1963), pp. 113–115.

9. Ibid., pp. 118, 125.

10. Unger, "Psychedelic Use of LSD," p. 202.

11. For uncontrolled research, see Albert A. Kurland, "Comparison of Chlorpromazine and Reserpine in Treatment of Schizophrenia: A Study of Four Hundred Cases," *A.M.A. Archives of Neurology and Psychiatry* 75, no. 5 (1956), pp. 510–513. For controlled research, see Albert A. Kurland et al., "The Comparative Effectiveness of Six Phenothiazine Compounds, Phenobarbital and Inert Placebo in the Treatment of Acutely Ill Patients: Global Measures and Severity of Illness," *Journal of Nervous and Mental Disease* 133, no. 1 (1961), pp. 1–18.

12. Kurland, "Curriculum Vitae."

13. John W. Shaffer et al., "Nialamide in the Treatment of Alcoholism," *Journal of Nervous and Mental Disease* 135, no. 3 (1962), pp. 222–232; John W. Shaffer et al., "A Controlled Comparison of Chlordiazepoxide (Librium) in the Treatment of Convalescing Alcoholics," *Journal of Nervous and Mental Disease* 137, no. 5 (1963), pp. 508–520.

14. *Drug Safety* (Part 5, Appendixes, and Index), Hearings before a Subcommittee on Government Operations, House of Representatives, 89th Congress, 2nd Session, March 9, 10; May 25, 26; June 7, 8, and 9, 1966 (Washington, DC: US Government Printing Office, 1966), p. 2209.

15. Jonathan O. Cole and Martin M. Katz, "The Psychotomimetic Drugs: An Overview," *JAMA* 187, no. 10 (1964), p. 760.

16. *Drug Safety*, p. 2209; *Organization and Coordination of Federal Drug Research and Regulatory Programs: LSD*, Hearings before the Subcommittee on Executive Reorganization of the Committee on Government Operations, United States Senate, 89th Congress, 2nd Session, May 24, 25, 26, 1966 (Washington: U.S. Government Printing Office, 1966), p. 23; Unger, "Curriculum Vitae."

17. Albert A. Kurland et al., "Psychedelic Therapy Utilizing LSD in the Treatment of the Alcoholic Patient: A Preliminary Report," *American Journal of Psychiatry* 123 (1967), p. 1203.

18. Ibid., p. 1206.

19. A. A. Kurland, J. W. Shaffer, and S. Unger, "Psychedelic Psychotherapy (LSD) in the Treatment of Alcoholism (an Approach to a Controlled Study)," in H. Brill (ed.), *Neuro-Psycho-Pharmacology* (Amsterdam: Excerpta Medica, 1967), p. 437.

20. Kurland et al., "Psychedelic Therapy," p. 1207

21. Kurland, Shaffer, and Unger, "Psychedelic Psychotherapy," p. 435; Albert A. Kurland and Sanford Unger, "The Present Status and Future Direction of Psychedelic LSD Research with Special Reference to the Spring Grove Studies," manuscript, n.d., folder 6, box 7, Savage Papers, p. 19.

22. Walter N. Pahnke et al., "The Experimental Use of Psychedelic (LSD) Psychotherapy," in James R. Zerkin and Edmund L. Gamage (eds.), *Hallucinogenic Drug Research: Impact on Science and Society* (Beloit, WI: STASH Press, 1970), p. 51.

23. Sanford Unger et al., "LSD-Type Drugs and Psychedelic Therapy," in John M. Shlien (ed.), *Research in Psychotherapy: Proceedings of the Third Conference* (Washington, DC: American Psychological Association, 1968), p. 522.

24. *Drug Safety*, p. 2212. Savage appears to have taken over the role of Spring Grove's director of research from Kurland by 1966, but the exact dates and nature of their positions are unclear. Nevertheless, Kurland remained above Savage, and in charge of the psychedelic research program, as director of research for the Department of Mental Hygiene.

25. J. Ross MacLean et al., "The Use of LSD-25 in the Treatment of Alcoholism and Other Psychiatric Problems," *Quarterly Journal of Studies on Alcohol* 22 (1961), pp. 34–45.

26. Charles Savage et al., "The Effects of Psychedelic (LSD) Therapy on Values, Personality, and Behavior," *International Journal of Neuropsychiatry* 2 (1966), pp. 241–254.

27. Albert A. Kurland to Charles Savage, 28 September 1964, folder 2, box 2, Savage Papers.

28. Albert A. Kurland and Charles Savage, "A Controlled Study of LSD Therapy with Neu-

rotics," application for research grant to U.S. Department of Health, Education, and Welfare, MH 11001-01, received 20 August 1964, folder 3, box 8, Savage Papers, p. 7.

29. Albert A. Kurland, "LSD-Assisted Psychotherapy in Terminal Cancer," application for research grant to Department of Health, Education and Welfare, MH CA 12916-01, received 1 February 1966, folder 4, box 9, Savage Papers, p. 3.

30. Eric C. Kast, "The Analgesic Action of Lysergic Acid Compared with Dihydromorphinone and Meperidine," *Bulletin on Drug Addiction and Narcotics*, Appendix 27 (1963), p. 3518.

31. Ibid., p. 3526. Drug doses employed in the comparison were: LSD 100 mcg, dihydromorphinone 2 mg, and meperidine 100 mg. For Kast's further work in this area, see Eric C. Kast, "Pain and LSD-25: A Theory of Attenuation of Anticipation," in David Solomon (ed.), *LSD: The Consciousness-Expanding Drug* (New York: G. P. Putnam's Sons, 1964), pp. 241–256; Eric Kast, "LSD and the Dying Patient," *Chicago Medical School Quarterly* 26 (1966), pp. 80–87.

32. Erika Dyck, *Psychedelic Psychiatry: LSD from Clinic to Campus* (Baltimore: Johns Hopkins University Press, 2008), p. 113. For more on the sensationalistic media coverage of LSD, see Stephen Siff, *Acid Hype: American News Media and the Psychedelic Experience* (Urbana: University of Illinois Press, 2015), pp. 151–155.

33. "A Remarkable Mind Drug Suddenly Spells Danger: LSD," *Life*, 25 March 1966, pp. 29, 30C. For other citations to this article, see Siff, *Acid Hype*, p. 170; Martin A. Lee and Bruce Shlain, *Acid Dreams: The Complete Social History of LSD; The CIA, the Sixties, and Beyond* (New York: Grove Press, 1985), p. 150.

34. Albert Rosenfeld, "The Vital Facts about the Drug and Its Effects," *Life*, 25 March 1966, p. 30A.

35. Ibid.

36. Barry Farrell, "Scientists, Theologian, Mystics Swept Up in a Psychic Revolution," *Life*, 25 March 1966, pp. 30D, 32–33.

37. Circulation and syndication details are for 1969; however, these are likely conservative for 1966: Stephen Siff has cited circulation for 1960 as thirteen million, and 1969 was the year that the magazine folded. See Henry Raymont, "This Week Magazine Ends Publication Nov. 2," *New York Times*, 14 August 1969, p. 27; Siff, *Acid Hype*, p. 105.

38. Cyril Solomon and Lester David, "The Nightmare Drug: Five Years Ago, Doctors Held High Hopes for LSD but Now They're Beginning to Wonder—and Worry," *This Week, Baltimore Sun*, 9 January 1966, pp. 6–7, 16, https://www.newspapers.com/image/219162730. Emphasis in original. Alfred Trembly of the Los Angeles Police Department's Narcotics Division submitted the article, as published in *This Week, Los Angeles Times*, to Thomas Dodd's 1966 congressional hearings on LSD (see chapter 2) as evidence for the dangers of LSD. The article was reproduced in the published proceedings. See *The Narcotic Rehabilitation Act of 1966*, Hearings before a Special Subcommittee of the Committee on the Judiciary, United States Senate, 89th Congress, 2nd Session, January 25, 26, and 27, May 12, 13, 19, 23, and 25, June 14 and 15, July 19, 1966 (Washington, DC: US Government Printing Office, 1966), pp. 219–222.

39. Charles C. Dahlberg, Ruth Mechaneck, and Stanley Feldstein, "LSD Research: The Impact of Lay Publicity," *American Journal of Psychiatry* 125, no. 5 (1968), pp. 685–689.

40. Charles Savage to Charles Clay Dahlberg, 30 June 1966, folder 2, box 3, Savage Papers.

41. Kurland is listed among the first seventeen researchers included under Sandoz's IND when submitted in 1963. See George P. Larrick to L. R. Fountain, 17 September 1963, box 3587, General Subject Files 1938–1974, Division of General Services, RG 88—Records of the Food and Drug Administration, National Archives at College Park, College Park, Maryland (hereafter RG 88).

42. Albert A. Kurland to Frances Kelsey, 14 April 1966, folder 6, box 2, Savage Papers; Albert A. Kurland to Frances Kelsey, 15 April 1966, folder 2, box 3, Savage Papers.

43. Savage to MacLean, 24 May 1966, folder 2, box 3, Savage Papers.

44. Memorandum of conference between representatives of Sandoz Pharmaceuticals, the NIMH, and the FDA, 7 December 1965, folder 521.6-525.091, box 3758, RG 88.

45. *Drug Safety*, pp. 2135–2136; *Organization and Coordination: LSD*, p. 57. For more on the regulation of LSD in this period, see chapter 2.

46. For material submitted in support of Kurland's IND application, see Albert A. Kurland to James L. Goddard, 21 June 1966, folder 4, box 9, Savage Papers.

47. *Drug Safety*, p. 2270.

48. For examples of newspaper coverage of the hearings, see John H. Averill, "Witnesses Tell of LSD Usage, Perils," *Los Angeles Times*, 14 May 1966, pp. 1, 15; Bruce Winters, "Senate Unit Probes LSD, Favors Strict Supervision," *Baltimore Sun*, 14 May 1966, pp. A2, A4; "Senators Baffled by LSD Exponent," *Arizona Daily Star*, 14 May 1966, p. A5. For more on the hearings, see chapter 2. For the television coverage, see Don Kirkley, "Look and Listen," *Baltimore Sun*, 16 May 1966, B6.

49. "LSD: The Spring Grove Experiment," *CBS Reports*, produced by John Sharnik and Harry Morgan, aired 17 May 1966 (New York: CBS News Archives, 2016), DVD.

50. In a 1998 follow-up interview, King continued to credit his psychedelic treatment for saving his life and marriage. See Richard Yensen and Donna Dryer, "Addiction, Despair, and the Soul: Successful Psychedelic Psychotherapy, a Case Study," in Michael J. Winkelman and Thomas Roberts (eds.), *Psychedelic Medicine: New Evidence for Hallucinogenic Drugs as Treatments*, vol. 2 (Westport, CT: Praeger, 2007), pp. 15–28.

51. "LSD: The Spring Grove Experiment."

52. Ibid.

53. Ibid.

54. Rick Du Brow, "Documentary on LSD Very Fine," *Cumberland (MD) Evening Times*, 18 May 1966, p. 13; Cynthia Lowry, "LSD Benefits Described on 'CBS Reports,'" *Santa Cruz (CA) Sentinel*, 18 May 1966, p. 12. For examples of the widespread publication of these reviews (under varying headlines), see Rick Du Brow, "LSD Documentary One of the Best," *Sandusky (OH) Register*, 18 May 1966, p. 26; Cynthia Lowry, "CBS Rates Plaudits for Report on LSD," *Ogden (UT) Standard-Examiner*, 18 May 1966, p. 9C.

55. Don Kirkley, "Look and Listen," *Baltimore Sun*, 20 May 1966, p. B6; Harry Harris, "Screening TV," *Philadelphia Inquirer*, 18 May 1966, p. 23.

56. Harold A. Abramson (ed.), *The Use of LSD in Psychotherapy and Alcoholism* (Indianapolis: Bobbs-Merrill, 1967); Brill, *Neuro-Psycho-Pharmacology*; Shlien, *Research in Psychotherapy*.

57. For their papers at these conferences, see Albert A. Kurland, Sanford Unger, and John W. Shaffer, "The Psychedelic Procedure in the Treatment of the Alcoholic Patient," in Abramson, *Use of LSD in Psychotherapy and Alcoholism*, pp. 496–503; Kurland, Shaffer, and Unger, "Psychedelic Psychotherapy," pp. 435–439; C. Savage and S. Wolf, "An Outline of Psychedelic Therapy," in Brill, *Neuro-Psycho-Pharmacology*, pp. 405–410; Unger et al., "LSD-Type Drugs," pp. 521–535; Charles Savage, "Psychedelic Therapy," in Shlien, *Research in Psychotherapy*, pp. 512–520.

58. *Drug Safety*, p. 2257; Sanford M. Unger to Rudolf Bircher, 24 September 1965, folder 1, box 3, Savage Papers.

59. "Visitors to Cottage #13" [1969], folder 11, box 10, Savage Papers.

60. *Drug Safety*, p. 2268.

61. Ibid., p. 2213, 2216.

62. Ibid., pp. 2240–2241, 2260–2262.

63. Ibid., p. 2269.

64. Ibid., pp. 2268–2271.

65. Maimon M. Cohen, Michelle J. Marinello, and Nathan Back, "Chromosomal Damage

in Human Leukocytes Induced by Lysergic Acid Diethylamide," *Science* 155, no. 3768 (1967), pp. 1417–1419.

66. Richard D. Lyons, "Genetic Damage is Linked to LSD," *New York Times*, 17 March 1967, p. 43.

67. Joe-Hin Tjio, Walter N. Pahnke, and Albert A. Kurland, "LSD and Chromosomes: A Controlled Experiment," *JAMA* 210, no. 5 (1969), pp. 849–856.

68. Norman I. Dihotsky et al., "LSD and Genetic Damage: Is LSD Chromosome Damaging, Carcinogenic, Mutagenic, or Teratogenic?," *Science* 172, no. 3982 (1971), pp. 431–440.

69. For more on the media coverage of the chromosome scare, see Siff, *Acid Hype*, pp. 155–158. For claims of deformities in babies due to LSD ingestion during pregnancy, see "First Birth Defect Attributed to Use of LSD by Mother," *New York Times*, 24 November 24, p. 45; Dihotsky et al., "LSD and Genetic Damage," pp. 438–439.

70. "A Demonstration Project of Psychedelic Therapy with Alcoholics," enclosed with Charles Savage to Robert Derbyshire, 9 January 1967, folder 5, box 3, Savage Papers. Emphasis in original.

71. Ibid.

72. Tuerk's positions at Spring Grove and in the Maryland Department of Mental Hygiene are acknowledged in Albert A. Kurland, "Psychiatric Research in a State Psychiatric Hospital," *Maryland State Medical Journal* 3, no. 11 (1954), p. 611; and Albert A. Kurland et al., "Comparative Studies of the Phenothiazine Tranquilizers: Methodological and Logistical Considerations," *Journal of Nervous and Mental Disease* 132, no. 1 (1961), p. 61. The date of Tuerk's appointment as commissioner of mental hygiene, as well as the details of Kurland's appointment as director of research in the department, are not clear. However, as Kurland took up his position in 1960, and Tuerk was in his role by 1961, it seems likely that Tuerk would have taken Kurland with him into the department.

73. Stanislav Grof, "The Great Awakening: Psychology, Philosophy and Spirituality in LSD Psychotherapy," in Roger Walsh and Charles S. Grob (eds.), *Higher Wisdom: Eminent Elders Explore the Continuing Impact of Psychedelics* (Albany: State University of New York Press, 2005), pp. 121–141; Stanislav Grof, "Curriculum Vitae," accessed 6 January 2018, http://www.stanislavgrof.com/page-6/. For his research prior to joining Spring Grove, see Stanislav Grof, "Use of LSD 25 in Personality Diagnostics and Therapy of Psychogenic Disorders," in Abramson, *LSD in Psychotherapy and Alcoholism*, pp. 154–190; Stanislav Grof, "Tentative Theoretical Framework for Understanding Dynamics of LSD Psychotherapy," in Shlien, *Research in Psychotherapy*, pp. 449–465.

74. See Stanislav Grof, *Realms of the Human Unconscious* (New York: Viking Press, 1975); Stanislav Grof and Joan Halifax, *The Human Encounter with Death* (New York: E. P. Dutton, 1977); Stanislav Grof, *LSD Psychotherapy* (Pomona: Hunter House, 1980).

75. "Curriculum Vita of Walter Norman Pahnke," n.d., William Richards Collection of Walter Pahnke Papers, 1952–1972, MSP 68, Archives and Special Collections, Purdue University Libraries, West Lafayette, Indiana.

76. Walter N. Pahnke, "Drugs and Mysticism: An Analysis of the Relationship between Psychedelic Drugs and Mystical Consciousness" (PhD diss., Harvard University, 1963), pp. 1–23. For Pahnke's acknowledgment of Leary's assistance in the "execution of the experiment," see ibid., p. ii. For Leary's account of the study and his participation in it, see Timothy Leary, *High Priest* (New York: College Notes and Texts, 1968), pp. 290–295, 304–318.

77. Pahnke, "Drugs and Mysticism," pp. 27–47.

78. Ibid., p. 47, 58, 60.

79. Ibid., pp. 60–62, 64, 67.

80. Ibid., pp. 70–81.

81. Ibid., pp. 87–96.

82. Ibid., pp. 105–107, 220–235.

83. Ibid., p. 236. The validity of Pahnke's study and the enduring positive effects of psilocybin on the participants were confirmed in a twenty-four-year follow-up conducted by Rick Doblin. However, Doblin also found that Pahnke had downplayed psychologically difficult periods in subjects' otherwise positive experiences and failed to report that one subject had been administered chlorpromazine after escaping the chapel—apparently on a mission to spread word of his insights—resisting efforts to bring him back, and becoming fearful and agitated. See Rick Doblin, "Pahnke's 'Good Friday Experiment': A Long-Term Follow-Up and Methodological Critique," *Journal of Transpersonal Psychology* 23, no. 1 (1991), pp. 1–28. For a description of this incident from one of the "guides" in the experiment, see Huston Smith, "The Good Friday Experiment," interview by Thomas Roberts, in Charles S. Grob (ed.), *Hallucinogens: A Reader* (New York: Jeremy P. Tarcher / Putnam, 2002), pp. 64–71.

84. "Curriculum Vita of Walter Norman Pahnke."

85. "Organizational Structure of Psychedelic Research: Specification of Project Directors and Assignment of Personnel," n.d., folder 2, box 11, Savage Papers.

86. Walter N. Pahnke et al., "LSD-Assisted Psychotherapy with Terminal Cancer Patients," in Hicks and Fink, *Psychedelic Drugs*, pp. 34, 39. Pahnke developed the Pahnke Mystical Experience Questionnaire to evaluate the completeness of psychedelic reactions. See Walter N. Pahnke, "Psychedelic Drugs and Mystical Experience," *International Psychiatry Clinics* 5, no. 4 (1967), pp. 149–162.

87. See Jerome Levine, Arnold M. Ludwig, and William H. Lyle, "The Controlled Psychedelic State," *American Journal of Clinical Hypnosis* 6, no. 2 (1963), pp. 163–164; Leo Hollister, Jack Shelton, and George Krieger, "A Controlled Comparison of Lysergic Acid Diethylamide (LSD) and Dextroamphetamine in Alcoholics," *American Journal of Psychiatry* 125, no. 10 (1969), pp. 1352–1357.

88. Yensen and Dryer, "Thirty Years of Psychedelic Research," p. 76.

89. Albert A. Kurland to John Walton, 18 December 1964, Savage Papers; Description of proposed Maryland Psychiatric Research Centre, n.d., Savage Papers.

90. "Description of Facilities," n.d., folder 3, box 11, Savage Papers; Yensen and Dryer, "Thirty Years of Psychedelic Research," p. 84.

91. Diagram of staff structure at Maryland Psychiatric Research Center, n.d., folder 7, box 11, Savage Papers; "Curriculum Vita of Walter Norman Pahnke"; Grof, "Curriculum Vitae."

92. In a 1968 document outlining the proposed study, the researchers used the term "narcotic" only when referring to the drugs that patients were addicted to. See "Narcotic Addiction—Psychedelic Therapy: Research Program," November 1968, folder 8, box 10, Savage Papers. "Narcotic" is a somewhat ambiguous term, as what drugs are considered narcotics can vary depending on the context (medical or legal) as well as the historical period. However, from later reports on the study, it is clear the Spring Grove researchers used the term to refer specifically to heroin. See Charles Savage and O. Lee McCabe, "Residential Psychedelic (LSD) Therapy for the Narcotic Addict: A Controlled Study," *Archives of General Psychiatry* 28 (June 1973), p. 808.

93. "Narcotic Addiction—Psychedelic Therapy." For Ludwig and Levine's research with narcotic addicts, see Arnold M. Ludwig and Jerome Levine, "A Controlled Comparison of Five Brief Treatment Techniques Employing LSD, Hypnosis, and Psychotherapy," *American Journal of Psychotherapy* 19 (1965), pp. 417–435.

94. Charles Savage et al., "Research with Psychedelic Drugs," in Hicks and Fink, *Psychedelic Drugs*, pp. 18–19.

95. Pahnke et al., "Terminal Cancer Patients," p. 36.

96. Walter N. Pahnke et al., "The Experimental Use of Psychedelic (LSD) Psychotherapy," *JAMA* 212, no. 11 (1970), pp. 1859–1860. Statistical significance was at the level of $p < 0.05$ (re-

sults would be produced by chance alone less than five times out of one hundred) for both drinking behavior and global adjustment in the treatment versus control group comparison.

97. "A Policy Statement Covering the Conduct of Psychedelic Research within the Department of Medical Research at Spring Grove State Hospital," 1965, folder 2, box 11, Savage Papers.

98. Albert A. Kurland, "Application to Amend IND-3250 for the Administration of LSD for Training Purposes," 7 March 1969, folder 9, box 1, Stanislav Grof Papers, MSP 1, Archives and Special Collections, Purdue University Libraries, West Lafayette, Indiana.

99. Yensen and Dryer, "Thirty Years of Psychedelic Research," p. 87. The only published Spring Grove study with mental health professionals was an exploration of the effects of methylenedioxyamphetamine (MDA) in ten staff members of the MPRC. See I. S. Turek, R. A. Soskin, and A. A. Kurland, "Methylenedioxyamphetamine (MDA) Subjective Effects," *Journal of Psychedelic Drugs* 6, no. 1 (1974), pp. 7–14.

100. Minutes—Psychedelic Research Staff Meeting, 27 January 1969, folder 2, box 11, Savage Papers.

101. Helen L. Bonny and Walter N. Pahnke, "The Use of Music in Psychedelic (LSD) Psychotherapy," *Journal of Music Therapy* 9 (1972), pp. 65–66.

102. Ibid., p. 79. For more on Bonny's research into music, LSD, and psychotherapy, see Helen L. Bonny, "Music and Psychotherapy: A Handbook and Guide Accompanied by Eight Music Tapes to Be Used by Practitioners of Guided Imagery and Music" (PhD diss., Union of Experimenting Colleges and Universities, 1976), William Richards Collection of Helen Bonny Materials, MSP 77, Archives and Special Collections, Purdue University Libraries, West Lafayette, Indiana.

Chapter 5 · Elusive Efficacy

Epigraph: [Charles Savage], "A Review of LSD and Alcoholism by Ludwig, Levine and Stark," unpublished manuscript, 1971, folder 3, box 6, Charles Savage Papers, MSP 70, Archives and Special Collections, Purdue University Libraries, West Lafayette, Indiana (hereafter Savage Papers), p. 8.

1. Charles Savage to Jonathan Cole, 2 March 1965, folder 3, box 2, Savage Papers. Savage first proposed this control design, but with a low dose of psilocybin instead of LSD, in a grant application for the International Foundation for Advanced Study. See Charles Savage, "A Controlled Study of LSD-25 and Alcoholism," draft application for research grant to the US Department of Health, Education, and Welfare, 27 December 1962, folder 3, box 8, Savage Papers. See also chapter 2 for a discussion of this proposed study. That it was Savage behind this idea, and that he also first proposed specifically using low-dose LSD, is further supported in [Charles Savage], untitled manuscript, n.d., folder 10, box 7, Savage Papers, p. 9.

2. Savage to Cole, 2 March 1965.

3. Ibid.

4. A. Kurland et al., "LSD in the Treatment of Alcoholics," *Pharmakopsychiatrie-Neuro-Psychopharmakologie* 4, no. 2 (1971), pp. 85–89.

5. Ibid., pp. 90–91. The patient follow-up rate, although considered very good, inevitably dropped over the study: 89 percent of treated patients participated in the six-month evaluation, dropping to 78 percent at eighteen months. This further decreased the statistical significance of the results.

6. For the common $p < 0.05$ standard level of significance in clinical research, see Daniel Carpenter, *Reputation and Power: Organizational Image and Pharmaceutical Regulation at the FDA* (Princeton: Princeton University Press, 2010), p. 518. This standard was used in significant trials such as the landmark 1960 Veterans Administration multihospital study of the efficacy of chlorpromazine. See Jesse F. Casey et al., "Drug Therapy in Schizophrenia: A Controlled Study

of the Relative Effectiveness of Chlorpromazine, Promazine, Phenobarbital, and Placebo," *A.M.A. Archives of General Psychiatry* 2, no. 2 (1960), pp. 210–220.

7. [Savage], untitled manuscript, p. 9.

8. Savage to Cole, 2 March 1965. Emphasis added.

9. [Savage], untitled manuscript, p. 9.

10. Ibid., p. 9. Emphasis original.

11. Walter N. Pahnke et al., "The Experimental Use of Psychedelic (LSD) Psychotherapy," *JAMA: The Journal of the American Medical Association* 212, no. 11 (1970), pp. 1859–1860. Patients' drug reactions were classed as "profound," "marked," or "minimal," with the percentage of patients "essentially rehabilitated" in each of these categories tabulated. For global adjustment, percentage scores for these categories were 61, 39, and 24, respectively, and, for drinking behavior, were 61, 48, and 36. For global adjustment, the statistical significance was at the level of $p < 0.025$.

12. Walker Pahnke made brief mention to the relationship between dose and the rate of peak experiences in a footnote to a 1969 paper that generally discussed the team's psychedelic research with cancer patients. Pahnke reported that in the Spring Grove alcoholic study, one in four high-dose patients had a profound mystical experience, while one in ten low-dose patients did. See Walter N. Pahnke, "The Psychedelic Mystical Experience in the Human Encounter With Death," *Harvard Theological Review* 62, no. 1 (1969), p. 11n9.

13. Kurland et al., "LSD in the Treatment of Alcoholics," p. 92.

14. [Savage], untitled manuscript, p. 9.

15. Ibid.

16. Kurland et al., "LSD in the Treatment of Alcoholics," pp. 91–92.

17. Charles Savage et al., "LSD-Assisted Psychotherapy in the Treatment of Severe Chronic Neurosis," *Journal of Altered States of Consciousness* 1, no. 1 (1973), pp. 31–47. Originally a fourth treatment group was planned, in which patients would undergo a regimen of psychedelic therapy tailored to their needs by their therapist. The therapist could vary the dosage, the timing of its administration, and administer repeat LSD sessions as desired. This approach was designed to assess "whether or not a 'no holds barred' treatment effort would produce more impressive results" than the standard psychedelic therapy procedure. For unknown reasons, this treatment group did not eventuate. See Albert A. Kurland and Charles Savage, "A Controlled Study of LSD Therapy with Neurotics," application for research grant to U.S. Department of Health, Education, and Welfare, MH 11001-01, received 20 August 1964, folder 3, box 8, Savage Papers, p. 6.

18. Savage et al., "LSD-Assisted Psychotherapy," pp. 38–42.

19. This dose-response relationship was statistically significant at the level of $p < 0.10$ at the six-month follow-up point. This was below the standard significance level of $p < 0.05$. The analysis simply indicated a trend, with further research needed to prove the dose-response relationship. At eighteen months the trend continued, but its significance had dropped further. Nevertheless, there was some significant corroborating evidence: female patients in the low-dose group improved more than those in the conventional treatment group to the level of $p < 0.05$, while there was no significant advantage for high-dose therapy for women. Ibid., pp. 38, 41–44.

20. Ibid., p. 43.

21. William Richards, email to author, 18 February 2013; S. Grof et al., "LSD-Assisted Psychotherapy in Patients with Terminal Cancer," *International Pharmacopsychiatry* 8 (1973), p. 144.

22. Grof et al., "LSD-Assisted Psychotherapy," pp. 136–143.

23. Charles Savage and O. Lee McCabe, "Residential Psychedelic (LSD) Therapy for the Narcotic Addict: A Controlled Study," *Archives of General Psychiatry* 28 (1973), pp. 809–810;

"Narcotic Addiction—Psychedelic Therapy: Research Program," November 1968, folder 8, box 10, Savage Papers.

24. Savage and McCabe, "(LSD) Therapy for the Narcotic Addict," pp. 808–814.

25. Ibid., p. 813. Twenty-nine of the thirty-six LSD patients (80 percent) achieved the psychedelic peak experience.

26. Charles Savage, O. Lee McCabe, and Albert A. Kurland, "LSD Therapy of Heroin Addicts: A Controlled Study," n.d., folder 3, box 9, Savage Papers, p. 4.

27. Savage and McCabe, "(LSD) Therapy for the Narcotic Addict," p. 813.

28. Jerome Levine, interview by Samuel Gershon, transcript, 10 December 1995, San Juan, Puerto Rico, American College of Neuropsychopharmacology Oral History Project, http://www.acnp.org/programs/history.aspx# (hereafter ACNP Oral History Project).

29. Arnold M. Ludwig and Jerome Levine, "Hypnodelic Therapy," *Current Psychiatric Therapies* 7 (1967), p. 131.

30. Ibid., pp. 134–135.

31. Arnold M. Ludwig and Jerome Levine, "A Controlled Comparison of Five Brief Treatment Techniques Employing LSD, Hypnosis, and Psychotherapy," *American Journal of Psychotherapy* 19 (1965), pp. 423–424. On volunteering for the trial, patients were told they might receive an "experimental" drug but were not given its name or told its effects.

32. Ibid., pp. 431–434.

33. J. Levine, "Models for Evaluating Therapies Employing LSD-Like Drugs," in H. Brill (ed.), *Neuro-Psycho-Pharmacology* (Amsterdam: Excerpta Medica Foundation, 1967), p. 422.

34. Jerome Levine, interview by William T. Carpenter Jr., transcript, 12 December 2007, Boca Raton, Florida, ACNP Oral History Project; Levine, interview by Gershon.

35. Arnold M. Ludwig, Jerome Levine, and Louis H. Stark, *LSD and Alcoholism: A Clinical Study of Treatment Efficacy* (Springfield, IL: Charles C. Thomas, 1970), pp. 19, 233. "Testimonial," as used here, was a particularly loaded term with a long history of use in derogating claims of efficacy based individual experience. At the time, research experts commonly used the term when supporting the need for controlled trials to determine treatment efficacy. See Scott H. Podolsky, *The Antibiotic Era: Reform, Resistance, and the Pursuit of a Rational Therapeutics* (Baltimore: Johns Hopkins University Press, 2015), pp. 51–55, 104–105.

36. Ludwig, Levine, and Stark, *LSD and Alcoholism*, p. 5.

37. Ibid., pp. 19, 25. Emphasis original.

38. Ibid., p. 71. The authors did not describe the nature of "industrial therapy" or "community therapy"; the former was likely occupational therapy, involving work assisting in the running of the hospital and its workshops.

39. Ibid., pp. 84–85, 80.

40. Ibid., pp. 74–76, 87, 164.

41. Ibid., pp. 46, 87–89.

42. Ibid., pp. 81, 90–96.

43. Ibid., pp. 128–145.

44. Ibid., pp. 101, 142.

45. Ibid., p. 9.

46. Leo Hollister, "From Hypertension to Psychopharmacology—a Serendipitous Career," interview by David Healy, in David Healy (ed.), *The Psychopharmacologists II* (London: Arnold, 1998), pp. 215–217; Leo E. Hollister, interview by Thomas A. Ban, transcript, 6 April 1999, Nashville, Tennessee, ACNP Oral History Project.

47. Casey et al., "Drug Therapy in Schizophrenia," pp. 210–220. For the details of this trial, see chapter 3.

48. Leo E. Hollister, "Drug-Induced Psychoses and Schizophrenic Reactions: A Critical Comparison," *Annals of the New York Academy of Sciences* 96 (1962), pp. 80–93.

49. Leo E. Hollister et al., "An Experimental Approach to Facilitation of Psychotherapy by Psychotomimetic Drugs," *Journal of Mental Science* 108 (1962), pp. 99–100. A total of twenty-two patients were administered LSD, psilocybin, mescaline, or a placebo during psychotherapy sessions. These sessions were then compared with control interviews with the same subjects, with ratings made of any changes that occurred in therapeutically desirable aspects of the interview, such as increased or decreased insight or rapport.

50. Leo E. Hollister, *Chemical Psychoses: LSD and Related Drugs* (Springfield, IL: Charles C. Thomas, 1968), pp. 124–125.

51. Leo Hollister, Jack Shelton, and George Krieger, "A Controlled Comparison of Lysergic Acid Diethylamide (LSD) and Dextroamphetamine in Alcoholics," *American Journal of Psychiatry* 125, no. 10 (1969), p. 1353.

52. Ibid.

53. Kurland et al., "LSD in the Treatment of Alcoholics," p. 85.

54. Hollister, Shelton, and Krieger, "Lysergic Acid Diethylamide (LSD) and Dextroamphetamine in Alcoholics," pp. 1355–1357.

55. Ibid., p. 1357.

56. See Colin M. Smith, "A New Adjunct to the Treatment of Alcoholism: The Hallucinogenic Drugs," *Quarterly Journal of Studies on Alcohol* 19 (1958), pp. 407, 414–415; J. Ross MacLean et al., "The Use of LSD-25 in the Treatment of Alcoholism and Other Psychiatric Problems," *Quarterly Journal of Studies on Alcohol* 22 (1961), pp. 34–45; and P. O. O'Reilly and A. Funk, "LSD in Chronic Alcoholism," *Canadian Psychiatric Journal* 9, no. 3 (1964), pp. 258–261. O'Reilly and Funk's treatment method is more clearly outlined in P. O. O'Reilly and Genevieve Reich, "Lysergic Acid and the Alcoholic," *Diseases of the Nervous System* 23 (1962), pp. 331–334.

57. Keith S. Ditman and John R. B. Whittlesey, "Comparison of the LSD-25 Experience and Delirium Tremens," *A.M.A. Archives of General Psychiatry* 1 (1959) pp. 47–57.

58. Keith S. Ditman, Max Hayman, and John R. B. Whittlesey, "Nature and Frequency of Claims Following LSD," *Journal of Nervous and Mental Disease* 134, no. 4 (1962), pp. 346–352.

59. See Keith S. Ditman, "The Value of LSD in Psychotherapy," in J. Thomas Ungerleider (ed.), *The Problems and Prospects of LSD* (Springfield, IL: Charles C. Thomas, 1968), pp. 45–60; and Keith S. Ditman et al., "Harmful Aspects of the LSD Experience," *Journal of Nervous and Mental Disease* 145, no. 6 (1967), pp. 464–474.

60. Keith S. Ditman et al., "Dimensions of the LSD, Methylphenidate and Chlordiazepoxide Experiences," *Psychopharmacologia* 14, no. 1 (1969), pp. 1–11. The design of the trial is also discussed in Keith S. Ditman et al., "Characteristics of Alcoholics Volunteering for Lysergide Treatment," *Quarterly Journal of Studies on Alcohol* 31, no. A (1970), pp. 414–422.

61. Kenneth E. Godfrey, "The Metamorphosis of an LSD Psychotherapist," in Harold A. Abramson (ed.), *The Use of LSD in Psychotherapy and Alcoholism* (Indianapolis: Bobbs-Merrill, 1967), pp. 458–471.

62. Ibid., pp. 460, 466.

63. K. E. Godfrey, R. A. Soskin, and H. M. Voth, "LSD Therapy Research Program," n.d., unit ID #291165, Menninger Foundation Archives, Kansas Historical Society, Topeka (hereafter Menninger Archives).

64. Godfrey, "Metamorphosis of an LSD Psychotherapist," p. 469. See also Kenneth E. Godfrey, "Evaluation of Psychedelic Drugs as Therapeutic Agents," in Richard E. Hicks and Paul Jay Fink (eds.), *Psychedelic Drugs* (New York: Grune & Stratton, 1969), pp. 226–233. Over the same years Godfrey was also conducting limited psycholytic therapy research with LSD. This, by its nature, involved extensive psychotherapy.

65. Godfrey, Soskin, and Voth, "LSD Therapy Research Program"; Phillip M. Rennick to Riley Gardner et al., memorandum, 16 May 1967, unit ID #291165, Menninger Archives; Gardner Murphy to Kenneth Godfrey, 27 April 1967, unit ID #291165, Menninger Archives.

66. Kenneth E. Godfrey, "LSD and Intensive Psychotherapy," application for research grant to U.S. Department of Health, Education, and Welfare, MH 18415-01, received 1 October 1969, unit ID #296002, Menninger Archives.

67. Kenneth Godfrey to Abram Hoffer, 29 October 1969, III. 106, S-A207, Abram Hoffer Fonds F 410, Provincial Archives of Saskatchewan, Saskatoon, Canada.

68. William T. Bowen, Robert A. Soskin, and John W. Chotlos, "Lysergic Acid Diethylamide as a Variable in the Hospital Treatment of Alcoholism," *Journal of Nervous and Mental Disease* 150, no. 2 (1970), p. 112.

69. Ibid., p. 113.

70. Ibid., p. 117.

71. Milan Tomsovic and Robert V. Edwards, "Lysergide Treatment of Schizophrenic and Nonschizophrenic Alcoholics: A Controlled Evaluation," *Quarterly Journal of Studies on Alcohol* 31 (1970), p. 937.

72. Ibid., pp. 935–937. The standard treatment routine of the hospital's Alcoholic Rehabilitation Program is not described in the report. It was likely similar to the milieu treatment programs that were the background ward conditions in many of the other studies, as described in this chapter.

73. Ibid., pp. 941–948. At twelve months, 44 percent of the LSD patients were completely abstinent, compared to 11 percent of the volunteer controls, and 31 percent of the standard treatment controls. These results were for nonschizophrenic patients. Schizophrenic patients who were not acutely psychotic had not initially been excluded from the study. However, the researchers soon found that LSD therapy had a negative effect on these patients; therefore, they considered the results for nonschizophrenic patients separately.

74. Wilson Van Dusen, "LSD and the Enlightenment of Zen," *Psychologia* 4 (1961), pp. 11, 14, 13.

75. Wilson Van Dusen et al., "Treatment of Alcoholism with Lysergide," *Quarterly Journal of Studies on Alcohol* 28, no. 2 (1967), pp. 295–297.

76. Ibid., p. 297, 296.

77. Ibid., p. 299.

78. Van Dusen, "LSD and the Enlightenment of Zen," p. 11.

79. Van Dusen et al., "Treatment of Alcoholism with Lysergide," pp. 300–301.

80. Ibid., p. 300.

81. Kurland et al., "LSD in the Treatment of Alcoholics," pp. 89–90.

82. Van Dusen et al., "Treatment of Alcoholism with Lysergide," p. 303.

83. Van Dusen's report did acknowledge that the treatment of women rendered their results not "directly comparable" with the Canadian studies, but the researchers did not speculate on whether gender may have played a role in treatment outcome. See ibid.

84. Kurland et al., "LSD in the Treatment of Alcoholics," p. 84. The Spring Grove researchers also described the work of Canadian researchers Reginald Smart and F. Gordon Johnson as psychedelic chemotherapy. Like their counterparts in the United States, in the mid-1960s these researchers challenged the work of the early Canadian psychedelic therapy researchers by performing controlled trials of a treatment method that differed significantly from psychedelic therapy. As well as incorporating little or no psychotherapy, these researchers restrained their patients to their beds. See R. G. Smart et al., *Lysergic Acid Diethylamide (LSD) in the Treatment of Alcoholism: An Investigation of Its Effects on Drinking Behaviour, Personality Structure and Social Functioning* (Toronto: University of Toronto Press, 1967); F. Gordon Johnson, "LSD in the Treatment of Alcoholism," *American Journal of Psychiatry* 126, no. 4 (October 1969), pp. 481–487. Unfortunately, the Spring Grove reports did not comment on the research of Van Dusen and colleagues, whose therapeutic method most closely resembled their own.

85. [Savage], "Review of *LSD and Alcoholism*," pp. 2, 7.

86. Ludwig, Levine, and Stark, *LSD and Alcoholism*, pp. 29, 88.

87. [Savage], "Review of *LSD and Alcoholism*," pp. 1–8.

88. Savage recounts Ludwig's description of his method at this conference in Hicks and Fink, *Psychedelic Drugs*, p. 51. The description is not included in Ludwig's paper in the conference proceedings. See Arnold M. Ludwig, "Relationship of Attitude to Behavior: Preliminary Results and Implications for Treatment Evaluation Studies," in John M. Shlien (ed.), *Research in Psychotherapy: Proceedings of the Third Conference* (Washington, DC: American Psychological Association, 1968), pp. 471–487.

89. Ludwig, Levine, and Stark, *LSD and Alcoholism*, p. 104, 107.

90. Quoted in [Savage], "Review of *LSD and Alcoholism*," p. 7. For the original discussion, see Ludwig, Levine, and Stark, *LSD and Alcoholism*, pp. 223–230.

91. [Savage], "Review of *LSD and Alcoholism*," p. 8. Truax used the phrase "for better or for worse" in his research reports exploring psychotherapy's potential for both positive and negative effects. See C. B. Truax and D. G. Wargo, "Psychotherapeutic Encounters that Change Behavior: For Better or for Worse," *American Journal of Psychotherapy* 20, no. 3 (1966), pp. 499–520; and Charles B. Truax et al., "Effects of Therapeutic Conditions in Child Therapy," *Journal of Community Psychology* 1, no. 3 (1973), p. 317.

92. Walter Pahnke et al., untitled manuscript, 22 June 1971, folder 3, box 6, Savage Papers. Nine members of the MPRC psychedelic research team signed this review, and while covering the same critique, it was written in a much more restrained tone than was Savage's review. While this suggests that it may have been intended for more widespread distribution, its actual distribution is not known.

93. Ludwig, Levine, and Stark, *LSD and Alcoholism*, p. 241.

94. [Savage], "Review of *LSD and Alcoholism*," p. 7.

95. Ludwig, Levine, and Stark, *LSD and Alcoholism*, p. 236.

96. [Savage], untitled manuscript, p. 10.

97. Richard Elliot Doblin, "Regulation of the Medical Use of Psychedelics and Marijuana" (PhD diss., Harvard University, 2000), p. 244.

98. Ludwig, Levine, and Stark, *LSD and Alcoholism*, pp. 236–237.

99. Kurland et al., "LSD in the Treatment of Alcoholics," p. 85.

100. Carl Salzman, "Controlled Therapy Research with Psychedelic Drugs: A Critique," in Hicks and Fink, *Psychedelic Drugs*, p. 28.

101. Hicks and Fink, *Psychedelic Drugs*, pp. 43–44.

102. Salzman, "Psychedelic Drugs: A Critique," pp. 26–27. He did acknowledge debate surrounding the treatment method of Reginald Smart and colleagues at the Addictions Research Foundation, Toronto. However, their use of physical restraints with patients made their method more obviously antitherapeutic.

103. Ludwig, Levine, and Stark, *LSD and Alcoholism*, dust jacket.

Chapter 6 · The Quiet Death of Research

Epigraph: O. Lee McCabe and Thomas E. Hanlon, "The Use of LSD-Type Drugs in Psychotherapy: Progress and Promise," in O. Lee McCabe (ed.), *Changing Human Behavior: Current Therapies and Future Directions* (New York: Grune & Stratton, 1977), p. 247.

1. Controlled Substances Act, 91 P.L. 513, 84 Stat. 1242, 27 October 1970, Sec. 202 (b) (1).

2. Quoted in Tom Huth, "Maryland Doctors Use LSD to Explore Minds," *Washington Post, Times Herald*, 19 November 1972, p. A22.

3. Jules Asher, "Whatever Happened to Psychedelic Research?," *APA Monitor* (November 1975), p. 4; National Institute of Mental Health Research Task Force, *Research in the Service of Mental Health: Report of the Research Task Force of the National Institute of Mental Health* (Rockville, MD: National Institute of Mental Health, 1975), p. 255.

4. For the background and passage of the Comprehensive Drug Abuse Prevention and Control Act of 1970, see Joseph F. Spillane, "Debating the Controlled Substances Act," *Drug and Alcohol Dependence* 76, no. 1 (2004), pp. 17–29; David T. Courtwright, "The Controlled Substances Act: How a 'Big Tent' Reform Became a Punitive Drug Law," *Drug and Alcohol Dependence* 76, no. 1 (2004), pp. 9–15; and David F. Musto and Pamela Korsmeyer, *The Quest for Drug Control: Politics and Federal Policy in a Period of Increasing Substance Abuse, 1963–1981* (New Haven: Yale University Press, 2002), pp. 15, 56–71.

5. Controlled Substances Act, Sec. 202 (b) (1).

6. Sidney Cohen's 1960 survey of LSD researchers for adverse reactions in treatment found that prolonged and serious adverse reactions were rare. See Sidney Cohen, "Lysergic Acid Diethylamide: Side Effects and Complications," *Journal of Nervous and Mental Disease* 130 (1960), pp. 30–40. Furthermore, no prolonged adverse reactions were found in the Spring Grove/MPRC research or reported in the other clinical trials discussed in the previous chapter.

7. *Part One, Drug Abuse Control Amendments—1970*, Hearings before the Subcommittee on Public Health and Welfare of the Committee on Interstate and Foreign Commerce, House of Representatives, 91st Congress, 2nd Session, February 8, 4, 17–20, 25–27, March 2 and 8, 1970 (Washington, DC: US Government Printing Office, 1970), pp. 165–167, 343.

8. Controlled Substances Act, Sec. 303 (f), Sec. 304 (a).

9. *Drug Abuse Control Amendments*, Hearings, pp. 195, 277, 313, 394–395, 423, 441, 455.

10. Walter Clark et al., "Psychedelic Research: Obstacles and Values," *Journal of Humanistic Psychology* 15, no. 3 (1975), p. 8.

11. Asher, "Psychedelic Research," p. 5.

12. Clark et al., "Psychedelic Research," p. 6, 8.

13. Ibid., pp. 13–14.

14. Ibid., p. 10.

15. According to the IND regulations, clinical studies were for the purpose of assessing a drug's safety, effectiveness, and optimum dosage "in the diagnosis, treatment, or prophylaxis of groups of subjects involving a given disease or condition." George P. Larrick, "Procedural and Interpretative Regulations; Investigational Use," *Federal Register* 28, no. 5 (8 January 1963), p. 180. The issue of INDs in the case of drugs investigated for purposes that were not directly medical was partly addressed by Frances Kelsey, chief of the FDA Investigational Drug Branch, in a 1963 speech to the Pharmaceutical Manufacturers Association. She specifically discussed the example of using LSD "to explore mental processes rather than to alleviate any mental disease." However, she pointed out that such research did have ultimate medical implications, as it could "contribute to the improvement of human welfare by adding to the sum knowledge of the functioning of the human body in health or disease." She therefore suggested that such research could proceed under an IND toward the goal of NDA approval for the drug as a research tool. This research example was thus still much more medically aligned than research areas such as those mentioned by the survey participants, which are harder to imagine fitting under the IND provisions. Frances O. Kelsey, "Problems Relating to Investigational Drugs," presentation to the Pharmaceutical Manufacturers Association, Clearwater, Florida, 20–22 March 1963, in FDA (comp.), *Speeches and Papers, 1963*, Part 1 (Rockville, MD: Food and Drug Administration, 1979), FDA Biosciences Library, Silver Spring, Maryland.

16. Food and Drug Administration, "FDA Lists Approved LSD Research Projects," *FDA Consumer* (September 1975), pp. 24–25.

17. Quoted in Asher, "Psychedelic Research," p. 5.

18. Clark et al., "Psychedelic Research," p. 7; Richard Ashley, "The Other Side of LSD," *New York Times*, 19 October 1975, https://nyti.ms/2mO6poN.

19. See Richard Elliot Doblin, "Regulation of the Medical Use of Psychedelics and Marijuana" (PhD diss., Harvard University, 2000), p. 54n312.

20. William A. Richards, *Sacred Knowledge: Psychedelics and Religious Experience* (New York: Columbia University Press, 2016), pp. 74–75.

21. Charles Savage, review of *Higher Wisdom: Eminent Elders Explore the Continuing Impact of Psychedelics*, by Roger Walsh and Charles S. Grob (eds.), *Journal of Nervous and Mental Disease* 194, no. 7 (2006), p. 552.

22. William Richards, email to author, 18 February 2013. For Unger's last author credit on an MPRC publication, see O. Lee McCabe et al., "Psychedelic (LSD) Therapy of Neurotic Disorders," *Journal of Psychedelic Drugs* 5, no. 1 (1972), pp. 18–28. For Savage's employment by 1973, see Charles Savage et al., "LSD-Assisted Psychotherapy in the Treatment of Severe Chronic Neurosis," *Journal of Altered States of Consciousness* 1, no. 1 (1973), p. 31.

23. Charles Savage, "Brief Bio," n.d., folder 10, box 1, Charles Savage Papers, MSP 70, Archives and Special Collections, Purdue University Libraries, West Lafayette, Indiana; "Obituary: Charles W. Savage," *Washington Post*, 20 December 2007.

24. Stanislav Grof, "The Great Awakening: Psychology, Philosophy and Spirituality in LSD Psychotherapy," in Roger Walsh and Charles S. Grob (eds.), *Higher Wisdom: Eminent Elders Explore the Continuing Impact of Psychedelics* (Albany: State University of New York Press, 2005), pp. 141–142; Richards, email to author, 18 February 2013. For Grof's post-MPRC publications, see Stanislav Grof, *Realms of the Human Unconscious* (New York: Viking Press, 1975); Stanislav Grof and Joan Halifax, *The Human Encounter with Death* (New York: E. P. Dutton, 1977); Stanislav Grof, *LSD Psychotherapy* (Pomona: Hunter House, 1980).

25. "Bill Richards: Curriculum Vitae," https://www.erowid.org/culture/characters/richards_bill/richards_bill_info1.shtml. See also Richards, *Sacred Knowledge*, pp. 73, xix, 16.

26. See Walter N. Pahnke et al., "LSD-Assisted Psychotherapy with Terminal Cancer Patients," in Richard E. Hicks and Paul Jay Fink (eds.), *Psychedelic Drugs* (New York: Grune & Stratton, 1969), pp. 33–42; William Richards et al., "LSD-Assisted Psychotherapy and the Human Encounter with Death," *Journal of Transpersonal Psychology* 4, no. 2 (1972), pp. 121–136; William A. Richards et al., "DPT as an Adjunct in Brief Psychotherapy with Cancer Patients," *Omega: Journal of Death and Dying* 10, no. 1 (1979), pp. 9–26; William A. Richards, "Counseling, Peak Experiences, and the Human Encounter with Death: An Empirical Study of the Efficacy of DPT-Assisted Counseling in Enhancing the Quality of Life of Persons with Terminal Cancer and their Closest Family Members" (PhD diss., Catholic University of America, 1975).

27. *Drug Safety* (Part 5, Appendixes, and Index), Hearings before a Subcommittee on Government Operations, House of Representatives, 89th Congress, 2nd Session, March 9, 10, May 25, 26, June 7, 8, and 9, 1966 (Washington, DC: US Government Printing Office, 1966), p. 2267. The psychoactive effects of DPT were first reported in 1967 by researchers at Saint Elizabeth's Hospital, Washington, DC. See Louis A. Faillace, Alkinoos Vourlekis, and Stephen Szara, "Clinical Evaluation of Some Hallucinogenic Tryptamine Derivatives," *Journal of Nervous and Mental Disease* 145, no. 4 (1967), pp. 306–313. The source of the MPRC researchers' DPT is unclear, but Faillace's paper cited the Upjohn Company of Michigan for supplies.

28. S. Grof et al., "DPT as an Adjunct in Psychotherapy of Alcoholics," *International Pharmacopsychiatry* 8 (1973), p. 106, 108; Robert A. Soskin, Stanislav Grof, and William A. Richards, "Low Doses of Dipropyltryptamine in Psychotherapy," *Archives of General Psychiatry* 28, no. 6 (1973), p. 817. DPT was not scheduled under the Controlled Substances Act; this could have influenced the researchers' decision to employ it. However, given that its effects fit with their long-held research plans and that as well as continuing to use LSD they also initiated studies with another Schedule I drug (methylenedioxyamphetamine), it seems unlikely that this was their primary motivation.

29. Grof et al., "DPT in Psychotherapy of Alcoholics," pp. 104–115.

30. Richards et al., "DPT with Cancer Patients," pp. 9–26.

31. Richard Yensen and Donna Dryer, "Thirty Years of Psychedelic Research: The Spring

Grove Experiment and Its Sequels," *Jahrbuch des Europäischen Collegiums für Bewußtseinsstudien / Yearbook of the European College for the Study of Consciousness* (1993–1994), pp. 81–82.

32. Soskin, Grof, and Richards, "Dipropyltryptamine in Psychotherapy," pp. 817–821. The sessions were not run according to a specific form of psychotherapy. The researchers described that the therapists focused on establishing a good therapeutic relationship and explored patients' past and present maladaptive behaviors and patterns of thinking, as well as their life philosophy, hierarchy of values, and religious beliefs. Despite the double-blind, therapists were usually able to correctly identify when patients received DPT.

33. MDA was first synthesized in 1930 by Los Angeles–based chemist Gordon Alles, who had also discovered amphetamine the previous year. Alles soon began working with the pharmaceutical company Smith, Kline, and French, where the drug was produced and further studied in the 1950s. This research, however, did not establish a therapeutic use, and the company did not develop the drug to market. See Nicolas Rasmussen, *On Speed: The Many Lives of Amphetamine* (New York: New York University Press, 2008), pp. 18–24, 226–231; Richard Yensen et al., "MDA-Assisted Psychotherapy with Neurotic Outpatients: A Pilot Study," *Journal of Nervous and Mental Disease* 163, no. 4 (1976), p. 234. The exact source of the MDA used at the MPRC is unclear.

34. Yensen et al., "MDA-Assisted Psychotherapy," pp. 233–245. See also I. S. Turek, R. A. Soskin, and A. A. Kurland, "Methylenedioxyamphetamine (MDA), Subjective Effects," *Journal of Psychedelic Drugs* 6, no. 1 (1974), pp. 7–14.

35. William A. Richards and Margaret Berendes, "LSD-Assisted Psychotherapy and Dynamics of Creativity: A Case Report," *Journal of Altered States of Consciousness* 3, no. 2 (1977–78), pp. 131–146; Margret Berendes, "Formation of Typical, Dynamic Stages in Psychotherapy before and after Psychedelic [*sic*] Drug Intervention," *Journal of Altered States of Consciousness* 5, no. 4 (1979–80), pp. 325–338. Berendes's reports focused on exploring the psychodynamic content and impact of the LSD sessions in a way reminiscent of much earlier LSD psychotherapy research, such as that of Harold Abramson.

36. John C. Rhead et al., "Psychedelic Drug (DPT)-Assisted Psychotherapy with Alcoholics: A Controlled Study," *Journal of Psychedelic Drugs* 9, no. 4 (1977), pp. 287–300.

37. Ibid., pp. 290–296.

38. Ibid., p. 297.

39. McCabe and Hanlon, "Use of LSD-Type Drugs in Psychotherapy," p. 245.

40. Barry Rascovar, "Group Abused State Hospital Aid, Audit Finds," *Baltimore Sun*, 24 January 1973, pp. C24, C5. In a 1997 interview, Kurland stated that the payout was compensation for performing his Friends work on his own time. Albert A. Kurland, interviewed by Leo E. Hollister, transcript, 15 April 1997, Washington DC, American College of Neuropsychopharmacology Oral History Project, http://www.acnp.org/programs/history.aspx#.

41. Barry C. Rascovar, "State Probing Charges about Psychiatric Unit," *Baltimore Sun*, 28 May 1973, p. C22.

42. "Conduct of State Psychiatric Center Is Criticized by a Second Scientist," *Baltimore Sun*, 30 May 1973, p. C15.

43. Mary Knudson, "Psychiatric Center Ousts Unit Director," *Baltimore Sun*, 26 June 1973, p. A11; Michael P. Weisskopf, "Psychiatric Center Held Badly Run," *Baltimore Sun*, 25 March 1974, A9; Michael P. Weisskopf, "Four Scientists Fired at State Center: Sought to Have Bosses Replaced," *Baltimore Sun*, 25 May 1974, p. B1; Anthony Barbieri Jr., "4 Fired State Researchers Sue for Jobs, $200,000," *Baltimore Sun*, 25 June 1974, p. C5; Robert A. Erlandson, "3 Ph.D.'s Get Jobs Back," *Baltimore Sun*, 2 August 1975, p. B1.

44. "Audit Critical of Center," *Baltimore Sun*, 4 March 1975, pp. C1–C2.

45. Barry C. Rascovar, "Plan to Shift Mental Center to UM Assailed," *Baltimore Sun*, 14 August 1975, p. C16; "Solomon Angers Delegates," *Baltimore Sun*, 19 February 1976, p. C2; "Judge

Finds No Retaliation in Dismissal of 3 Scientists," *Baltimore Sun*, 9 July 1977, p. B2; 1976 Laws of Maryland, chapter 677, House Bill 767; Legislative Services Bill File for House Bill 767 (MD, 1976).

46. American Psychiatric Association, *Maryland Department of Health and Mental Hygiene: A Study by the Consultation and Evaluation Services Board of the American Psychiatric Association* (Washington, DC: American Psychiatric Association, 1976), p. 29.

47. "No Retaliation in Dismissal," p. B2.

48. Richards, email to author, 18 February 2013; William Richards, email to author, 13 September 2012.

49. "UM Tied to LSD Testing," *Baltimore Sun*, 17 July 1975, pp. C1, C2. See also "The CIA's Shocking LSD Experiments," *Baltimore Sun*, 13 July 1975, p. K4; David Zielenziger, "Army Admits LSD Test," *Baltimore Sun*, 18 July 1975, pp. C1, C2; David Zielenziger, "Army Saw LSD as Tool, Researcher Says," *Baltimore Sun*, 21 July 1975, pp. A1, A4; "Army Says LSD Testing Ignored Rights," *Baltimore Sun*, 9 September 1975, p. A6; "CIA Studies Gave LSD to 200 in Mass.," *Baltimore Sun*, 9 August 1977, p. A6. For an overview of the CIA and military research, see John Marks, *The Search for the "Manchurian Candidate": The CIA and Mind Control* (New York: Times Books, 1979).

50. "The Nation's LSD Trip," *Baltimore Sun*, 31 July 1975, p. A16. See also Robert P. Wade, "State Unit Still Gives LSD Tests," *Baltimore Sun*, 29 July 1975, pp. C1, C4.

51. "Psychedelic Research," *Baltimore Sun*, 22 October 1975, p. A14. See also "100 Got LSD at Center," *Baltimore Sun*, 4 August 1975, p. C14; "End of Psychedelic Research?," *Baltimore Sun*, 8 August 1975, p. A12; and "LSD Worked a Miracle for Him, Man Testifies," *Baltimore Sun*, 18 August 1975, p. A3.

52. Acknowledgment of sponsorship or assistance from Sandoz is made in the proceedings of the following conferences: Louis S. Cholden (ed.), *Lysergic Acid Diethylamide and Mescaline in Experimental Psychiatry* (New York: Grune & Stratton, 1956), p. xi; Harold A. Abramson (ed.), *The Use of LSD in Psychotherapy* (New York: Josiah Macy, Jr. Foundation, 1960), title page; and in the 1960 symposium *LSD, Transcendence and the New Beginning.* See James Terrill, "The Nature of the LSD Experience," *Journal of Nervous and Mental Disease* 135 (1962), p. 425.

53. For the patent expiration date, see Albert Hofmann, *LSD: My Problem Child; Reflections on Sacred Drugs, Mysticism and Science*, trans. Jonathan Ott (Santa Cruz: Multidisciplinary Association for Psychedelic Studies, 2009), p. 86.

54. Drug Amendments of 1962, 87 P.L. 781, 76 Stat. 780, 10 October 1962, Title 1, Part A, Sec. 102 (c). Emphasis added.

55. Peter Temin, *Taking Your Medicine: Drug Regulation in the United States* (Cambridge, MA: Harvard University Press, 1980), p. 127.

56. As discussed in chapter 5, Ditman's trial assessed outcome through a comparison of LSD and active placebo treatment sessions for experiences usually deemed therapeutic, such as increased insight. See Keith S. Ditman et al., "Dimensions of the LSD, Methylphenidate and Chlordiazepoxide Experiences," *Psychopharmacologia* 14, no. 1 (1969), pp. 1–11.

57. Herbert L. Ley Jr., "Disulfiram: Drugs for Human Use; Drug Efficacy Study Implementation," *Federal Register* 34, no. 175 (12 September 1969), p. 14340. Antabuse was originally approved in 1951, before proof of efficacy was required in a New Drug Application. The quoted labeling and efficacy determination were the result of the drug's efficacy review as part of the FDA's Drug Efficacy Study Implementation, which brought drugs approved between 1938 and 1962 into line with the new regulatory requirements.

58. Edward Shorter, *Before Prozac: The Troubled History of Mood Disorders in Psychiatry* (New York: Oxford University Press, 2009), pp. 65–68; David Healy, *The Antidepressant Era* (Cambridge, MA: Harvard University Press, 1997), pp. 122–128.

Epilogue

Epigraph: Anthony K. Busch and Warren C. Johnson, "L.S.D. 25 as an Aid in Psychother-apy," *Diseases of the Nervous System* 11, no. 8 (August 1950), p. 243; Albert A. Kurland, "Debate and Discussion: Psychedelic Therapy," *Baltimore Sun*, 24 February 1979, p. A18.

1. Sidney Cohen, "Lysergic Acid Diethylamide: Side Effects and Complications," *Journal of Nervous and Mental Disease* 130 (1960), p. 30.

2. Richard Yensen and Donna Dryer, "Thirty Years of Psychedelic Research: The Spring Grove Experiment and Its Sequels," *Jahrbuch des Europäischen Collegiums für Bewußtseinsstudien/ Yearbook of the European College for the Study of Consciousness* (1993–1994), p. 90.

3. A 1997 international bibliography of psychotherapy research with psychedelic drugs listed 687 entries, the vast majority of which were published between the 1950s and 1970s. See Torsten Passie, *Psycholytic and Psychedelic Therapy Research 1931–1995: A Complete International Bibliography* (Hannover: Laurentius, 1997).

4. Kurland, "Debate and Discussion," p. A18.

5. Yensen and Dryer, "Thirty Years of Psychedelic Research," p. 91: Ronald Kartzinel to Albert Kurland, 20 June 1979, folder "IND 3250," Orenda Institute, Cortes Island, British Columbia, Canada (hereafter Orenda Institute); "Biographical Information: Albert A. Kurland, M.D.," n.d., folder "IND 3250," Orenda Institute; Richard Yensen, personal communication, December 2016.

6. Albert Kurland, "Psychedelic Research—the Administrative Challenge," unpublished manuscript, n.d., folder "Al Kurland Cancer Project," Orenda Institute. Leber was the acting director of the FDA's Division of Neuropharmacological Drug Products, of the Office of New Drug Evaluation.

7. Paul Leber to Albert Kurland, n.d. [1982], folder "Al Kurland: Letters," Orenda Institute.

8. "Psychedelic Research and the Administrative Dragons," unpublished manuscript, n.d., folder "Al Kurland Cancer Book," Orenda Institute, pp. 10–11.

9. [Charles Savage], untitled manuscript, n.d., folder 10, box 7, Charles Savage Papers, MSP 70, Archives and Special Collections, Purdue University Libraries, West Lafayette, Indiana.

10. Edward Shorter, *Before Prozac: The Troubled History of Mood Disorders in Psychiatry* (New York: Oxford University Press, 2009), p. 5.

11. *Drug Industry Act of 1962*, Senate Report No. 1744, Calendar No. 1703, 87th Congress, 2nd Session (Washington, DC: US Government Printing Office, 1962), p. 16.

12. Drug-assisted psychotherapy, as considered here, should not be confused with the concurrent employment of drug therapy and psychotherapy. Drug-assisted psychotherapies, such as forms of LSD psychotherapy and narcosynthesis, featured an attempt to harness the acute, subjective effects of a drug to facilitate a psychotherapeutic process. Aside from a recent resurgence in psychedelic research (see discussion later in the chapter), drug-assisted psychotherapy effectively vanished from US psychiatry in the 1970s. Research reporting benefits for concurrent drug therapy and psychotherapy (primarily cognitive and behavioral forms) over drug therapy alone has increased in recent decades. However, here, as one major meta-analysis concluded, "The effects of psychotherapy and pharmacotherapy may be largely independent from each other and additive, not interfering with each other." See Pim Cuijpers et al., "Adding Psychotherapy to Antidepressant Medication in Depression and Anxiety Disorders: A Meta-analysis," *World Psychiatry* 13, no. 1 (2014), p. 64.

13. For a discussion of the biological turn in psychiatry in the late twentieth century, including the loss of interest in the "meaning" of patients' inner lives, see Andrew Scull, *Madness in Civilization: A Cultural History of Insanity from the Bible to Freud, from the Madhouse to Modern Medicine* (Princeton: Princeton University Press, 2015), pp. 383–405. See also Leon Eisenberg and Laurence B. Guttmacher, "Were We All Asleep at the Switch? A Personal Reminiscence of Psychiatry from 1940 to 2010," *Acta Psychiatrica Scandinavica* 122, no. 2 (2010),

pp. 89–102. For an account that discusses many of the influences in psychoanalysis's fall from dominance yet that largely portrays this fall simply as a triumph of science over a belief system, see Joel Paris, *The Fall of an Icon: Psychoanalysis and Academic Psychiatry* (Toronto: University of Toronto Press, 2005). For the role of the *DSM-III* in the biological turn and in the discipline's increasing focus on overt symptoms over a detailed and nuanced assessment of the patients' lives and psychopathologies, see Hannah S. Decker, *The Making of "DSM-III": A Diagnostic Manual's Conquest of American Psychiatry* (New York: Oxford University Press, 2013), pp. 324–327. For the narrow focus on symptom reduction in psychotherapy research since the 1990s, see Glenn Shean, "Limitations of Randomized Control Designs in Psychotherapy Research," *Advances in Psychiatry* (2014), doi:10.1155/2014/561452.

14. "Orenda Institute: Administrative History Regarding LSD Project," appendix to Albert Kurland, "The Psychedelic (LSD) Peak," unpublished manuscript, 1997, Orenda Institute. The DEA was established in 1973 as a successor organization to the Bureau of Narcotics and Dangerous Drugs in the Department of Justice.

15. DEA import license, 15 December 1996, Orenda Institute.

16. Cynthia McCormick to Richard Yensen, 28 October 1997, folder "Orenda Cancer Protocol," Orenda Institute; Draft letter to Cynthia McCormick, 13 December 1999, folder "Orenda Cancer Protocol," Orenda Institute. McCormick was director of the Division of Anesthetic, Critical Care, and Addiction Drug Products.

17. Richard Leiby, "The Magical Mystery Cure," *Esquire* 128, no. 3 (September 1997), p. 98, EBSCOhost (9709295464); Yensen, personal communication, December 2016.

18. Transcript of teleconference between FDA and Orenda Institute, 22 August 2001, folder "Orenda Cancer Protocol," Orenda Institute.

19. Cynthia McCormick to Albert Kurland, n.d. [c. 2001], folder "Orenda Cancer Protocol," Orenda Institute.

20. Yensen, personal communication, December 2016.

21. Bruce T. Taylor, "Obituary: Albert Kurland," *Neuropsychopharmacology* 34, no. 13 (2009), p. 2780.

22. Rick Strassman, *DMT: The Spirit Molecule* (Rochester, VT: One Park Press, 2001), pp. xv–xvi.

23. Amy Emerson et al., "History and Future of the Multidisciplinary Association for Psychedelic Studies (MAPS)," *Journal of Psychoactive Drugs* 46, no. 1 (2014), pp. 27–36.

24. Michael C. Mithoefer et al., "The Safety and Efficacy of $\pm$3,4-Methylenedioxymethamphetamine-Assisted Psychotherapy in Subjects with Chronic, Treatment-Resistant Posttraumatic Stress Disorder: The First Randomized Controlled Pilot Study," *Journal of Psychopharmacology* 25, no. 4 (2011), pp. 439–452.

25. Emerson et al., "History and Future," pp. 30–32; Yensen, personal communication, December 2016.

26. "MAPS Email Newsletter: December 9, 2016," http://www.maps.org/news/update/64 79-newsletter-december-9-2016.

27. David Nichols, "The Heffter Research Institute: Past and Hopeful Future," *Journal of Psychoactive Drugs* 46, no. 1 (2014), pp. 20–26; Francisco A. Moreno et al., "Safety, Tolerability, and Efficacy of Psilocybin in 9 Patients With Obsessive-Compulsive Disorder," *Journal of Clinical Psychiatry* 67, no. 11 (2006), pp. 1735–1740.

28. Roland Griffiths, "Psilocybin Studies and the Religious Experience: An Interview with Roland Griffiths, Ph.D.," interview by David Jay Brown and Louise Reitman, *MAPS Bulletin* 20, no. 1 (2010), p. 22, http://www.maps.org/news-letters/v20n1/v20n1–22t025.pdf; William A. Richards, *Sacred Knowledge: Psychedelics and Religious Experience* (New York: Columbia University Press, 2016), p. 4. For an overview of the Johns Hopkins psilocybin research program through 2014, see Robert Jesse and Roland R. Griffiths, "Psilocybin Research at Johns Hop-

kins: A 2014 Report," in J. Harold Ellens (ed.), *Seeking the Sacred with Psychoactive Substances: Chemical Paths to Spirituality and to God*, vol. 2 (Santa Barbara, CA: Praeger, 2014), pp. 29–43.

29. R. R. Griffiths et al., "Psilocybin Can Occasion Mystical-Type Experiences Having Substantial and Sustained Personal Meaning and Spiritual Significance," *Psychopharmacology* 187, no. 3 (2006), pp. 268–283.

30. Ibid.; Roland R. Griffiths et al., "Psilocybin Occasioned Mystical-Type Experiences: Immediate and Persisting Dose-Related Effects," *Psychopharmacology* 218, no. 4 (2011), pp. 649–665.

31. Roland R. Griffiths et al., "Psilocybin Produces Substantial and Sustained Decreases in Depression and Anxiety in Patients with Life-Threatening Cancer: A Randomized Double-Blind Trial," *Journal of Psychopharmacology* 30, no. 12 (2016), pp. 1181–1197.

32. Matthew W. Johnson et al., "Pilot Study of the 5-HT2AR Agonist Psilocybin in the Treatment of Tobacco Addiction," *Journal of Psychopharmacology* 28, no. 11 (2014), pp. 983–992; Michael P. Bogenschutz et al., "Psilocybin-Assisted Treatment for Alcohol Dependence: A Proof of Concept Study," *Journal of Psychopharmacology* 29, no. 3 (2015), pp. 289–299.

33. Stephen Ross et al., "Rapid and Sustained Symptom Reduction Following Psilocybin Treatment for Anxiety and Depression in Patients with Life-Threatening Cancer: A Randomized Controlled Trial," *Journal of Psychopharmacology* 30, no. 12 (2016), pp. 1165–1180. For the failure of blinding, see "Supplementary Appendix" (online only), ibid., doi:10.1177/0269881116675512.

34. Richard A. Friedman, "LSD to Cure Depression? Not So Fast," *New York Times*, 13 February 2017, https://nyti.ms/2l6moMh.

35. Griffiths et al., "Psilocybin Produces Decreases in Depression and Anxiety," p. 1182; Ross et al., "Symptom Reduction Following Psilocybin Treatment," pp. 1168, 1166; "Supplementary Appendix" (online only), ibid. Patients in the Spring Grove cancer study received six to twelve hours of preparation, less than the approximately twenty hours in the alcoholic and other studies. See S. Grof et al., "LSD-Assisted Psychotherapy in Patients with Terminal Cancer," *International Pharmacopsychiatry* 8 (1973), p. 135. Patients in the Heffter-sponsored tobacco study received six hours of preparation, and patients in the alcoholism study received four preparatory sessions, although the duration of these sessions is not given. See Johnson et al., "Treatment of Tobacco Addiction," p. 985; and Bogenschutz et al., "Treatment for Alcohol Dependence," *Journal of Psychopharmacology* 29, no. 3 (2015), p. 291.

36. Alexandra Sifferlin, "Just One Dose of This Psychedelic Drug Can Ease Anxiety," *Time*, 30 November 2016, http://time.com/4586333/psilocybin-cancer-anxiety-depression/; Olga Khazan, "The Life-Changing Magic of Mushrooms," *Atlantic*, 1 December 2016, https://www.the atlantic.com/health/archive/2016/12/the-life-changing-magic-of-mushrooms/509246/.

37. Charles S. Grob, "Psychiatric Research with Hallucinogens: What Have We Learned?," *Heffter Review of Psychedelic Research* 1 (1998), p. 15.

38. Grob did recognize that reports of LSD's efficacy were criticized on the grounds of poor research methodology in the 1960s and that some researchers (including Ludwig, Levine, and Stark) conducted controlled trials that reported negative results. However, he portrays these trials as deliberately "designed to refute" the efficacy of LSD therapy and does not discuss the difficulties that researchers who had a positive outlook on psychedelic therapy (such as those at Spring Grove) faced when attempting to demonstrate the efficacy of their treatments though controlled research. See ibid., pp. 16–17.

39. Charles S. Grob et al., "Pilot Study of Psilocybin Treatment for Anxiety in Patients with Advanced-Stage Cancer," *Archives of General Psychiatry* 68, no. 1 (2011), pp. 71–78.

40. Grob, "Research with Hallucinogens," p. 15.